Diabetes and Aging-related Complications

Sho-ichi Yamagishi
Editor

Diabetes and Aging-related Complications

Springer

Editor
Sho-ichi Yamagishi
Department of Pathophysiology and Therapeutics
of Diabetic Vascular Complications
Kurume University School of Medicine
Kurume
Fukuoka
Japan

ISBN 978-981-10-4375-8 ISBN 978-981-10-4376-5 (eBook)
https://doi.org/10.1007/978-981-10-4376-5

Library of Congress Control Number: 2017955825

Printed on acid-free paper

This Springer imprint is published by Springer Nature
The registered company is Springer Nature Singapore Pte Ltd.
The registered company address is: 152 Beach Road, #21-01/04 Gateway East, Singapore 189721, Singapore

Preface

According to the recent report of Diabetes Atlas in 2015, diabetes affects 415 million people worldwide, that is, one in every 11 adults is estimated to have diabetes, and half of them are undiagnosed. Further, it is expected that the number of diabetic patients will increase to 642 million by 2040. Diabetes and its associated metabolic derangements are one of the most important risk factors for aging-related and life-threatening disorders, such as atherosclerotic cardiovascular disease, chronic kidney disease, cancer, Alzheimer's disease, and osteoporosis. Indeed, atherosclerotic cardiovascular disease accounts for about 60% of death in diabetic patients, and microvascular complications are leading causes of end-stage renal failure, acquired blindness, and foot amputations. In addition, hazard ratios of death from any cause, non-cardiovascular disease, and several cancers in diabetic patients are 1.8, 1.7, and 1.25, respectively, compared with nondiabetic individuals. Moreover, Alzheimer's disease and osteoporotic bone fractures are highly prevalent in diabetes, and average life span and healthy life expectancy of diabetic patients are about 10–15 years shorter than those of nondiabetic subjects. These observations suggest that diabetes and its numerous complications are a global health burden and that early detection and treatment of various diabetes-related complications are urgently needed for slowing the aging process and achieving a successful life in diabetic patients. This book entitled *Diabetes and Aging-Related Complications* deals with why and how aging process is accelerated under diabetes, providing valuable and comprehensive information for management of various types of diabetes- and aging-related disorders. I organized a symposium on diabetes and aging in the 58th Annual Meeting of Japan Geriatrics Society in 2016. I selected the contributors of chapters mainly from scientists who presented their updated data in the symposium. I think that the book helps most of the researchers and clinicians in the field of diabetes and its related complications acquire more updated knowledge about a diverse range of topics.

Recently, there is accumulating evidence that cumulative hyperglycemic exposure has contributed to the development and progression of diabetes- and aging-related disorders. In the Diabetes Control and Complications Trial-Epidemiology of Diabetes Interventions and Complications (DCCT-EDIC) trials, former intensive therapy has been shown to be associated with the reduced risk of all-cause mortality over 27 years' mean follow-up. The phenomenon is called as metabolic memory, thus suggesting that past hyperglycemic exposure may persistently cause chronic damage in numerous organs and tissues of diabetes that are not easily reversed, even by subsequent, relatively good glycemic control. In other words, the observations suggest that beneficial influence of early glycemic control on the risk of vascular complications and death is sustained in patients with diabetes. The readers of this book will also get information on underlying molecular mechanisms of the metabolic memory in diabetes.

I hope that the book inspires readers to take various actions on behalf of diabetic patients.

Kurume, Japan Sho-ichi Yamagishi, M.D., Ph.D.

Contents

Chapter 1
Diabetic Kidney Disease

Mai Sugahara, Tetsuhiro Tanaka, Reiko Inagi, and Masaomi Nangaku

Abstract Renal senescence is accompanied by a gradual decrease in its function. Although it rarely causes clinical problems per se, superimposition of various diseases, such as diabetes, may accelerate this functional decline. Recent research has revealed some of the complex mechanisms of how diabetes promotes the aging process in the kidney, including the pathogenic roles of hemodynamic changes, tubulointerstitial hypoxia, oxidative stress, advanced glycation end-products, and impaired autophagy. Diabetes also modulates aging-related signaling pathways, such as sirtuins and mammalian target of rapamycin. Current therapeutic strategy for diabetic kidney disease consists of glycemic control and antihypertensive treatment with renin-angiotensin system inhibitors. However, they fail to fully prevent the progression of diabetic kidney disease, raising an urgent need for novel therapeutic methods. Some pharmacological agents are being developed based on the knowledge of hemodynamic and molecular basis of diabetes- and aging-related kidney function decline.

Keywords Diabetic kidney disease • Hypoxia • Oxidative stress • Advanced glycation end-products • Autophagy

1.1 Introduction

Aging is a universal process that affects all organs including the kidney. Even in healthy individuals, glomerular filtration rate (GFR) starts to decline at 30 years of age and proceeds at the rate of approximately 8 ml/min/1.73 m^2 per decade [1]. This loss in renal function is largely attributed to hemodynamic changes within the kidney and age-related vulnerability to physiological stress, such as hypoxia and oxidative stress.

M. Sugahara • T. Tanaka (✉) • R. Inagi • M. Nangaku
Division of Nephrology and Endocrinology, The University of Tokyo Graduate School of Medicine, 7-3-1 Hongo, Bunkyo-ku, Tokyo 113-8655, Japan
e-mail: tetsu-tky@umin.ac.jp

S.-i. Yamagishi (ed.), *Diabetes and Aging-related Complications*,
https://doi.org/10.1007/978-981-10-4376-5_1

The rate of kidney function decline may increase with superimposition of various diseases. Diabetes is one of the strong drivers of this decline, and it accelerates the process of aging through several different mechanisms, such as hemodynamic changes, endothelial dysfunction, tubulointerstitial hypoxia, oxidative stress, accumulation of advanced glycation end-products (AGEs), and impaired autophagy. Diabetes also modulates some aging-related signaling pathways including sirtuins and mammalian target of rapamycin (mTOR). This chapter discusses the pathogenesis of diabetic kidney disease (DKD) in relation to aging process and introduces some potential therapeutic methods to cope with diabetes-related kidney function decline.

1.2 Hemodynamic Changes and Chronic Hypoxia at the Center of Aging Kidney and DKD

1.2.1 Vasculature of the Kidney (Fig. 1.1) [2]

The kidney has a unique spatial arrangement of vasculature; it has two capillary networks that run in series. The renal artery bifurcates into interlobar arteries, arcuate arteries, interlobular arteries, and afferent arterioles. The afferent arterioles give

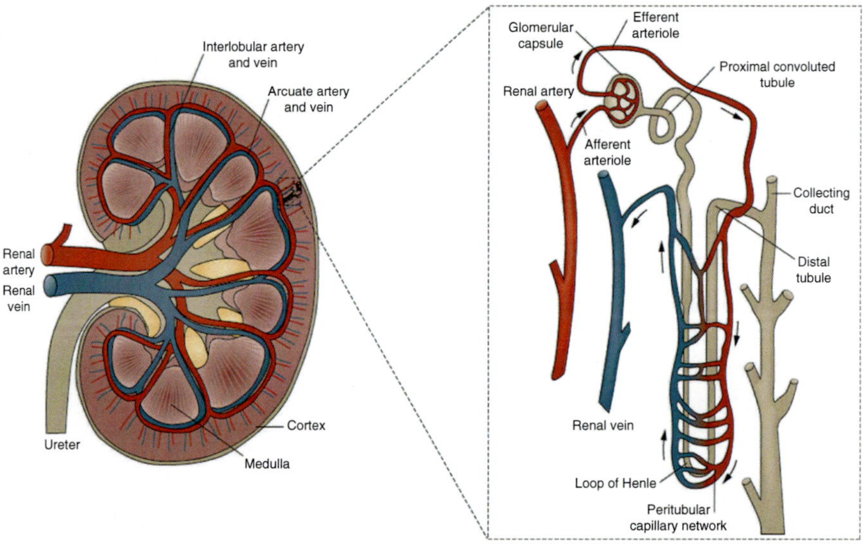

Fig. 1.1 Vasculature of the kidney. The renal artery bifurcates into interlobar arteries, arcuate arteries, interlobular arteries, and afferent arterioles. The afferent arterioles give rise to the first capillary network, the glomerulus, and they merge again at the vascular pole to form efferent arterioles. The efferent arterioles enter the second capillary network, the peritubular capillaries, which surround tubules and offer oxygen and nutrients to tubular and interstitial cells. The enlargement shows the architecture of a nephron with arrows indicating the direction of blood flow. Reprinted by permission from Macmillan Publishers Ltd.: Nat Rev. Nephrol 6: 667–78, © 2010

rise to the first capillary network, the glomerulus, and they merge again at the vascular pole to form efferent arterioles. The efferent arterioles enter the second capillary network, the peritubular capillaries (PTCs), which surround tubules and offer oxygen and nutrients to tubular and interstitial cells.

Although this anatomy is crucial for the regulation of renal blood flow (RBF), GFR, urine concentration, and other specialized kidney functions, arterial and venous vessels running in close parallel to each other gives rise to a diffusional oxygen shunt, which results in comparatively low oxygen tensions in the renal tissue. The renal medulla is especially prone to hypoxia, because its blood supply depends on vasa recta which emerge from juxtamedullary glomeruli and travel along the long loop of Henle.

1.2.2 Morphological and Hemodynamic Changes of Aging Kidney

Histological observations of kidneys from autopsies and nephrectomies have revealed some universal changes associated with aging (Table 1.1), not only in the glomerulus and tubules but also in the vessels. After 40 years of age, atherosclerotic changes become evident in the pre-glomerular arteries, i.e., interlobar arteries, arcuate arteries, and interlobular arteries, causing RBF to decrease at a rate of approximately 10% per decade [3]. This decrease is most profound in the renal cortex, resulting in cortical atrophy. The degree of atherosclerosis correlates with the degree of glomerulosclerosis [3], which is a common finding in the aging kidney, suggesting a hemodynamic role in the aging process.

In the arterioles, hyaline deposition within the vascular wall leads to obliteration of the lumen and is also related to glomerulosclerosis. There are two types of structural changes associated with arteriolopathy; it results in complete atrophy of the cortical glomeruli, whereas it forms a shunt between the afferent and efferent arterioles in the juxtamedullary nephrons (Fig. 1.2) [4]. The latter change increases the

Table 1.1 Histological changes in DKD and aging kidney

	DKD	Aging kidney
Glomerulus	Mesangial matrix expansion Uniform thickening of capillary wall Nodular lesion Diffuse lesion Exudative lesion (hyalinosis)	Focal and segmental glomerulosclerosis Hyaline deposition Thickening of glomerular basement membrane
Tubulointerstitium	Thickening of tubular basement membrane Tubular atrophy Fibrosis	Tubular atrophy Fibrosis
Vessels	Hyaline deposition in arterioles Atherosclerosis Loss of PTCs New vessel formation near the hilus	Hyaline deposition in arterioles Atherosclerosis Loss of PTCs Aglomerular arterioles

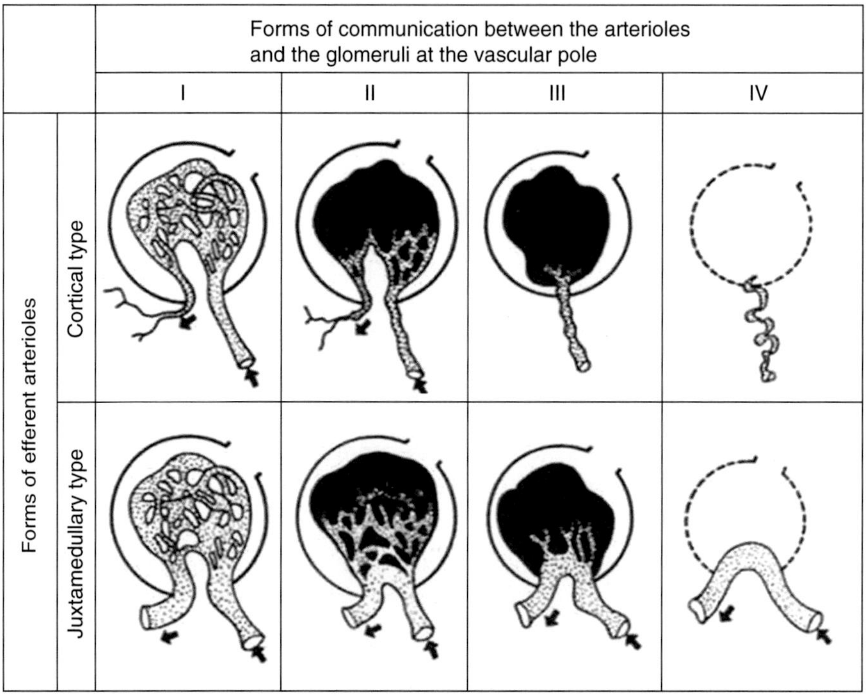

Fig. 1.2 Two types of structural changes associated with arteriolopathy. There are two types of structural changes associated with arteriolopathy; it results in complete atrophy of the cortical glomeruli, whereas it forms a shunt between the afferent and efferent arterioles in the juxtamedullary nephrons, resulting in aglomerular arterioles. Reprinted by permission from Elsevier: Kidney Int 2: 224–30, © 1972

blood flow to the medulla, resulting in a redistribution of blood flow from the cortex to the medulla.

As a consequence of glomerulosclerosis, the aging kidney fails to maintain PTCs, causing hypoxia in the tubulointerstitial area. Hypoxia has now been recognized as a common mediator to progressive kidney diseases [2, 5], and the same scenario also applies to the process of physiological aging. Experimentally, the kidneys from old rats were indeed exposed to extensive degrees of hypoxia [6].

1.2.3 Hemodynamic Changes of DKD

Diabetes is the leading cause of end-stage kidney disease (ESKD) and is associated with increased cardiovascular mortality. The earliest sign of DKD is persistent albuminuria, and even with appropriate glycemic control and antihypertensive treatment, a certain number of patients progress to overt proteinuria and eventually to renal failure. Histological changes typically observed in DKD are listed in Table 1.1.

As DKD is often referred to as one of the "microvascular" complications of diabetes, vascular dysfunction plays an important role in the pathogenesis of DKD.

Both arteries and arterioles invariably show the typical changes of arteriosclerosis and arteriolosclerosis, respectively. The arteries exhibit intimal thickening accompanied by reduplication of elastic lamina [7], the finding also observed in the aging kidney. Hyaline arteriolosclerosis is also a frequent and early manifestation of DKD. Arteriolopathy results in a maladaptive autoregulation that permits the transmission of systemic hypertension to glomerular capillaries. Moreover, diabetes disturbs vasoactive humoral systems which control the glomerular circulation. The balance between factors influencing the afferent arteriolar tone is shifted toward vasodilation, whereas opposite changes may occur on the efferent arterioles, resulting in glomerular hypertension and subsequent hyperfiltration [8].

Glomerular hypertension causes mechanical damage to the capillary wall, eventually leading to glomerulosclerosis and loss of PTCs. Elevated glomerular pressure also increases filtration of proteins to tubular lumen. Consequently, enhanced tubular reabsorption induces synthesis of pro-inflammatory and profibrotic factors, further resulting in tubulointerstitial inflammation and fibrosis. Fibrosis and loss of PTCs generate hypoxic state in associated tubulointerstitial areas, which is known as the common final pathway of progressive kidney diseases [2, 5]. These insights indicate that arterio- and arteriolosclerosis underlie the pathogenesis of both diabetic and aging kidney. This would further imply that diabetes accelerates the process of aging through hemodynamic changes and associated tubulointerstitial injury in the kidney.

1.3 Cellular and Molecular Biology of DKD in Relation to Aging

Hyperglycemia alters metabolic pathways and cellular environments; many of these changes are involved not only in the pathogenesis of DKD but also in renal senescence. The altered metabolism further contributes to the progression of hemodynamic changes and tubulointerstitial injury described above. In these regards, understanding the molecular basis of DKD may also help to unveil the aging process in the kidney.

1.3.1 Reactive Oxygen Species (ROS)

It has been generally accepted that the imbalance between antioxidant defense mechanism and ROS production leads to oxidative stress and subsequent pathological conditions including diabetic and aging kidney. ROS are chemically reactive molecules containing oxygen. Several ROS with unpaired electrons, such as superoxide, hydroxyl radicals, and lipid radicals, are considered as free radicals. Hydrogen peroxide (H_2O_2), peroxynitrite ($ONOO^-$), and hydrochlorous acid (HOCl) are not free radicals but possess an oxidizing effect. ROS are usually considered cytotoxic, because they oxidize important macromolecules including proteins, lipids, carbohydrates, and nucleic acids, disrupting their physiological functions.

One pathogenic mechanism of ROS in relation to DKD and aging kidney is through inducing endothelial dysfunction and subsequent atherosclerosis [9]. For example, superoxide anions inactivate endothelium-derived NO by converting it to peroxynitrite. NO has important anti-atherosclerotic properties which include regulation of vascular tone and vessel wall permeability, suppression of leukocyte adhesion to the endothelial surface, inhibition of vascular smooth muscle cell migration, and proliferation; its inactivation inevitably results in atherosclerosis. In the kidney, reduced levels of NO leads to vasoconstriction and a subsequent decrease in PTC blood flow [2, 5]. Furthermore, ROS elicit inflammatory pathway, another important contributor in the pathogenesis of atherosclerosis.

Within the mammalian cell, there are mainly three sources of ROS; mitochondrion, endoplasmic reticulum (ER), and the enzyme systems in the cytosol, such as xanthine oxidase, lipoxygenase, and nicotinamide adenine dinucleotide phosphatase oxidase (NOX) [10]. The traditional view has been that production of ROS would generate harmful effects, regardless of the cell types or their source. However, recent findings revealed that some ROS are essential in specific intracellular signaling pathways and actually function in a beneficial manner.

The ROS molecules whose functions are extensively reevaluated include superoxide produced in mitochondria. It has been assumed that excess glucose uptake would lead to an increase in pyruvate entry into mitochondria and an increased flux of substrates to the electron transport chain, resulting in hyperpolarization of the mitochondrial membrane and accumulation of electrons at complex III and coenzyme Q, which donate electrons to molecular oxygen and generate superoxide anions. This pathway has been considered as the central source of ROS in the pathogenesis of DKD. However, a new *in vivo* method of measuring superoxide via *in vivo* administration of dihydroethidium (DHE) to mice revealed that superoxide was actually reduced in the kidney in both streptozotocin (STZ)-induced diabetic mice and Ins2-Akita mice [11]. Mice with reduced superoxide dismutase (SOD) 2, an antioxidant enzyme, did show increased renal superoxide production, but the degrees of mesangial expansion or albuminuria were comparable to the wild-type mice when they were made diabetic. Furthermore, a stimulation of mitochondrial biogenesis with adenosine monophosphate kinase (AMPK) activation resulted in an increased superoxide production, accompanied by reduced mesangial matrix and albuminuria in STZ-induced diabetic mice [11].

These observations led to the proposal of a new theory, "mitochondrial hormesis," whereby a "physiological" increase in mitochondrial superoxide is actually beneficial, whereas excessively high levels of superoxide and/or decreased superoxide may contribute to the disease progression or be a permissive factor for inflammation and fibrosis [10]. The same applies to the process of aging. It has been proposed that ROS in general contributed to chronic organ damage in the elderly, but some recent studies provided compelling results. For example, exposure of *Caenorhabditis elegans* to 2-deoxyglucose (DOG), an inhibitor of glycolysis, increased mitochondrial ROS and increased life span. In the same study, co-administration of N-acetylcysteine with 2-DOG reduced ROS production and the benefit in life span extension [12].

Overall, the way oxidative stress contributes to the pathogenesis of DKD and aging kidney might be more complex than initially thought. A further investigation is required to unveil these two sides of ROS.

1.3.2 AGEs

AGEs are a heterogeneous group of bioactive molecules that are formed by the nonenzymatic glycation of proteins, lipids, and nucleic acids. In diabetes, hyperglycemia and oxidative stress promote the reversible glycation of target substrates, forming Schiff bases. The following chemical rearrangement forms the more stable early glycated product, Amadori product. Then, the slow complex rearrangement finally proceeds to the formation of AGEs. This final process is irreversible, resulting in the accumulation of AGEs in diabetes [7, 8] (Fig. 1.3a).

AGEs contribute to the pathogenesis of DKD in both receptor-independent and dependent manners [8] (Fig. 1.3b). The former includes modification of extracellular matrix (ECM) structure by cross-linking of proteins such as collagen and elastin. This process increases ECM rigidity and its resistance to proteolytic degradation, leading to mesangial matrix accumulation and interstitial fibrosis. Cross-linking of matrix proteins also increases permeability of glomerular basement membranes.

In addition to altering the structure of extracellular proteins, AGEs exert their effects through various specific cell surface receptors, collectively referred to as "RAGE," receptor for AGEs. The AGE-RAGE interaction stimulates multiple intracellular signaling pathways which contribute to the pathophysiology of DKD; for example, it activates NOX and increases cytosolic production of ROS. It also activates several nuclear transcription factors, such as nuclear factor kappa-B (NF-κB). The subsequent cellular responses include production of cytokines, growth factors, and cell adhesion molecules, promoting inflammation and fibrosis [8].

Recent evidence suggests that AGEs are also involved in renal senescence. A cross-sectional study of older community-dwelling women showed that higher levels of serum carboxymethyl-lysine (CML), a common AGE, correlated with reduced GFR [13]. Experimentally, overexpression of glyoxalase I (GLO1), an enzyme which detoxifies precursors of AGEs, was shown to ameliorate age-related interstitial thickening as well as serum creatinine increase in aged rats [14]. A part of this anti-aging effect arises from preserved endothelial function. In GLO1 transgenic rats, NO production in endothelial cells was well maintained even at 53 weeks of age [15]. Therefore, AGEs may be a novel therapeutic target of both DKD and aging kidney.

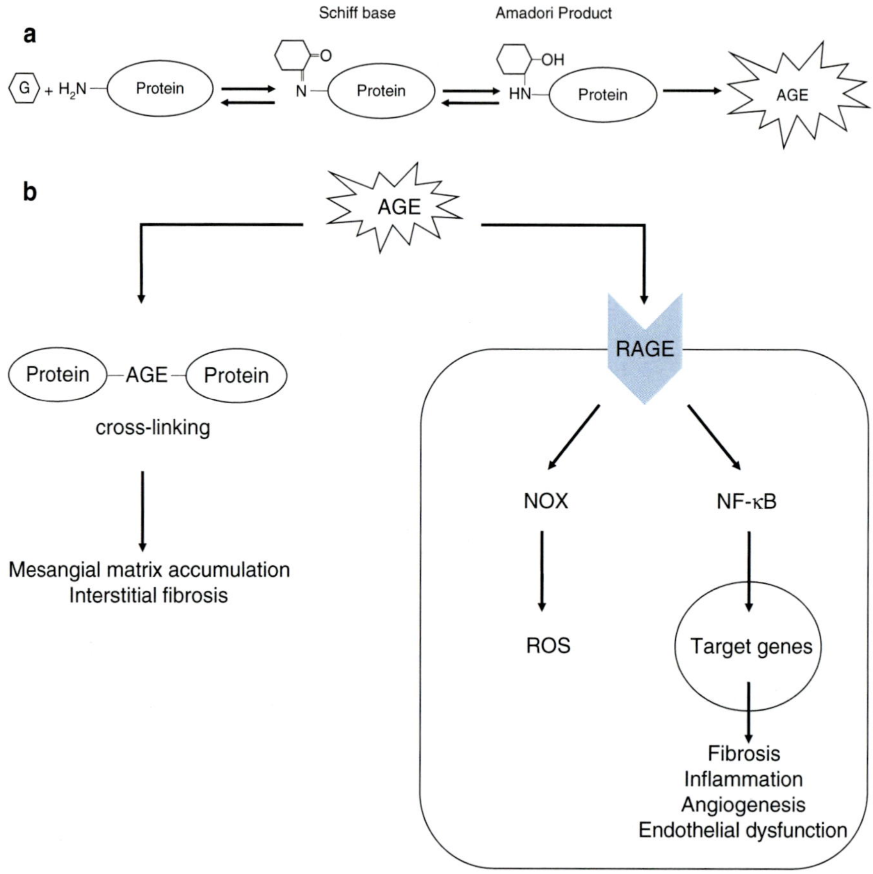

Fig. 1.3 (**a**) AGE formation. AGEs are formed by nonenzymatic Maillard reaction between carbonyl groups of reducing sugars and amino groups on proteins, lipids, or nucleic acids. The rates of these reactions are slow under physiological conditions, but are accelerated under persistent hyperglycemia, dyslipidemia, and oxidative stress. (**b**) Effects of AGEs. AGEs contribute to the pathogenesis of DKD in both receptor-independent and dependent manners. AGEs form cross-links between ECM proteins, which increase ECM rigidity and its resistance to proteolytic degradation, leading to mesangial matrix accumulation and interstitial fibrosis. AGEs also modulate cellular activities through RAGE. The AGE-RAGE interaction activates NOX and increases cytosolic production of ROS. It also activates several nuclear transcription factors, including NF-κB. However, this drawing shows only a part of the complex mechanism of how AGEs contribute to the pathogenesis of DKD

1.3.3 Impaired Autophagy

Autophagy is a "self-eating" pathway by which cells degrade macromolecules and organelles to maintain intracellular homeostasis. It has two major physiological roles; one is to recycle intracellular resources in response to conditions of nutrient deficiency, and the other is to remove damaged proteins and organelles under various stress conditions [16]. Accumulating evidence has shown that autophagy is impaired in both diabetic and aging kidney, making renal cells more vulnerable to pathological stresses such as ROS, AGEs, and hypoxia.

Transgenic mice systemically expressing green fluorescent protein (GFP)-labeled LC-3, a marker protein for autophagosomes, revealed a high basal level of autophagy in podocytes [17], and its inhibition was detrimental to podocytes' cytoskeleton [18]. Hyperglycemia was shown to reduce autophagic activity [18], indicating a pathogenic role of impaired autophagy in DKD. Indeed, mice with podocyte-specific deletion of autophagy-related 5 (*Atg5*) developed podocyte loss and massive proteinuria in a high-fat diet-induced diabetic model [19].

Autophagy is also essential in maintaining homeostasis in renal tubular cells. Unlike podocytes, the basal autophagic activity in proximal tubular cells is low [16]. However, insults to the kidney, such as ischemia-reperfusion and cisplatin, resulted in increased autophagy [20, 21]. In these studies, mice lacking *Atg5* specifically in proximal tubular cells exhibited severer acute kidney injury (AKI), suggesting renoprotective effects of autophagy. Proteinuria is also known to exert nephrotoxic stress on tubular cells, stimulating autophagy. However, in animal models of diabetes, autophagy was suppressed in proximal tubules, which was accompanied by exacerbation of proteinuria-induced tubulointerstitial damage [22]. The investigation of human kidney biopsy also revealed lower autophagic activity in type 2 diabetic patients [22]. These findings may indicate that insufficient upregulation of autophagy underlies the tubulointerstitial injury in DKD.

The association of autophagy with aging has also been extensively studied; it is generally considered that autophagic activity declines with aging, leading to accumulation of damaged proteins and organelle within cells, which subsequently results in functional deterioration in the elderly. In the field of nephrology, mice with podocyte-specific deletion of *Atg5* were shown to develop a higher level of albuminuria and a significant increase in glomerulosclerosis at the age of 20–24 months compared with control littermates [23]. Moreover, accumulating body of evidence has revealed that some life span-related signaling pathways, including mTOR and sirtuins, regulate autophagy in the kidney, casting an influence on the progression of DKD and renal senescence (discussed in the next section).

1.4 Signaling Pathways Related to DKD and Aging Kidney

Research into the aging process has revealed some key signaling pathways associated with life span, such as mTOR-, sirtuin-, insulin-like growth factor (IGF)-, and Klotho-related pathways. Diabetes may shorten patients' lives by modulating these pathways [24]. This section describes some of the proposed relationships between mTOR or sirtuin signaling and kidney aging in diabetic patients.

1.4.1 mTOR Signaling Pathways

mTOR is an evolutionarily conserved serine-threonine kinase that regulates cell growth, proliferation, and metabolism. mTOR forms at least two distinct functional complexes, called mTOR complex 1 (mTORC1) and mTOR complex 2 (mTORC2) [25]. Inhibition of mTOR increases life span of animals, and calorie restriction (CR) is considered to induce longevity by downregulating mTOR [24].

Although both mTORC1 and mTORC2 regulate a number of different downstream pathways, the most extensively studied in relation to DKD is mTORC1's effect on autophagy. mTORC1 negatively regulates autophagy by inhibiting the activity of the Unc-51-like kinase 1 (ULK1), one of the autophagy initiating kinases, through direct phosphorylation [26]. Enhanced mTORC1 activity is observed in human patients and animal models of diabetes [26], which may be one of the causes of impaired autophagy discussed above. Interestingly, nondiabetic mice with podocyte-specific activation of mTORC1 also manifested mesangial expansion, glomerular basement membrane thickening, and proteinuria, all of which resemble DKD [27]. Moreover, treatment with rapamycin, an inhibitor of mTORC1, suppressed the development of DKD in STZ-induced diabetic rats and db/db mice, suggesting the important pathogenic role of mTORC1 in DKD [26].

1.4.2 Sirtuins

Sirtuins are another family of molecules associated with life span of organisms. One of the members, silent information regulator 2 (SIR2), was originally found to promote longevity in yeast. There are seven mammalian homologues of SIR2, SIRT1–7, of which SIRT1 most closely resembles SIR2. SIRT1 was initially recognized as an NAD-dependent histone deacetylase, which induces chromatin silencing and transcriptional repression. However, recent studies have revealed that its targets are not confined to histones; SIRT1 regulates a wide variety of cellular processes, including glucose and lipid metabolism, mitochondrial biogenesis, inflammation, and autophagy, which are largely organ protective [28].

SIRT1 is also considered to have an anti-aging effect in the kidney. Kume et al. reported a decreased expression of SIRT1 in 24-month-old mice, which was recovered by long-term CR, attenuating hypoxia-associated mitochondrial damage [29]. SIRT1 deacetylases forkhead box O3 (FOXO3), a transcription factor regulating the expression of BCL2/adenovirus E1B 19-kDa interacting protein 3 (Bnip3), which is an essential component of autophagy. Taken together, SIRT1 deficiency underlies the impaired autophagic activity in the aging kidney, resulting in decreased cellular resistance to stress conditions, such as hypoxia. Furthermore, an accumulating body of evidence has shown anti-apoptotic, anti-inflammatory, and anti-fibrotic effects of SIRT1, suggesting multiple pathways by which SIRT1 deficiency promotes the process of kidney aging [28].

A decrease in SIRT1 protein expression has also been observed in both type 1 and type 2 diabetic animal models [26]. In addition to its effect on renal cells, SIRT1 modulates glucose and lipid metabolism through various mechanisms; it promotes insulin secretion, improves insulin resistance, and increases adiponectin excretion [30]. Therefore, activation or upregulation of SIRT1 may serve as an effective therapeutic strategy against DKD.

1.5 Potential Renoprotective Treatments for DKD

Current therapeutic strategy for DKD consists of glycemic control and antihypertensive treatment with renin-angiotensin system (RAS) inhibitors. However, they fail to fully prevent the progression of kidney function decline, emphasizing the need for novel therapies. This section explains how RAS inhibitors slow the progression of DKD and introduces some potential therapeutic methods that are being developed based on new knowledge of the pathogenesis of DKD.

1.5.1 RAS Inhibitors

RAS blockade induces vasodilation of glomerular arterioles; the degree of dilatation is greater in the efferent arterioles, resulting in reduced intraglomerular pressure and, thus, less damage to the capillary walls. RAS inhibitors also restore PTC blood flow and subsequently improve oxygenation of the tubulointerstitium. In addition, RAS inhibitors have an important role as antioxidants, ameliorating oxidative stress induced by hyperglycemia [2, 5]. Furthermore, RAS inhibitors contribute to reorganization of functional molecules composing the slit diaphragm, which maintains the barrier function of glomerular capillary walls and reduces proteinuria [31].

1.5.2 Sodium-Glucose Cotransporter-2 (SGLT2) Inhibitors

SGLT2 inhibitors are another family of drugs that may slow the progression of DKD by restoring intrarenal hemodynamics. SGLT2 is located in the early proximal tubule and couples glucose reabsorption to sodium reabsorption. Since it reabsorbs 80–90% of filtered glucose, SGLT2 blockade results in glucose excretion into urine and a subsequent decrease in blood glucose levels.

Although developed as a new class of antidiabetic agent, SGLT2 inhibitors slow the progression of DKD possibly by a mechanism independent of their blood glucose lowering effects. In a randomized controlled trial, EMPA-REG OUTCOME trial, patients treated with empagliflozin revealed a significantly smaller decrease in estimated GFR (eGFR) during the 192-week interventional period compared to the placebo-treated group [32]. It has been postulated that SGLT2 inhibition results in increased sodium delivery to the juxtaglomerular apparatus, which subsequently leads to vasoconstriction of afferent arterioles and lowering of intraglomerular pressure through the mechanism of tubuloglomerular feedback. Other effects, such as those on arterial stiffness, vascular resistance, serum uric acid levels, and the systemic and renal neurohormonal systems may also contribute to the renoprotective effects of SGLT2 inhibitors [32]. Additionally, some studies point to an increasing trend in serum erythropoietin (EPO) levels by SGLT2 inhibitors [33], which may also contribute to the protective effect. At cellular levels, hyperglycemia accelerates tubular senescence through upregulation of p21 expression; this upregulation was also attenuated by SGLT2 knockdown in an *in vitro* experiment [34].

1.5.3 Prolyl Hydroxylase Domain (PHD) Inhibitors

As mentioned earlier, tubulointerstitial hypoxia underlies the pathogenesis of progressive kidney diseases, including DKD. On the other hand, cells possess several mechanisms for adapting themselves to hypoxic conditions. Facilitating these responses may mitigate detrimental consequences of hypoxia and possibly induce renoprotective effects.

Hypoxia-inducible factor (HIF) lies at the center of these adaptive responses to hypoxia. HIF is a heterodimeric transcription factor composed of an oxygen-dependent α-subunit and a constitutively expressed β-subunit. In hypoxic conditions, HIF upregulates its target genes, which are involved in angiogenesis, erythropoiesis, glycolysis, and cell survival. Cells continuously synthesize HIF-α subunits, and their transcriptional activity is primarily controlled by the rate of degradation. Under normoxic conditions, oxygen-dependent HIF-α degradation is initiated by PHD enzymes. They use molecular oxygen to hydroxylate HIF-α at specific proline residues, and these proline-hydroxylated HIF-α is recognized by the von Hippel-Lindau (VHL)-E3 ubiquitin ligase complex, resulting in ubiquitination of HIF-α. Ubiquitinated HIF-α is then destroyed by the proteasome. Under hypoxic conditions, hydroxylation of HIF-α is inhibited, allowing it to translocate to the nucleus where it dimerizes with HIF-β and enhances transcription of target genes (Fig. 1.4) [2, 5].

Inhibition of PHD enzymes, therefore, would increase the expression of HIF-target genes including EPO. Based on these findings, small-molecule inhibitors of PHDs have been developed as a new therapeutic method for anemia in chronic kidney disease (CKD) patients. At least six compounds are currently tested in clinical trials, most of them showing promising results [35]. There are some expectations that these PHD inhibitors would also ameliorate CKD; however, preclinical studies present inconclusive results. HIF activation by cobalt reduced proteinuria and tubulointerstitial damage in STZ-induced diabetic rats [36], while proximal tubular deletion of HIF-1α ameliorated fibrosis in the unilateral ureteral obstruction model, suggesting a profibrotic role of HIF [37]. Along similar lines, overexpression of

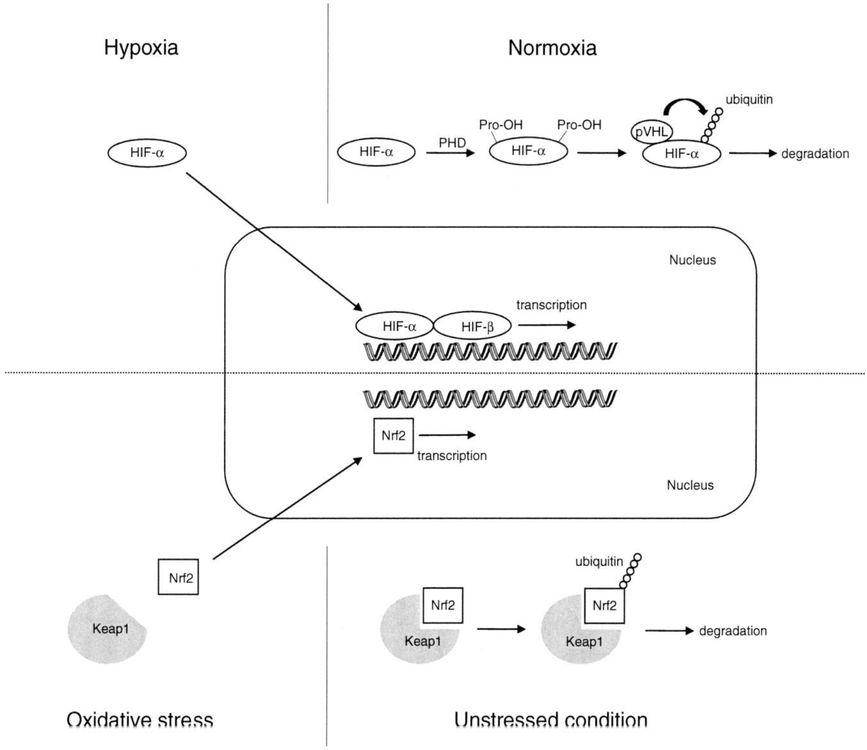

Fig. 1.4 Cellular defense mechanisms against hypoxia and oxidative stress. (*Upper panel*) Under normoxic conditions, HIF-α is hydroxylated at specific proline residues by PHD enzymes. Proline-hydroxylated HIF-α is recognized by VHL proteins, resulting in ubiquitination of HIF-α. Ubiquitinated HIF-α is then destroyed by the proteasome. Under hypoxic conditions, hydroxylation of HIF-α is inhibited, allowing them to translocate to the nucleus where they dimerize with HIF-β and induces transcription of target genes. (*Lower panel*) Under unstressed conditions, Nrf2 is continuously ubiquitinated by Keap1 and degraded within the proteasome. Under oxidative stress, ubiquitination of Nrf2 is inhibited, allowing it to translocate to the nucleus where it enhances transcription of target genes

HIF-2α in distal tubules using an ectopic promoter resulted in fibrogenesis [38]. Further studies are required to clarify the optimal timing and cell types of HIF activation as well as the specific PHD subtypes to inhibit, which would generate desirable renoprotective effects in CKD including DKD.

1.5.4 Bardoxolone Methyl

Oxidative stress, another key player in the pathogenesis of DKD, is also a target of new therapeutic strategy. Similar to the PHD-HIF axis against hypoxic stress, cells have antioxidant mechanism called the Keap1-Nrf2 pathway (Nrf2: nuclear factor-erythroid

2-related factor 2). Nrf2 is a transcription factor which regulates the expression of several antioxidant and cytoprotective genes. Its level is primarily regulated by the rate of degradation by Keap1. Under unstressed conditions, Nrf2 is continuously ubiquitinated by Keap1 and degraded within the proteasome. Under oxidative stress, on the other hand, ubiquitination of Nrf2 is inhibited, allowing it to translocate to the nucleus where it enhances transcription of target genes (Fig. 1.4) [39].

Bardoxolone methyl is a potent inducer of Nrf2 originally developed as an anticancer drug. In two phase I clinical trials with 81 oncology patients, however, it showed unexpected improvement in eGFR and was further developed as a renal drug [39, 40]. In a phase II clinical trial with 20 patients whose eGFR were between 15 and 45 ml/min/1.73 m^2, bardoxolone methyl did improve renal function with only mild side effects [40]. Unfortunately, the subsequent phase III BEACON trial enrolling patients with stage 4 CKD and type 2 diabetes had to be terminated prematurely because of a higher rate of cardiovascular events in the drug-treated group [41]. However, secondary analysis revealed that the elevated baseline B-type natriuretic peptide and previous hospitalization for heart failure were the risk factors for cardiovascular events related to bardoxolone methyl; for patients without these baseline characteristics, the risk was in fact similar between the bardoxolone methyl- and placebo-treated patients [42]. In addition, the prevalence of cardiovascular diseases in the Japanese population tends to be lower than that in the American and other Western populations, suggesting that it is relatively safe to continue a clinical trial in Japan, provided that patients at risk are excluded from the study. A phase II clinical trial involving patients with stage 3 CKD and type 2 diabetes is currently underway (TSUBAKI study).

1.6 Conclusion

Although numerous efforts have been made to find a new therapeutic method to treat DKD, it continues to be the leading cause of ESKD worldwide. Recent research into pathogenesis of DKD has revealed that much of its molecular mechanism is shared with that of renal senescence. In addition, diabetes induces atherosclerosis and subsequent hemodynamic changes, which also accelerate the aging process within the kidney. This highlights the importance of unveiling the influence of both diabetes and aging in the field of nephrology, especially in a highly aging society.

References

1. Weinstein JR, Anderson S. The aging kidney: physiological changes. Adv Chronic Kidney Dis. 2010;17:302–7. doi:10.1053/j.ackd.2010.05.002.
2. Mimura I, Nangaku M. The suffocating kidney: tubulointerstitial hypoxia in end-stage renal disease. Nat Rev Nephrol. 2010;6:667–78. doi:10.1038/nrneph.2010.124.

3. Kasiske BL. Relationship between vascular disease and age-associated changes in the human kidney. Kidney Int. 1987;31:1153–9.
4. Takazakura E, Sawabu N, Handa A, Shinoda A, Takeuchi J. Intrarenal vascular changes with age and disease. Kidney Int. 1972;2:224–30.
5. Nangaku M. Chronic hypoxia and tubulointerstitial injury: a final common pathway to end-stage renal failure. J Am Soc Nephrol. 2006;17:17–25.
6. Tanaka T, Kato H, Kojima I, Ohse T, Son D, Kawakami T, et al. Hypoxia and expression of hypoxia-inducible factor in the aging kidney. J Gerontol A Biol Sci Med Sci. 2006;61:795–805.
7. Olson JL, Laszik ZG. Diabetic nephropathy. In: Jennette JC, Olson JL, Schwartz MM, Silva FG, editors. Heptinstall's pathology of the kidney. 6th ed. Philadelphia: Lippincott Williams & Wilkins; 2007.
8. Vallon V, Komers R. Pathophysiology of the diabetic kidney. Compr Physiol. 2011;1:1175–232. doi:10.1002/cphy.c100049.
9. Panth N, Paudel KR, Parajuli K. Reactive oxygen species: a key hall mark of cardiovascular disease. Adv Med. 2016. doi: 10.1155/2016/9152732.
10. Coughlan MT, Sharma K. Challenging the dogma of mitochondrial reactive oxygen species overproduction in diabetic kidney disease. Kidney Int. 2016;90:272–9. doi:10.1016/j.kint.2016.02.043.
11. Dugan LL, You YH, Ali SS, Diamond-Stanic M, Miyamoto S, DeCleves AE, et al. AMPK dysregulation of superoxide and mitochondrial function. J Clin Invest. 2013;123:4888–99. doi:10.1172/JCI66218.
12. Schulz TJ, Zarse K, Voigt A, Urban N, Birringer M, Ristow M. Glucose restriction extends *Caenorhabditis elegans* life span by inducing mitochondrial respiration and increasing oxidative stress. Cell Metab. 2007;6:280–93. doi:10.1016/j.cmet.2007.08.011.
13. Semba RD, Ferrucci L, Fink JC, Sun K, Beck J, Dalal M, et al. Advanced glycation end products and their circulating receptors and level of kidney function in older community-dwelling women. Am J Kidney Dis. 2009;53:51–8. doi:10.1053/j.ajkd.2008.06.018.
14. Ikeda Y, Inagi R, Miyata T, Nagai R, Arai M, Miyashita M, et al. Glyoxalase I retards renal senescence. Am J Pathol. 2011;179:2810–21. doi:10.1016/j.ajpath.2011.08.023.
15. Jo-Watanabe A, Ohse T, Nishimatsu H, Takahashi M, Ikeda Y, Wada T, et al. Glyoxalase I reduces glycative and oxidative stress and prevents age-related endothelial dysfunction through modulation of endothelial nitric oxide synthase phosphorylation. Aging Cell. 2014;13:519–28. doi:10.1111/acel.12204.
16. Kume S, Koya D. Autophagy: a novel therapeutic target for diabetic nephropathy. Diabetes Metab J. 2015;39:451–60. doi:10.4093/dmj.2015.39.6.451.
17. Mizushima N, Yamamoto A, Matsui M, Yoshimori T, Ohsumi Y. In vivo analysis of autophagy in response to nutrient starvation using transgenic mice expressing a fluorescent autophagosome marker. Mol Biol Cell. 2004;15:1101–11.
18. Fang L, Zhou Y, Cao H, Wen P, Jiang L, He W, et al. Autophagy attenuates diabetic glomerular damage through protection of Hyperglycemia-induced podocyte injury. PLoS One. 2013;8:360546.
19. Tagawa A, Yasuda M, Kume S, Yamahana K, Nakazawa J, Chin-Kanasaki M, et al. Impaired podocyte autophagy exacerbates proteinuria in diabetic nephropathy. Diabetes. 2016;65:755–67. doi:10.2337/db15-0473.
20. Kimura T, Takabatake Y, Takahashi A, Kaimori J, Matsui I, Namba T, et al. Autophagy protects the proximal tubule from degeneration and acute ischemic injury. J Am Soc Nephrol. 2011;22:902–13. doi:10.1681/ASN.2010070705.
21. Takahashi A, Kimura T, Takabatake Y, Namba T, Kaimori J, Kitamura H, et al. Autophagy guards against cisplatin-induced acute kidney injury. J Am Pathol. 2012;180:517–25. doi:10.1016/j.ajpath.2011.11.001.
22. Yamahara K, Kume S, Koya D, Yanaka Y, Morita Y, Chin-Kanasaki M, et al. Obesity-mediated autophagy insufficiency exacerbates proteinuria-induced tubulointerstitial lesions. J Am Soc Nephrol. 2013;24:1769–81. doi:10.1681/ASN.2012111080.

23. Hartleben B, Gödel M, Meyer-Schwesinger C, Liu S, Ulrich T, Köbler S, et al. Autophagy influences glomerular disease susceptibility and maintains podocyte homeostasis in aging mice. J Clin Invest. 2010;120:1084–96. doi:10.1172/JCI39492.
24. Bitzer M, Wiggins J. Aging biology in the kidney. Adv Chronic Kidney Dis. 2016;23:12–8. doi:10.1053/j.ackd.2015.11.005.
25. Fantus D, Rogers NM, Grahammer F, Huber TB, Thomson AW. Roles of mTOR complexes in the kidney: implications for renal disease and transplantation. Nat Rev Nephrol. 2016;12:587–609. doi:10.1038/nrneph.2016.108.
26. Ding Y, Choi ME. Autophagy in diabetic nephropathy. J Endocrinol. 2015;224:R15–30. doi:10.1530/JOE-14-0437.
27. Inoki K, Mori H, Wang J, Suzuki T, Hong S, Yoshida S, et al. mTORC1 activation in podocytes is a critical step in the development of diabetic nephropathy in mice. J Clin Invest. 2011;121:2181–96. doi:10.1172/JCI44771.
28. Kitada M, Kume S, Takeda-Watanabe A, Kanasaki K, Koya D. Sirtuins and renal diseases: relationship with aging and diabetic nephropathy. Clin Sci. 2013;124:153–64. doi:10.1042/CS20120190.
29. Kume S, Uzu T, Horiike K, Chin-Kanasaki M, Isshiki K, Araki S, et al. Calorie restriction enhances cell adaptation to hypoxia through Sirt1-dependent mitochondrial autophagy in mouse aged kidney. J Clin Invest. 2010;120:1043–55. doi:10.1172/JCI41376.
30. Kitada M, Koya D. SIRT1 in type 2 diabetes: mechanisms and therapeutic potential. Diabetes Metab J. 2013;37:315–25. doi:10.4093/dmj.2013.37.5.315.
31. Suzuki K, Han GD, Miyauchi N, Hashimoto T, Nakatsue T, Fujioka Y, et al. Angiotensin II type 1 and type 2 receptors play opposite roles in regulating the barrier function of kidney glomerular capillary wall. Am J Pathol. 2007;170:1841–53. doi:10.2353/ajpath.2007.060484.
32. Wanner C, Inzucchi SE, Lachin JM, Fitchett D, von Eynatten M, Mattheus M, et al. Empagliflozin and progression of kidney disease in type 2 diabetes. N Engl J Med. 2016;375:323–34. doi:10.1056/NEJMoa1515920.
33. Lambers Heerspink HJ, de Zeeuw D, Wie L, Leslie B, List J. Dapagliflozin a glucose-regulating drug with diuretic properties in subjects with type 2 diabetes. Diabetes Obes Metab. 2013;15:853–62. doi:10.1111/dom.12127.
34. Kitada K, Nakano D, Ohsaki H, Hitomi H, Minamino T, Yatabe J, et al. Hyperglycemia causes cellular senescence via a SGLT2- and p21-dependent pathway in proximal tubules in the early stage of diabetic nephropathy. J Diabetes Complicat. 2014;28:604–11. doi:10.1016/j..jdiacomp.2014.05.010.
35. Maxwell PH, Eckardt KU. HIF prolyl hydroxylase inhibitors for the treatment of renal anaemia and beyond. Nat Rev Nephrol. 2016;12:157–68. doi:10.1038/nrneph.2015.193.
36. Nordquist L, Friederich-Persson M, Fasching A, Liss P, Shoji K, Nangaku M, et al. Activation of hypoxia-inducible factors prevents diabetic nephropathy. J Am Soc Nephrol. 2015;26:328–38. doi:10.1681/ASN.2013090990.
37. Higgins DF, Kimura K, Bernhardt WM, Shrimanker N, Akai Y, Hohenstein B, et al. Hypoxia promotes fibrogenesis in vivo via HIF-1 stimulation of epithelial-to-mesenchymal transition. J Clin Invest. 2007;117:3810–20. doi:10.1172/JCI30487.
38. Schietke RE, Hackenbeck T, Tran M, Günther R, Klanke B, Warnecke CL, et al. Renal tubular HIF-2α expression requires VHL inactivation and causes fibrosis and cysts. PLoS One. 2012;7:e31034. doi:10.1371/journal.pone.0031034.
39. Miyata T, Suzuki N, van Ypersele de Strihou C. Diabetic nephropathy: are there new and potentially promising therapies targeting oxygen biology? Kidney Int. 2013;84:693–702. doi:10.1038/ki.2013.74.
40. Pergola PE, Krauth M, Huff JW, Ferguson DA, Ruiz S, Meyer C, Warnock DG. Effect of bardoxolone methyl on kidney function in patients with T2D and stage 3b-4 CKD. Am J Nephrol. 2011;33:469–76. doi:10.1159/000327599.

41. de Zeeuw D, Akizawa T, Audhya P, Bakris GL, Chin M, Christ-Schmidt H, et al. Bardoxolone methyl in type 2 diabetes and stage 4 chronic kidney disease. N Engl J Med. 2013;369:2492–503. doi:10.1056/NEJMoa1306033.
42. Chin MP, Wrolstad D, Barkris G, Chertow GM, de Zeeuw D, Goldsberry A, et al. Risk factors for heart failure in patients with type 2 diabetes mellitus and stage 4 chronic kidney disease treated with bardoxolone methyl. J Card Fail. 2014;20:953–8. doi:10.1016/j.cardfail.2014.10.001.

Chapter 2
Diabetic Eye Disease

Yuichi Kaji

Abstract More than 50 million people are suffering from blindness worldwide. In addition, the number of blinded patients is increasing. Cataract, diabetic retinopathy, age-related macular degeneration, and corneal disorders are major causes of blindness. Advanced glycation end products (AGEs) have a central role in the development of the above ocular diseases. Understanding the mechanism of AGE formation will be a clue to the prevention and treatment of major causes of blindness.

Keywords Advanced glycation end products (AGEs) • Receptor for AGEs (RAGE) • Diabetic retinopathy • Diabetic keratopathy • Cataract • Age-related macular degeneration • Diabetic keratopathy

2.1 Causes of Blindness

Humans receive more than 90% of information using their eyes. With advance of our technology, we receive various information from many informative devices such as computers, TVs, tablets, and smartphones, and good vision is therefore important. This means that vision loss would result in severe difficulty in daily life. The World Health organization (WHO) estimates that more than 50 million people are suffering from decreased vision or blindness [1]. Figure 2.1 shows the main causes of blindness worldwide. Even with the progression of modern medicine, the prevalence of blindness is increasing worldwide. The main causes of blindness are closely related to the Maillard reaction. The accumulation of products of the Maillard reaction in the body, or a reaction to these products, are involved in the development of severe ocular disorders. Understanding the Maillard reaction, and its regulation, is therefore a potential target for the prevention and treatment of blindness.

The causes of blindness differ considerably from country to country. In most of the developing countries, blinded patients with cataract are increasing. For example,

Y. Kaji
Department of Ophthalmology, University of Tsukuba, 1-1-1 Tennoudai, Tsukuba, Ibaraki 305-8575, Japan
e-mail: kajiyuichi@gmail.com

S.-i. Yamagishi (ed.), *Diabetes and Aging-related Complications*,
https://doi.org/10.1007/978-981-10-4376-5_2

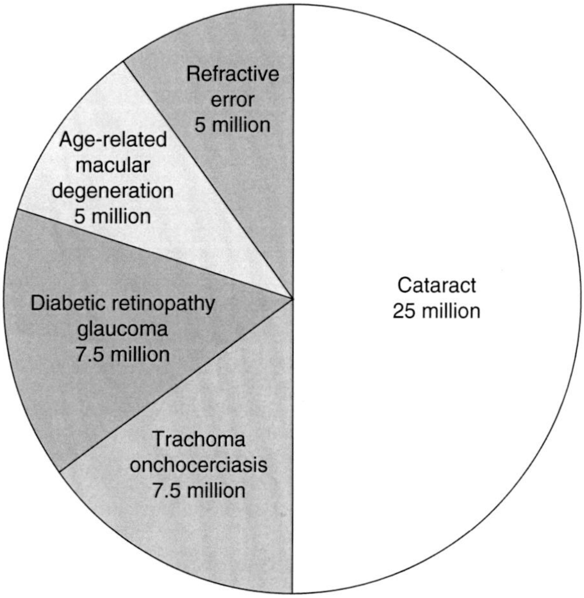

Fig. 2.1 Cause of blindness worldwide. Among the major causes of blindness, the Maillard reaction is closely related to cataracts, diabetic retinopathy, and age-related macular degeneration

cataracts are the cause of 86% cases of blindness in Nigeria [2]. As one ages, cataracts (clouded lenses) may develop; cataract surgery can restore good eyesight. However, the number of patients who can undergo cataract surgery is very limited in some developing countries. Ultimately, cataracts are now the cause of 50% cases of blindness worldwide [1]. If cataract formation could be reduced through the inhibition of the Maillard reaction, the number of blind patients may decreases considerably. In contrast, age-related macular degeneration is the leading cause of blindness in most developed countries. The Maillard reactions are known to play an important role in the development of age-related macular degeneration. The Maillard reaction could therefore be a candidate of therapeutic targets to prevent and treat age-related macular degeneration.

2.2 Cataracts and the Maillard Reaction

Cataract is a condition in which the lens in the eye becomes clouded with age (Fig. 2.2). Cataracts cause 50% of the cases of blindness worldwide, making cataracts the most important ocular disease leading to blindness.

The prevalence and the severity of the cataract increases with age, as the age-related changes of the lens accumulate in the lens itself. Accumulation of age-related materials in the lens is related to its histological character. In the tissue with epithelial cells, old cells are removed and replaced by new cells. This renewal system prevents age-related changes accumulating in the organ. However, the lens has quite a unique structure; the basement membrane covers the entire surface of the lens, and the older lens cells are pushed toward the center of the lens (Fig. 2.3). Old lens cells are

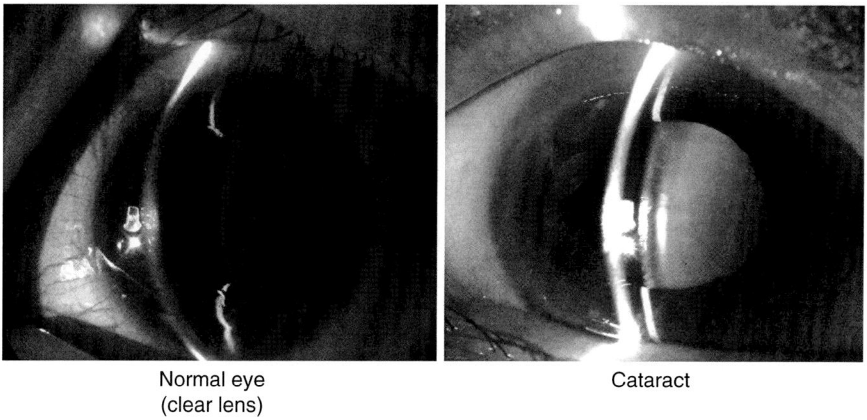

Fig. 2.2 Patient image of cataract. The lens is originally translucent. However, during the aging process, the lens becomes clouded, and the patient cannot capture a clear image

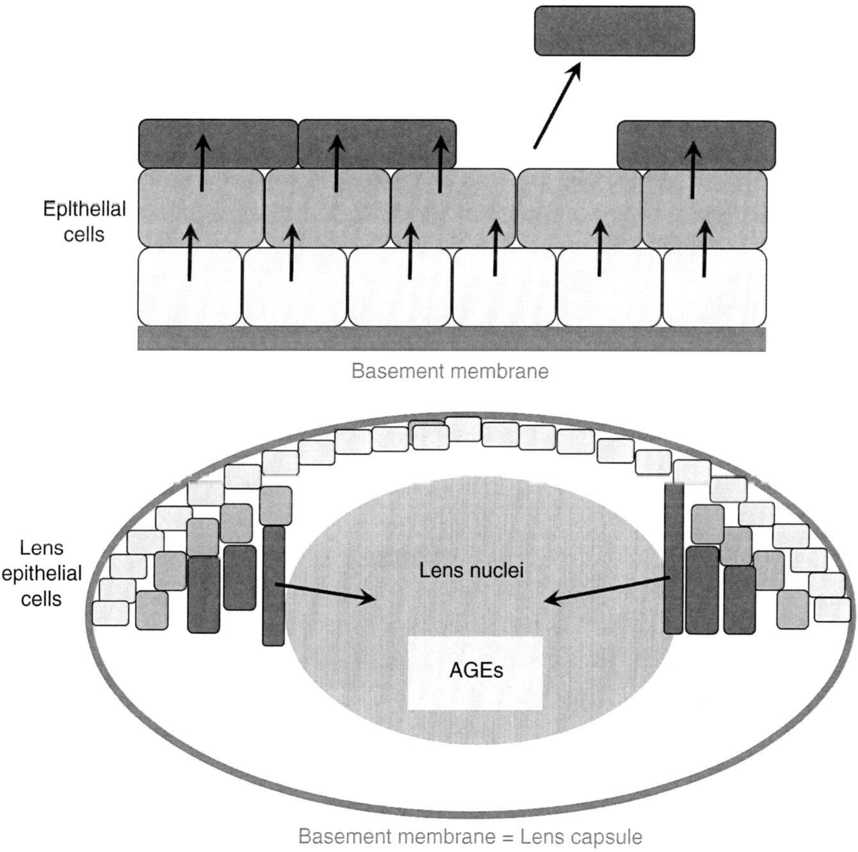

Fig. 2.3 Renewal system of epithelial cells and the lens epithelium. In the skin, old epithelial cells exfoliate from the surface of the epithelium. However, in the lens epithelium, the old epithelial cells accumulate toward the center of the lens

therefore not removed but accumulate at the center of the lens. The central part of the lens is one of the parts of the body most affected by the aging changes of tissue.

Etiological studies have reported ultraviolet irradiation, smoking, diabetes, alcohol intake, and oxidative stresses are risk factors in the development of cataracts [3–5]. These factors are known to accelerate the Maillard reaction and the advanced glycation end products. In fact, the lens is one of the first organs in which advanced glycation end products have been detected in vivo. In a cataract lens, various advanced glycation end products, including CML, pentosidine, and pyrraline, have been detected [6–8]. Advanced glycation in lens proteins, such as crystalline, induces intra- and intermolecular cross-linking, leading to the aggregation of abnormal proteins and lens clouding.

2.3 Age-Related Macular Degeneration and the Maillard Reaction

Age-related macular degeneration affects the central section of the retina and is a major cause of blindness, especially in United States, Australia, and a number of European countries [9, 10]. A major risk factor of age-related macular degeneration is the increase in age of the patient. Therefore, the number of the patients with age-related macular degeneration is increasing as the life expectancy increases, particularly in most of the developed countries. The prevalence of age-related macular degeneration is roughly 10% in patients over the age of 75 years [9, 10]. However, a precursor lesion develops more often. Early degenerative changes of macula, the central section of the retina, are seen in 30% of 70–80-year-old individuals, and 50% in those individuals are over the age of 80 years. It is important to prevent or limit the degenerative changes and the progression to the final stages of age-related macular degeneration.

In the end stages of the age-related macular degeneration, uncontrolled proliferation of the blood vessels extends from the choroid into the retina (Fig. 2.4). The

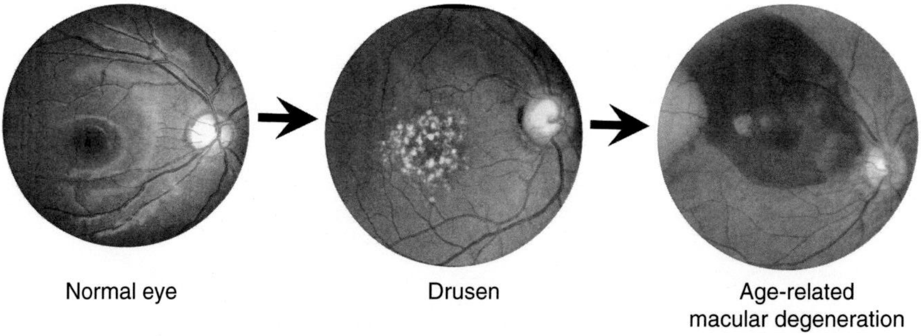

Fig. 2.4 Progression of age-related macular degeneration. In the early stage of age-related macular degeneration, drusen are seen in the retina. In the advanced stage, neovascularization and hemorrhage lead to visual loss

structure of the normal retina is completely destroyed and severe bleeding ensues. Generally, a lesion called a druse precedes these severe retinal changes. Histologically, drusen are lesions with an abnormal accumulation of various proteins such as amyloid beta, immunoglobulin, and complement factors [11]. Even though the abnormal accumulation of proteins is observed in the early stages of macular degeneration, the visual acuity is generally not affected at this stage. With an unknown mechanism, the expression of VEGF is upregulated, and neovascularization occurs in the latter stage of age-related macular degeneration.

The inhibition of the progression from the early stage (drusen) to the late stage (neovascularization) is an important strategy in the prevention of blindness. Recently, inhibition of VEGF with intravitreous injection of neutralizing antibody is utilized as a first choice of treatment for age-related macular degeneration. However, the effect of the anti-VEGF treatment is temporary because the treatment cannot stop the expression of VEGF in the retinal lesion. However, there are some supporting data that drusen in the retina induces neovascularization by increased expression of VEGF. Ishibashi et al. have reported that drusen contain advanced glycation end products (Fig. 2.5) [12]. In addition, retinal epithelial cells express receptor for AGE (RAGE). This constant interaction between AGE and RAGE is seen in the retinal pigment epithelial cells of patients with age-related macular degeneration. The AGE-RAGE axis may increase the expression of various cytokines, including VEGF, and increase oxidative stress in the retinal pigment epithelial cells. This constant interaction of AGE and RAGE in the retinal pigment epithelial cells may play a central role in the pathogenesis of age-related macular degeneration [13–15].

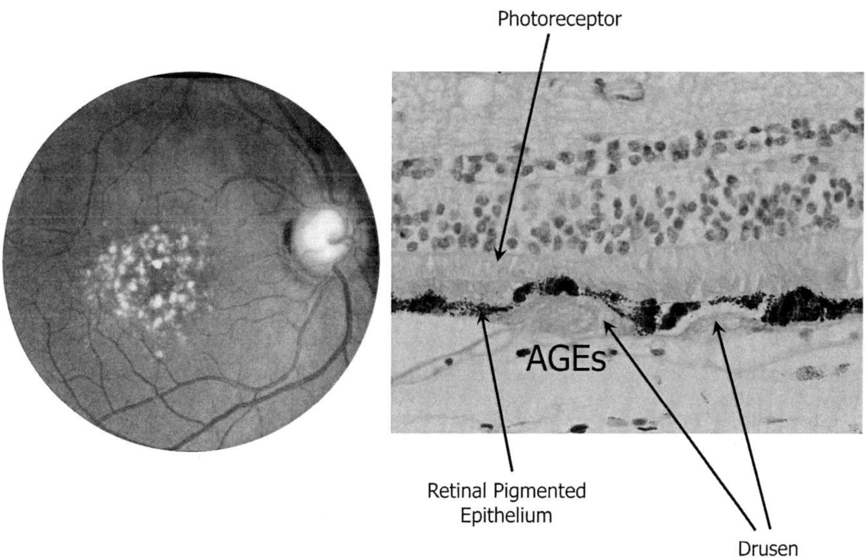

Fig. 2.5 AGEs in drusen. AGEs are detected in the drusen, an abnormal aggregation of proteins in age-related macular degeneration

2.4 Diabetic Retinopathy and the Maillard Reaction

The number of patients with diabetes is increasing not only in the developed but also developing countries. The WHO has reported that the number of people with diabetes has risen from 108 million in 1980 to 422 million in 2014 [16]. With the improvement of medical care and the medication on offer, life expectancy of patients is increasing. With an increased duration of diabetes, severe complications may develop in the retina, kidney, nerves, blood vessels, and heart.

Diabetic retinopathy first affects blood vessels in the retina. The retina has a fine structure of capillary vessels to meet the high demand of oxygen and glucose to change the light into the electric signal of nerves. However, with the increase of the duration of diabetes, retinal capillaries are obstructed, and severe ischemia is induced in the retina. This ischemic change induces the expression of VEGF and induces neovascular vessel formation in the retina. The neovascular vessels bleed easily, and the proliferation of the vessels is uncontrolled, which causes the eyeball to fill with blood (Fig. 2.6).

The most important risk factor for diabetic retinopathy is [17–19] the duration of the diabetes. Diabetic retinopathy is seen in roughly 20% of patients with a 5-year duration of diabetes, which increases to 60% in a 20-year duration. Poor glycemic control, increased blood pressure, smoking, and alcohol are also risk factors for diabetic retinopathy. The Maillard reaction is known to be involved in the development of diabetic retinopathy (Fig. 2.7). In diabetic patients, the blood sugar level is increased, and the proteins in the body are constantly exposed to this high glucose level. The proteins in the body and the blood sugar react to form a Schiff base and initiate the Maillard reaction. An example of glycated proteins is glycated hemoglobin in blood. Hemoglobin A_{1c} is now clinically used as a reference for the average blood sugar level of diabetic patients [20–23]. Increased blood sugar levels also induce the glycation of proteins in the retina. Increased accumulation of the Maillard reaction products and advanced glycation end products are seen in experimental animals, as well as diabetic patients. An increased interaction of advanced glycation end products and RAGE

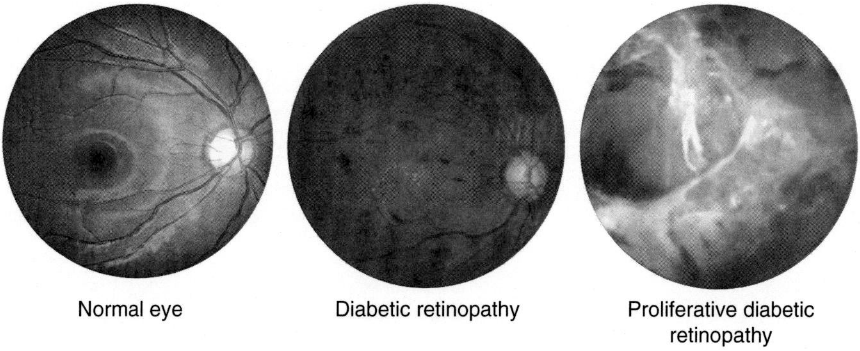

Fig. 2.6 Clinical picture of diabetic retinopathy. In diabetic retinopathy, numerous hemorrhages, retinal edema, and neovascularization are the major pathways of visual loss in diabetic retinopathy

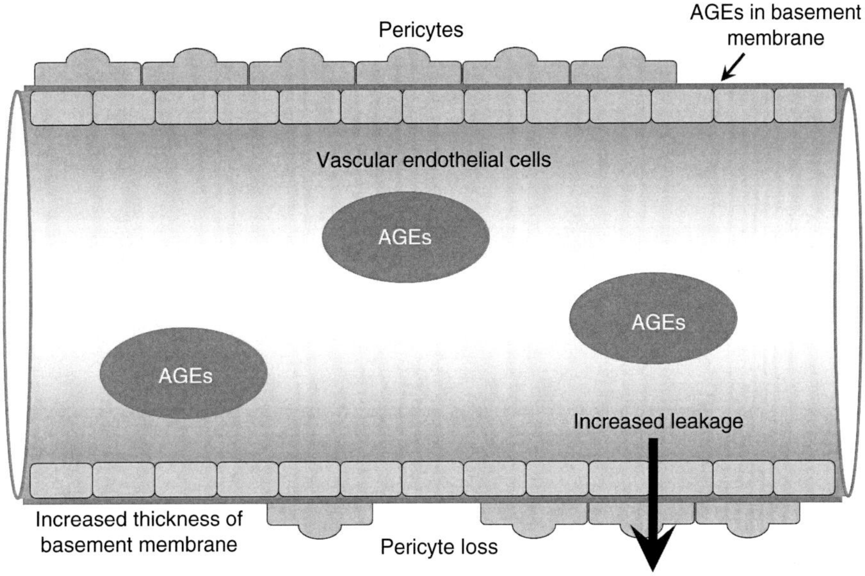

Fig. 2.7 AGE-induced diabetic retinopathy. In diabetic retinopathy, AGEs in the blood or blood vessel walls induce an increased leakage of the vessels (inducing retinal edema), increased thickness of the basement membrane, and pericytes loss (inducing capillary loss and the resulting ischemia)

expressed in vessel endothelial cells and pericytes is speculated to play an important role in the development of diabetic retinopathy [13, 20, 21, 24, 25].

Retinal photocoagulation is widely applied to treat diabetic retinopathy. In addition, blockage of VEGF by intravitreous injection of neutralizing antibody to VEGF is recently applied to treat diabetic retinopathy. In the end stage of diabetic retinopathy, surgical removal of proliferative tissue with retinal photocoagulation is the only treatment. Even with the advance in the treatment of diabetic retinopathy, the number of blinded patients with diabetic retinopathy is increasing. So new treatment strategy based on the molecular mechanism is needed. Experimentally, blocking the interaction of AGE and RAGE has inhibited the development of diabetic retinopathy in animal model [13, 20, 21, 24, 25]. However, no drug targeting the AGE and RAGE axis is clinically available to treat or to prevent diabetic retinopathy. An alternative target of treatment in the treatment and inhibition of diabetic retinopathy is required, and we believe the AGE and RAGE axis will be a promising target.

2.5 Diabetic Keratopathy and the Maillard Reaction

Diabetic retinopathy is not the only cause of visual loss in patients with diabetes. Diabetic keratopathy is also the important causes of poor vision in diabetes. Diabetic keratopathy comprises several symptomatic corneal conditions inducing superficial

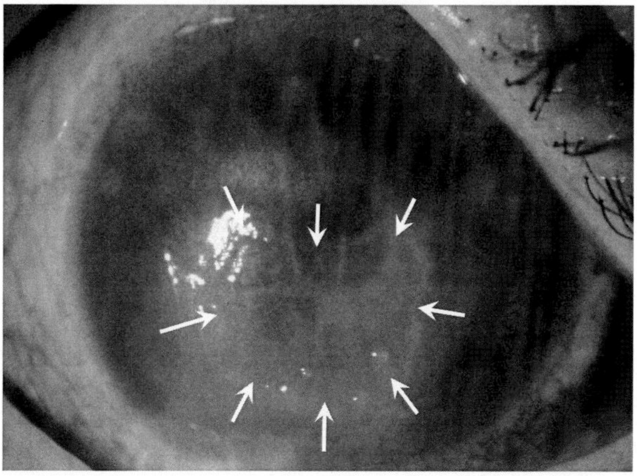

Fig. 2.8 Clinical picture of diabetic keratopathy. In diabetes, AGEs in the blood or blood vessel walls induce an increased leakage of the vessels (inducing retinal edema), increased thickness of the basement membrane, and pericytes loss (inducing capillary loss and the resulting ischemia)

punctate keratopathy and persistent corneal epithelial erosion (Fig. 2.8). Especially, persistent corneal erosion in diabetic patients is often resistant to routine clinical management of corneal erosions including topical medication and bandage contact lenses. These poorly healing epithelial surfaces have compromised defenses against general microbial attack predisposing these patients to corneal infection. In addition, we cannot observe inside the eyes with diabetic keratopathy. This means that eye doctors cannot conduct the evaluation as well as treatment of diabetic keratopathy.

Various molecular mechanisms have been proposed for the development of diabetic keratopathy including accumulation of polyols in epithelial cells [26–28], reduced sensation with reduced neurotrophic factors [29, 30], alteration in basement membrane components, and advanced glycation in the basement membrane [31]. Advanced glycation end products (AGEs) have been implicated in the development of diabetic keratopathy and may explain some of the structural changes noted. We have found AGEs deposit in the basement membrane of the corneal epithelial cells of diabetic patients. When this happens, the molecular structure of basement membrane components changes, and they lose adhesive property. In our previous study, advanced glycation end products in laminin induce the decreased attachment of corneal epithelial cells (Fig. 2.9) [31]. In this way, the corneal epithelial cells lose a clue for the attachment on the basement membrane.

Prevention and treatment of diabetic keratopathy are difficult with the conventional ocular therapy. New treatment based on the molecular mechanism of diabetic keratopathy is needed. Inhibition of aldose reductase inhibitor exerts some prophylactic effect on the diabetic keratopathy [26–28]. In addition, topical application of substance P and insulin-like growth factor-1 peptide has the potential to treat diabetic keratopathy as well as neurotrophic corneal ulcer [29, 30]. We have shown that aminoguanidine, an antioxidant, was effective in inhibiting AGE formation in vitro and thus ameliorated the attachment of corneal epithelial cells to the basement membrane [31]. However, the in vivo effect of aminoguanidine on diabetic keratopathy remains unknown.

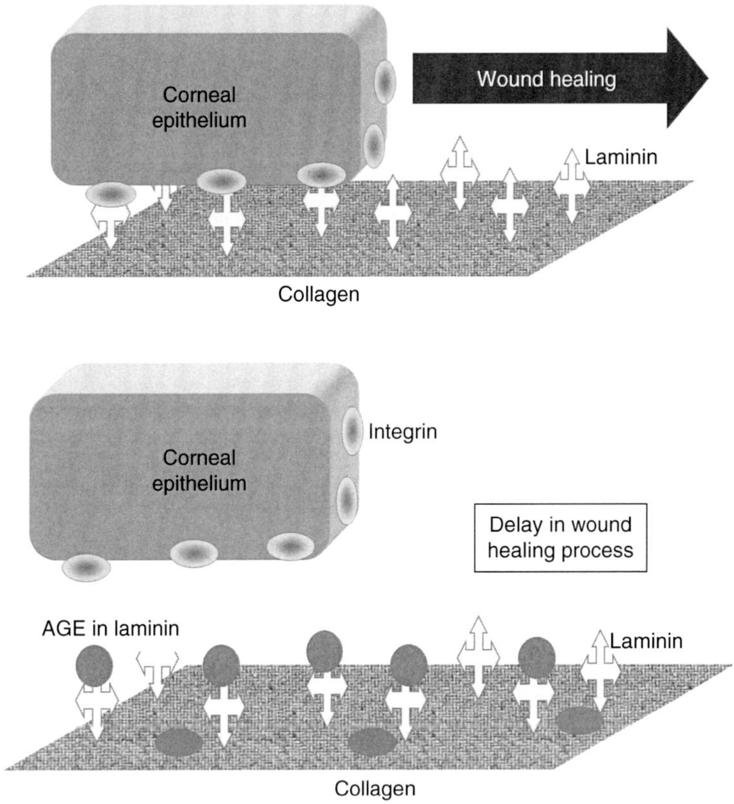

Fig. 2.9 AGEs induce diabetic keratopathy. Association of corneal epithelial cells with basement membrane components including collagen and laminin is important in the wound healing. However, in diabetes, AGE formation especially in laminin inhibits the attachment of corneal epithelial cells to the basement membrane

References

1. World Health Organization. Global initiative for the elimination of avoidable blindness. An informal cunsultation. WHO/PBL/9761. Geneva: WHO; 1997.
2. Ezepue UF. Magnitude and causes of blindness and low vision in Anambra State of Nigeria (results of 1992 point prevalence survey). Public Health. 1997;111:305–9.
3. Klein R, Klein BE, Jensen SC, Moss SE, Cruickshanks KJ. The relation of socioeconomic factors to age-related cataract, maculopathy, and impaired vision. The Beaver Dam Eye Study. Ophthalmology. 1994;101:1969–79.
4. Leske MC, Connell AM, Wu SY, Hyman L, Schachat A. Prevalence of lens opacities in the Barbados Eye Study. Arch Ophthalmol. 1997;115:105–11.
5. Mitchell P, Cumming RG, Attebo K, Panchapakesan J. Prevalence of cataract in Australia: the Blue Mountains eye study. Ophthalmology. 1997;104:581–8.
6. Ahmed MU, Brinkmann Frye E, Degenhardt TP, Thorpe SR, Baynes JW. N-epsilon-(carboxyethyl)lysine, a product of the chemical modification of proteins by methylglyoxal, increases with age in human lens proteins. Biochem J. 1997;324(Pt 2):565–70.

7. Dyer DG, Blackledge JA, Katz BM, Hull CJ, Adkisson HD, Thorpe SR, et al. The Maillard reaction in vivo. Z Ernahrungswiss. 1991;30:29–45.
8. Monnier VM, Cerami A. Nonenzymatic browning in vivo: possible process for aging of long-lived proteins. Science. 1981;211:491–3.
9. Attebo K, Mitchell P, Smith W. Visual acuity and the causes of visual loss in Australia. The Blue Mountains Eye Study. Ophthalmology. 1996;103:357–64.
10. Munoz B, West SK, Rubin GS, Schein OD, Quigley HA, Bressler SB, et al. Causes of blindness and visual impairment in a population of older Americans: The Salisbury Eye Evaluation Study. Arch Ophthalmol. 2000;118:819–25.
11. Crabb JW, Miyagi M, Gu X, Shadrach K, West KA, Sakaguchi H, et al. Drusen proteome analysis: an approach to the etiology of age-related macular degeneration. Proc Natl Acad Sci U S A. 2002;99:14682–7. doi:10.1073/pnas.222551899.
12. Ishibashi T, Murata T, Hangai M, Nagai R, Horiuchi S, Lopez PF, et al. Advanced glycation end products in age-related macular degeneration. Arch Ophthalmol. 1998;116:1629–32.
13. Glenn JV, Stitt AW. The role of advanced glycation end products in retinal ageing and disease. Biochim Biophys Acta. 1790;2009:1109–16. doi:10.1016/j.bbagen.2009.04.016.
14. Howes KA, Liu Y, Dunaief JL, Milam A, Frederick JM, Marks A, et al. Receptor for advanced glycation end products and age-related macular degeneration. Invest Ophthalmol Vis Sci. 2004;45:3713–20. doi:10.1167/iovs.04-0404.
15. Park SW, Kim JH, Park SM, Moon M, Lee KH, Park KH, et al. RAGE mediated intracellular Abeta uptake contributes to the breakdown of tight junction in retinal pigment epithelium. Oncotarget. 2015;6:35263–73. doi:10.18632/oncotarget.5894.
16. World Health Organization. Global report on diabetes. Geneva: WHO; 2016.
17. Klein R, Klein BE, Moss SE, Davis MD, DeMets DL. The Wisconsin epidemiologic study of diabetic retinopathy. III. Prevalence and risk of diabetic retinopathy when age at diagnosis is 30 or more years. Arch Ophthalmol. 1984;102:527–32.
18. Klein R, Klein BE, Moss SE, Davis MD, DeMets DL. The Wisconsin epidemiologic study of diabetic retinopathy. II. Prevalence and risk of diabetic retinopathy when age at diagnosis is less than 30 years. Arch Ophthalmol. 1984;102:520–6.
19. West SK, Klein R, Rodriguez J, Munoz B, Broman AT, Sanchez R, et al. Diabetes and diabetic retinopathy in a Mexican-American population: Proyecto VER. Diabetes Care. 2001;24:1204–9.
20. Barile GR, Pachydaki SI, Tari SR, Lee SE, Donmoyer CM, Ma W, et al. The RAGE axis in early diabetic retinopathy. Invest Ophthalmol Vis Sci. 2005;46:2916–24. doi:10.1167/iovs.04-1409.
21. Chen M, Curtis TM, Stitt AW. Advanced glycation end products and diabetic retinopathy. Curr Med Chem. 2013;20:3234–40.
22. Monnier VM, Sun W, Sell DR, Fan X, Nemet I, Genuth S. Glucosepane: a poorly understood advanced glycation end product of growing importance for diabetes and its complications. Clin Chem Lab Med. 2014;52:21–32. doi:10.1515/cclm-2013-0174.
23. Sharma Y, Saxena S, Mishra A, Saxena A, Natu SM. Advanced glycation end products and diabetic retinopathy. J Ocul Biol Dis Infor. 2012;5:63–9. doi:10.1007/s12177-013-9104-7.
24. Kaji Y, Usui T, Ishida S, Yamashiro K, Moore TC, Moore J, et al. Inhibition of diabetic leukostasis and blood-retinal barrier breakdown with a soluble form of a receptor for advanced glycation end products. Invest Ophthalmol Vis Sci. 2007;48:858–65. doi:10.1167/iovs.06-0495.
25. Moore TC, Moore JE, Kaji Y, Frizzell N, Usui T, Poulaki V, et al. The role of advanced glycation end products in retinal microvascular leukostasis. Invest Ophthalmol Vis Sci. 2003;44:4457–64.
26. Jacot JL, Hosotani H, Glover JP, Lois N, Robison WG Jr. Diabetic-like corneal sensitivity loss in galactose-fed rats ameliorated with aldose reductase inhibitors. J Ocul Pharmacol Ther. 1998;14:169–80. doi:10.1089/jop.1998.14.169.
27. Kador PF, Wyman M, Oates PJ. Aldose reductase, ocular diabetic complications and the development of topical Kinostat((R)). Prog Retin Eye Res. 2016;54:1–29. doi:10.1016/j.preteyeres.2016.04.006.

28. Ohashi Y, Matsuda M, Hosotani H, Tano Y, Ishimoto I, Fukuda M, et al. Aldose reductase inhibitor (CT-112) eyedrops for diabetic corneal epitheliopathy. Am J Ophthalmol. 1988;105:233–8.
29. Chikamoto N, Chikama T, Yamada N, Nishida T, Ishimitsu T, Kamiya A. Efficacy of substance P and insulin-like growth factor-1 peptides for preventing postsurgical superficial punctate keratopathy in diabetic patients. Jpn J Ophthalmol. 2009;53:464–9. doi:10.1007/s10384-009-0693-4.
30. Nakamura M, Kawahara M, Morishige N, Chikama T, Nakata K, Nishida T. Promotion of corneal epithelial wound healing in diabetic rats by the combination of a substance P-derived peptide (FGLM-NH2) and insulin-like growth factor-1. Diabetologia. 2003;46:839–42. doi:10.1007/s00125-003-1105-9.
31. Kaji Y, Usui T, Oshika T, Matsubara M, Yamashita H, Araie M, et al. Advanced glycation end products in diabetic corneas. Invest Ophthalmol Vis Sci. 2000;41:362–8.

Chapter 3
Diabetic Neuropathy

Soroku Yagihashi and Hiroki Mizukami

Abstract Neuropathy is the most common and earliest to occur among a variety of vascular complications of diabetes. In contrast to its popularity, it seems that attention has not been sufficiently paid to this complication. This may have been ascribed to the difficulty in understanding of the pathophysiology of neuropathy or lack of effective treatment regimen due in part to the complicated etiology. Nevertheless, there are slow but steady advances in clinical management of diabetic neuropathy involving the proposal of diagnostic criteria or clinical staging of neuropathy for an early detection of nerve deficits and direction of the treatment. Emergence of pain-relieving agents has also contributed to the improvement of quality of life in patients with symptomatic neuropathy. Notwithstanding, there still needs clarification of the pathogenesis for the development of diabetic neuropathy, clinical indices for nerve deficits, and for the prediction of prognosis. In this communication, recent progress in the pathogenesis of diabetic neuropathy will be summarized and its underlying pathology will be introduced.

Keywords Diabetic neuropathy • Pathology • Pathogenesis

3.1 Introduction

Importance of neuropathy is well understood in clinical practice of diabetes management. It is not always the case, however, that clinical care for this common complication is satisfactory. The reason for the insufficiency of clinical attention may be ascribed to the difficulty in the understanding of the clinical status of neuropathy or

---

S. Yagihashi (✉)
Department of Pathology and Molecular Medicine, Hirosaki University Graduate School of Medicine, 5 Zaifu-cho, Hirosaki 036-8562, Japan

Nukada Institute for Medical and Biological Research, 5-18 Inage-machi, Inage, Chiba 263-0035, Japan
e-mail: yagihasi@hirosaki-u.ac.jp, soroku@nukada.or.jp

H. Mizukami
Department of Pathology and Molecular Medicine, Hirosaki University Graduate School of Medicine, 5 Zaifu-cho, Hirosaki 036-8562, Japan

S.-i. Yamagishi (ed.), *Diabetes and Aging-related Complications*,
https://doi.org/10.1007/978-981-10-4376-5_3

lack of effective treatment regimens for neuropathy. Alternatively, it may also be attributed to the lack of established criteria for the evaluation of the treatment effects. In this review, we will refer to the current consideration on the basic pathology and pathogenetic mechanisms of diabetic neuropathy and attempt to correlate the pathologic basis with clinical signs and symptoms.

3.2 Basic Pathology of Diabetic Polyneuropathy

3.2.1 Nerve Fiber Degeneration and Fiber Loss

Most dramatic changes in diabetic nerve in humans are represented by loss of nerve fibers with distal predominance (Table 3.1) [1]. Axonal degeneration and Schwann cell changes are characteristic. Demyelination also appears where there is a local pressure or local ischemia/reperfusion injury. Distal axonal degeneration starts in the most distal portion of the axon processes, and degeneration will ascend with progression of the disease. In diabetes, all three types of degenerative fibers may be encountered. However, most prevalent are fibers with distal axonal degeneration. Reduction of small nerve fibers in the distal foot occurs in early stage of diabetes, even in prediabetic stage [2]. The loss of intraepidermal nerve fibers well parallels with progression of neuropathy [3]. Currently, evaluation of intraepidermal nerve fibers by skin biopsy becomes world standard indicative of presence of neuropathy.

Table 3.1 Pathologic features of diabetic neuropathy

	Large fiber lesions	Small fiber lesions	Microvessel changes
Somatic nerves			
(Sural nerve)	Distal nerve fiber loss (focal and diffuse) Axonal degeneration Demyelination	Loss of small fibers	Luminal occlusion Swollen endothelial cells Thickened basement membrane
(Skin)		Loss and disruption of nerve fibers	Fenestration
(Cornea)		Loss of nerve fibers	
		Loss of branching	
Autonomic nerves			
(Parasympathetic)		Postganglionic	
		Nerve fiber loss	
(Sympathetic)		Axonal dystrophy	
		Loss of synapses	
Clinical phenotype	Ankle jerk↓	Thermal sensation↓	
	Perception↓	Pain sensation↓	
	Vibration sense↓	Spontaneous pain	
	Nerve conduction↓		
	Amplitudes↓		

However, as skin biopsy is claimed to be still invasive, alternative noninvasive observation of small fibers on the cornea (corneal confocal microscopy, CCM) has been established as a diagnostic tool for the small fiber neuropathy. With this method, regeneration of small fibers could be detected earlier in cornea than in the skin in patients with diabetes who undertook pancreas transplantation [4].

Distal axonal degeneration is known to occur in cases of metabolic neuropathies including vitamin deficiencies and alcoholism [1]. In diabetes, in addition to metabolic aberration, altered blood flow with hypoxia/ischemia or reperfusion perturbs the integrity of peripheral axons and Schwann cells and thereby induces the degeneration starting in the most distal part [5]. Axons with small diameter are preferentially affected because of limited supporting system due to its small size. Consequently, symptoms transmitted by small-sized nerve fibers commence with pain and alterations of thermal sensations, followed by paresthesia as well as sensory loss.

3.2.2 *Role of Microangiopathy*

Vascular supply is sparse in the peripheral nerve compared to other tissues. Neural regulation of blood flow is limited to the arteriole at the entry in the nerve which is controlled by sympathetic or peptidergic nerve endings. Consequently, endoneurial area of the nerve is extremely susceptible to ischemia/hypoxia [6]. It was repeatedly shown that ischemia/hypoxia greatly contributes to the development of neuropathy. In fact, endoneurial microvessels show swollen endothelial cells, narrowing of the lumen, and thickening/duplication of basement membranes of the vascular walls [7]. The vascular changes well correlated with the severity of neuropathy, indicating that microangiopathy promotes the progression of neuropathy in diabetes. In fact, there is a close correlation between basement membrane thickening and nerve fiber loss.

3.3 Relationship Between Neuropathological Changes and Clinical Syndrome

Despite of considerable variability for the clinical signs and symptoms, recent studies slowly but steadily shed light on the relationship between clinical features and pathologic changes.

3.3.1 *Subjective Symptoms*

The most prominent symptom in diabetic neuropathy may be pain as a positive symptom. Pain in diabetic polyneuropathy is roughly divided into inflammatory pain and neuropathic pain. The latter of which is ascribed to nerve degeneration and nerve fiber loss and occurs in progressive stage of neuropathy. In this setting, small nerve fibers are responsible to convey pain signals, but in the lower extremities, such fibers are largely lost in distal site. Thus, the pain may be accounted for by a reflection of phantom pain [8]. Under such circumstances, degenerated nerve fibers that attempt to regenerate send pain signals to dorsal column of the spinal cord through dorsal root ganglia. Ascending nerve fibers from dorsal column to the central nervous system also carry pain to the brain. A variety of factors are also involved in pain induction such as acute vascular occlusion, rapid changes of blood glucose, or acute energy imbalance. Thin fibers (C fibers) usually transmit dull pain while sharp pain is conveyed by relatively thick fibers (Aδ). Recently, pain threshold of the skin was found to be increased and related to decreased density of intraepidermal small nerve fibers. It is still open to question, however, whether the density of skin small nerve fibers is in fact related to the occurrence of spontaneous pain.

With advancement of the disease, as loss of nerve fibers becomes more prominent, loss of sensation is a cardinal sign which is a strong risk for foot gangrene or ulcer. Since patients do not complain on this sign, every effort should be made to educate the importance of foot care to the patients (Fig. 3.1).

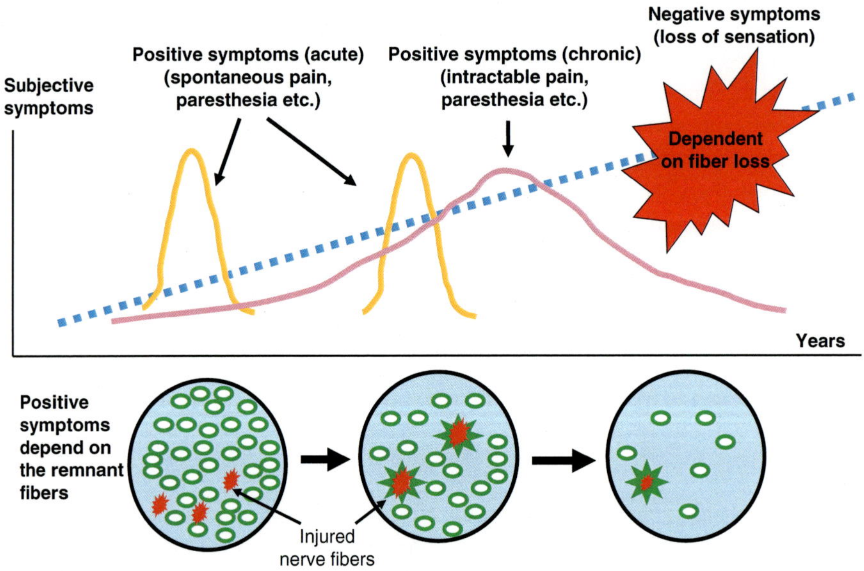

Fig. 3.1 Natural history of diabetic neuropathy and its relationship to positive and negative symptoms. With background of progressive decline of nerve fibers, patients with diabetes complain pain and paresthesia in the foot which are triggered by injured nerve fibers. Acute pain is induced by rapid metabolic deterioration or vascular impairments that cause rapid processes of nerve fiber degeneration which sends pain signals. Pain also appears chronically as consequence of long-term nerve injury. Such positive symptoms are caused by remnant nerve fibers that convey pain signals. On the other hand, negative symptoms of loss of sensation are caused by loss of nerve fibers and patients usually do not complain. Therefore, this condition is more serious for prognosis

3.3.2 Objective Signs and Symptoms; Ankle Jerk and Vibration Perception

Ankle jerk and vibration perception test are useful for the diagnosis of neuropathy. Loss of ankle jerk is dependent on the involvement of small unmyelinated afferent nerve fibers that surround muscle spindles. Spiral afferent nerve fibers of the muscle spindle were found to be disrupted in animals with diabetes [9], possibly resulting in abnormal ankle jerk.

Vibration perception test or pressure test are sensed by Meissner and Pacini corpuscles distributed in the dermis. These corpuscles send afferent nerve fibers of Aβ size to spinal dorsal root ganglion cells and then central axons extend to the brain through dorsal fascicle of the spinal cord. It is known that aging is associated with decreased large nerve fiber function. In fact, the number of Pacini corpuscles is decreased with aging [10], resulting in increased threshold of vibration perception.

3.3.3 Autonomic Nerve Symptoms

Connection of autonomic signs and symptoms with pathologic alterations is challenging in diabetic neuropathy. There are only a few pathologic studies on autonomic nervous systems in human diabetes. In their studies, distal axonal degeneration of postganglionic nerve fibers was reported to correlate with abnormal function of gastrointestinal tract, cardiovascular system, and urogenital tracts. Loss of afferent sensory nerve fibers is relevant to painless myocardial ischemia or gastroparesis or atonic bladder.

Most distinct changes in sympathetic nerves are axonal and dendritic dystrophy which is swollen axon or dendrite containing aggregates of cytoplasmic organelles, mitochondria, endoplasmic reticula, and ribosomes in the axon terminals or dendrites [11]. Dystrophic changes are frequent in diabetes but also found in normal aging although less frequently. The frequency of dystrophy was well correlated with loss of synapses.

3.4 Risk Factors for Diabetic Neuropathy

It is well established from Diabetes Control and Complications Trial (DCCT) studies and subsequent Epidemiology of Diabetes Interventions and Complications (EDIC) studies that blood glucose control is critical to the onset and progression of neuropathy in patients with type 1 diabetes. Also in Europe, epidemiologic prospective study on neuropathy in type 1 diabetes for consecutive 5 years demonstrated that long-term blood glucose control (HbA1c), hypertension, lipidemia, smoking, and obesity were found to be risk factors for the progression of neuropathy

Table 3.2 Risk factors of neuropathy development in patients with type 1 diabetes[a]

Risk factors	Odd's ratio (CI)	*p* value
Model 1		
Duration of diabetes	1.40 (1.21–1.63)	$p < 0.001$
HbA1c	1.48 (1.23–1.79)	$p < 0.001$
HbA1c (Δ)	1.36 (1.14–1.62)	$p = 0.001$
Triglyceride	1.21 (1.02–1.40)	$p = 0.03$
Total cholesterol	1.15 (0.98–1.35)	$p = 0.08$
BMI	1.27 (1.08–1.47)	$p < 0.001$
Smoking history	1.38 (1.03–1.85)	$p = 0.03$
Hypertension	1.57 (1.03–2.39)	$p = 0.03$
Albumin excretion rate	1.01 (0.88–1.14)	$p = 0.93$
Model 2		
Duration of diabetes	1.25 (1.03–1.51)	$p = 0.02$
HbA1c	1.64 (1.33–2.03)	$p < 0.001$
HbA1c(Δ)	1.44 (1.17–1.77)	$p = 0.001$
Triglyceride	1.17 (0.97–1.41)	$p = 0.10$
Total cholesterol	1.11 (0.93–1.54)	$p = 0.25$
BMI	1.20 (1.01–1.43)	$p = 0.04$
Smoking history	1.68 (1.20–2.36)	$p = 0.003$
Hypertension	1.54 (0.96–2.47)	$p = 0.07$
Cardiovascular disease	2.12 (1.16–3.86)	$p = 0.01$
Retinopathy	1.45 (0.98–2.13)	$p = 0.06$
Albumin excretion rate	1.02 (0.89–1.18)	$p = 0.75$

Model 1 was the result of 1101 cases with inclusion of albumin excretion rate but without cardiovascular disease, and Model 2 was the result of 932 cases with inclusion of cardiovascular diseases and retinopathy but without albumin excretion rate
[a]Modified from Reference [12]

(Table 3.2) [12]. In contrast to type 1 diabetes, however, it is yet to be established whether long-term hyperglycemia is a critical determinant for the development of neuropathy by UKPDS study. Recent studies disclosed possible implication of hyperlipidemia and hypertension as contributing factors for neuropathy [13].

3.5 Biochemical Mechanisms for Peripheral Nerve Damage in Diabetes

It is yet to be clear how hyperglycemia leads to peripheral nerve damage. Basically, increased flux of glucose into collateral glycolytic pathway is a major process which is still complicated. In this review, we will introduce several key metabolic pathways which are known to be activated in chronic hyperglycemia, contributing to the development of neuropathy (Fig. 3.2).

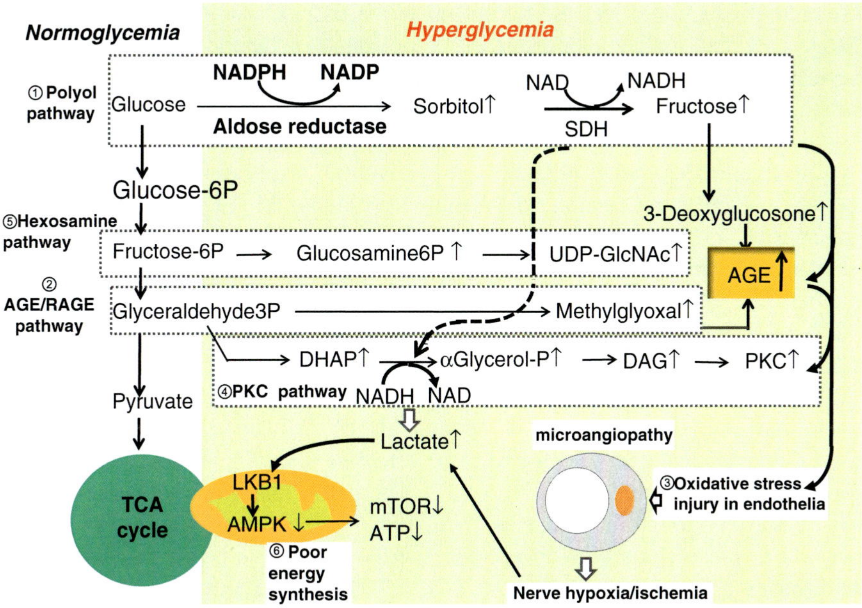

Fig. 3.2 Proposed mechanisms of how hyperglycemia affects the peripheral nerve. In normoglycemia, intracellular glucose undergoes glycolysis through TCA cycle in mitochondria to produce ATP. Once hyperglycemia occurs, polyol pathway is activated (*1*) to produce sorbitol and fructose. Hyperglycemia also elicits nonenzymatic glycation and AGE formation via intermediate glycation products like 3-deoxyglucosone and methylglyoxal (*2*). AGE binds with receptor for AGE (RAGE) releasing NADPH oxidase and activation of NF-κB. These pathways exert oxidative stress damage to the endothelial cells and nerve tissues (*3*). Hyperglycemia also elicits activation of protein kinase C via production of diacylglycerol (*4*). It was also pointed out that increased fructose-6-P and glutamate-6-P undergo excessive glycosylation of nuclear, membranous proteins leading to O-GlcNAc glycosylation of cellular proteins, thus modifying cellular function (*5*). Recently, excessive lactate production in the nerve was found to associate with reduced AMPkinase (AMPK) with suppression of mTOR and ATP synthesis (*6*)

3.5.1 Polyol Pathway (Aldose Reductase Pathway)

The first collateral pathway of glycolysis in hyperglycemia is polyol pathway. Excessive flux of glucose is converted to sorbitol mediated by aldose reductase (AR) [14]. Sorbitol is impermeable and thereby accumulates in the cell. Then the sorbitol is converted into fructose via sorbitol dehydrogenase (SDH). As the first step of this pathway progresses, there occurs much consumption of nicotinamide adenine dinucleotide phosphate (NADPH) acting as coenzyme of AR. NADPH is also utilized for the production of reduced glutathione (GSH) as a scavenger of oxygen radicals and for the production of nitric oxide (NO) which is derived from L-arginine. Following the consumption of NADPH, as a consequence of deficient GSH and NO, excessive oxygen radicals and insufficient NO with impaired endoneurial function affect the peripheral nerve tissues, resulting in neuropathic changes. Recent studies also disclosed complicated metabolic interplay between impaired mitochondrial energy production and redox alteration incurred by increased flux of polyol pathway [15]. In this setting, excessive lactate production suppresses AMP-activated protein kinase (AMPK) to inhibit serine-threonine kinase (mTOR, mammalian target of rapamycin) activation, resulting in poor energy production. It is intriguing that mice deficient in liver kinase B1 (LKB1) as an upstream molecule of AMPK develop sensory neuropathy reminiscent of typical diabetic neuropathy in humans [16]. Further investigation is expected to solve the relationship between LKB1-AMPK and diabetic neuropathy.

Clinical application of AR-inhibitors (ARI) showed benefits for improvement of delayed nerve conduction velocity (NCV) and promotion of nerve fiber regeneration. Although ARI developed in Western countries were given up to develop on the market because of potential adverse effects or insufficient efficacy, epalrestat marketed in Japan was found to be effective showing significant suppression of the progressive delay of NCV [17]. The failure of the clinical trial of ARI may be ascribed to the inappropriate inclusion of subjective symptoms as clinical endpoint because symptoms do not necessarily parallel with the progression of the disease.

3.5.2 Nonenzymatic Glycation (AGE/RAGE) Pathway

Superfluous glucose is likely to bind with amino acid base of structural proteins in the body forming Amadori products of intermediate glycated proteins. Glycated proteins further cross-link with each other to aggregate as insoluble large molecules, called advanced glycation endproducts (AGE). There are plenty of suggested mechanisms that account for the implication of protein glycation in the development of neuropathy in diabetes. As early glycation products, intermediate glycation products such as methylglyoxal (MG) and 3-deoxyglucosone (3-DG) are shown to be toxic to neural tissues. These intermediate glycation metabolites produce oxygen radicals to exert cell death or dysfunction. It was also found that MG mediates pain induction in diabetic neuropathy [18]. During the course of AGE formation, there also occur concurrent vitamin deficiency and metabolic imbalance [19]. In addition to intermediate glycation products, AGE accumulate in various components of peripheral nerve tissues to induce cell damage and degeneration of structural proteins. Long-lived proteins such as basement membrane proteins are likely to undergo AGE accumulation, resulting in nerve fiber degeneration and impaired nerve fiber regeneration. Furthermore, bindings of AGE and their receptors (RAGE, receptor for AGE) also elicit cell biological reactions to cause cell damage [20]. RAGE is expressed diffusely in the peripheral nerve, in particular cell membranes of neuronal cells, Schwann cells, and endothelial cells [21]. Following the attachment of AGE with RAGE, NADPH oxidase is activated to release OH radicals (NADPH activation). As a consequence, NF-κB is activated to exert proinflammatory reaction [22].

When RAGE is transgenetically overexpressed in endothelial cells, nerve conduction delay is further worsened in diabetic mice [21], whereas NCV delay and nerve fiber atrophy were mitigated in RAGE-deficient diabetic mice compared to wild diabetic mice, thus implicating in the AGE/RAGE role in the development of neuropathy [23]. Administration of AGE was recently found to induce NCV delay and nerve fiber atrophy in normal rats, similar to those found in diabetic animals, confirming a pathogenic role of AGE in the development of neuropathy [24]. AGE is known to be elevated in the serum of patients with end-stage renal failure who show the delay of NCV.

There have been attempts of inhibition of glycation process and AGE/RAGE action for the prevention and treatment of diabetic complications. Treatment with aminoguanidine demonstrated the inhibition of AGE accumulation in the nerve, improvement of nerve blood flow, and NCV delay as well as nerve fiber lesions [25]. More recently, benfotiamine, a derivative of vitamin B1, and pyridoxamine, a vitamin B6 derivative, are examined for their efficacy on the neuropathy by clinical trials [19]. No definite clinical efficacy was obtained in these trials.

3.5.3 *Protein Kinase C Pathway*

Protein kinase C (PKC) plays a central role in the protein synthesis and Ca metabolism in nerve cells. There are many isoforms of PKC such as α, β, δ, γ, and so on. In hyperglycemic condition, there is an increase in the expression of PKCβ in the eye and renal tissues of diabetic animals with increased vascular permeability, perturbed vascular supply, and ischemia, thus contributing to the development of retinopathy and nephropathy in diabetes. Experimental trials with PKCβ inhibitor successfully improved pathological alterations in the eye or kidney. Also in neuropathy, there was improvement of NCV and nerve blood flow in STZ-induced diabetic rats treated with PKCβ inhibitor. However, phase III clinical trial of PKCβ inhibitor was unsuccessful.

It is of note that there is a difference in PKC changes between neural and vascular tissues. While vascular tissues were associated with increased expression of PKCβ and increased PKC activity, neural tissues showed decreased expression of PKCα and lowered PKC activity [26]. It is therefore likely that targeting the tissues with specific PKC-isoform inhibitor may be essential to obtain better efficacy.

3.5.4 *Hexosamine Pathway*

There is an increasing interest in the hexosamine pathway as a causative mechanism for the development of diabetic complications [27]. When excessive glucose enters the cell, it is converted to glucose-6-phosphate and then fructose-6-phosphate. Fructose-6-phosphate is converted to glucosamine 6-phosphate (GlcN6-P) by the enzyme glutamine/fructose-6-phosphate-amido-transferase (GFAT). GlcN6P is further attached with glycosyl chain to modify the molecules of nucleus, cytoplasm, and cell membrane, resulting in altered cell function and cell injury. In fact, hyperglycemia induced activation of GFAT and glycosylation of crucial cellular proteins. When GFAT was inhibited by a specific inhibitor, glycosylation was suppressed and cell injury was prevented. Animals given glucosamine developed NCV delay and cultured neuronal cells exposed to glucosamine underwent apoptosis [28]. Since precise metabolic pathway of hexosamine is yet to be clear, role of this pathway in neuropathy is still unknown.

3.5.5 Oxidative Stress

Oxidative stress has long been regarded as a main contributor to the pathogenesis of diabetic complications. In fact, its role in vascular complications or effect on endothelial cells or smooth muscle cells is well established by preclinical studies. There still remain many unsolved issues, however, on neurological complications in diabetes. There is a controversy on the source of oxidative stress. Recent studies disclosed decreased energy production (ATP production) in nerve mitochondria and less production of oxygen stress in diabetic nerve [15]. In Germany, based on the premise that oxidative stress is a major cause of neuropathy, alpha-lipoic acid, as an anti-oxidant, is clinically applied to the treatment of neuropathy. In short-term study, there was an improvement of subjective symptoms. No definite improvement was confirmed, however, by double-blind clinical trials; as such it is still not approved as an effective treatment.

3.5.6 Cytokine and Neurotrophic Factors

There is an enhancement of inflammatory process in diabetic tissues. Also in the peripheral nerve, there is an increased infiltration of macrophages with excessive production of inflammatory cytokines. It was also found that TNF-α, IL-1α, and IL-1β were all increased in diabetic nerve where they affected the nerve as cytotoxic, thereby causing neurodegeneration [29]. Based on the data, TNF-α antagonist or cyclooxygenase (COX)-2 inhibitor was found to be effective for amelioration of experimental diabetic neuropathy in animals, but confirmation in humans is yet to be complete.

On the other hand, several studies demonstrated that production and release of nerve growth factor, neurotrophin 3, and ciliary neurotrophic factor (CNTF) were deficient in diabetic animals. Erythropoietin derivative was found to be effective for functional and structural deficits in animals with diabetes [30]. It is yet to be determined, however, whether the deficit of neurotrophic factors is the cause of neuropathy or merely the consequence of nerve damage in diabetes.

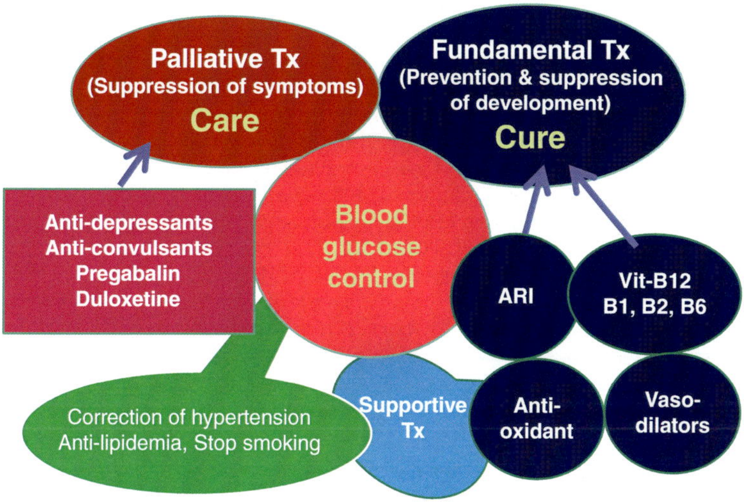

Fig. 3.3 Management of diabetic neuropathy with consideration of "care" and "cure." The treatment of diabetic neuropathy should separately be considered to be "care" and "cure." For the relief of positive symptoms such as pain, drugs can be prescribed only as a relief. It should be of note, however, that such "care" does not prevent the progression of neuropathy. In contrast, fundamental treatment that attempts to halt the disease is based on the pathogenetic mechanisms. Since precise mechanisms are yet to be clear, multiple treatment regimens are required for the better management of neuropathy

3.6 Direction of Treatment

Final goal of diabetes treatment may be the maintenance of good quality of life and healthy life expectancy. To this end, it is essential to prevent the clinical onset of neuropathy and to inhibit the progression of symptomatic neuropathy. To achieve this goal, precise pathogenesis of neuropathy should be clarified to establish the fundamental treatment. For the management of diabetic neuropathy, care and cure should be separately taken into account (Fig. 3.3). Currently, there is no consensus on the treatment for the patients who already have an established neuropathy. To alleviate the symptoms, care is the main purpose, though palliative, in which pain control is the major problem. Recent development of analgesics or antidepressants improved the quality of pain control, but there still needs further development. In contrast to symptomatic therapy, means to prevent the progression or reversal of neuropathy is still immature. To develop effective treatment for the cure, clarification of natural history of neuropathy and establishment of appropriate clinical endpoint is crucial. Otherwise, candidate compounds based on the pathogenetic mechanisms may again be only effective for the animals, but not for humans.

Acknowledgment The authors greatly acknowledge previous collaborators who conducted studies cited in this review. Our research was supported by grants in aid from the Ministry of Health and Welfare and the Ministry of Education, Culture, Sports, Science and Technology, Japan.

DOI: There is no duality of interest for the authors.

References

1. Dyck PJ, Giannini C. Pathologic alterations in the diabetic neuropathies of humans: a review. J Neuropathol Exp Neurol. 1996;55(12):1181–93.
2. Smith AG, Russell J, Feldman EL, Goldstein J, Peltier A, Smith S, et al. Lifestyle intervention for pre-diabetic neuropathy. Diabetes Care. 2006;29(6):1294–9.
3. Arimura A, Deguchi T, Sugimoto K, Uto T, Nakamura T, Arimura Y, et al. Intraepidermal nerve fiber density and nerve conduction study parameters correlate with clinical staging of diabetic polyneuropathy. Diabetes Res Clin Pract. 2013;99(1):24–9.
4. Tavakoli M, Mitu-Pretorian M, Petropoulos IN, Fadavi H, Asghar O, Alam U, et al. Corneal confocal microscopy detects early nerve regeneration in diabetic neuropathy after simultaneous pancreas and kidney transplantation. Diabetes. 2013;62(1):254–60. doi:10.2337/db12-0574.
5. Low PA, Lagerlund TD, McManis PG. Nerve blood flow and oxygen delivery in normal, diabetic, and ischemic neuropathy. Int Rev Neurobiol. 1989;31:355–438.
6. Malik RA. The pathology of human diabetic neuropathy. Diabetes. 1997;46(Suppl 2):S50–3.
7. Yagihashi S. Pathology and pathogenetic mechanisms of diabetic neuropathy. Diabetes Metab Rev. 1995;11(3):193–225.
8. Malik RA, Veves A, Walker D, Siddique I, Lye RH, Schady W, et al. Sural nerve fibre pathology in diabetic patients with mild neuropathy: relationship to pain, quantitative sensory testing and peripheral nerve electrophysiology. Acta Neuropathol. 2001;101(4):367–74.
9. Muller KA, Ryals JM, Feldman EL, Wright DE. Abnormal muscle spindle innervation and large-fiber neuropathy in diabetic mice. Diabetes. 2008;57(6):1693–701.
10. Decorps J, Saumet JL, Sommer P, Sigaudo-Roussel D, Fromy B. Effect of ageing on tactile transduction processes. Ageing Res Rev. 2014;13:90–9.
11. Schmidt RE. Neuropathology and pathogenesis of diabetic autonomic neuropathy. Int Rev Neurobiol. 2002;50:257–92.
12. Tesfaye S, Chaturvedi N, Eaton SE, Ward JD, Manes C, Ionescu-Tirgoviste C, et al.; EURODIAB Prospective Complications Study Group. Vascular risk factors and diabetic neuropathy. N Engl J Med. 2005;352(4):341–50.
13. Vincent AM, Hinder LM, Pop-Busui R, Feldman EL. Hyperlipidemia: a new therapeutic target for diabetic neuropathy. J Peripher Nerv Syst. 2009;14(4):257–67.
14. Yagihashi S, Mizukami H, Sugimoto K. Mechanism of diabetic neuropathy: where are we now and where to go? J Diabetes Investig. 2011;2(1):18–32.
15. Fernyhough P. Mitochondrial dysfunction in diabetic neuropathy: a series of unfortunate metabolic events. Curr Diab Rep. 2015;15(11):89. doi:10.1007/s11892-015-0671-9.
16. Beirowski B, Babetto E, Golden JP, Chen YJ, Yang K, Gross RW, et al. Metabolic regulator LKB1 is crucial for Schwann cell-mediated axon maintenance. Nat Neurosci. 2014;17(10):1351–61.
17. Hotta N, Akanuma Y, Kawamori R, Matsuoka K, Oka Y, Shichiri M, et al. Long-term clinical effects of epalrestat, an aldose reductase inhibitor, on diabetic peripheral neuropathy: the 3-year, multicenter, comparative Aldose Reductase Inhibitor-Diabetes Complications Trial. Diabetes Care. 2006;29(7):1538–44.
18. Bierhaus A, Fleming T, Stoyanov S, Leffler A, Babes A, Neacsu C, et al. Methylglyoxal modification of Nav1.8 facilitates nociceptive neuron firing and causes hyperalgesia in diabetic neuropathy. Nat Med. 2012;18(6):926–33.
19. Thornalley PJ. Glycation in diabetic neuropathy: characteristics, consequences, causes, and therapeutic options. Int Rev Neurobiol. 2002;50:37–57.
20. Yamamoto Y, Yamamoto H. Controlling the receptor for advanced glycation end-products to conquer diabetic vascular complications. J Diabetes Investig. 2012;3(2):107–14.
21. Wada R, Yagihashi S. Role of advanced glycation end products and their receptors in development of diabetic neuropathy. Ann N Y Acad Sci. 2005;1043:598–604.
22. Haslbeck KM, Schleicher E, Bierhaus A, Nawroth P, Haslbeck M, Neundörfer B, et al. The AGE/RAGE/NF-κB pathway may contribute to the pathogenesis of polyneuropathy in impaired glucose tolerance (IGT). Exp Clin Endocrinol Diabetes. 2005;113(5):288–91.

23. Juranek JK, Geddis MS, Song F, Zhang J, Garcia J, Rosario R, et al. RAGE deficiency improves postinjury sciatic nerve regeneration in type 1 diabetic mice. Diabetes. 2013;62(3):931–43.
24. Nishizawa Y, Wada R, Baba M, Takeuchi M, Hanyu-Itabashi C, Yagihashi S. Neuropathy induced by exogenously administered advanced glycation end-products in rats. J Diabetes Investig. 2010;1(1–2):40–9.
25. Yagihashi S, Kamijo M, Baba M, Yagihashi N, Nagai K. Effect of aminoguanidine on functional and structural abnormalities in peripheral nerve of STZ-induced diabetic rats. Diabetes. 1992;41(1):47–52.
26. Yamagishi S, Uehara K, Otsuki S, Yagihashi S. Differential influence of increased polyol pathway on protein kinase C expressions between endoneurial and epineurial tissues in diabetic mice. J Neurochem. 2003;87(2):497–507.
27. Slawson C, Copeland RJ, Hart GW. O-GlcNAc signaling: a metabolic link between diabetes and cancer? Trends Biochem Sci. 2010;35(10):547–55.
28. Lim JG, Lee JJ, Park SH, Park JH, Kim SJ, Cho HC, et al. Glucagon-like peptide-1 protects NSC-34 motor neurons against glucosamine through Epac-mediated glucose uptake enhancement. Neurosci Lett. 2010;479(1):13–7.
29. Pop-Busui R, Ang L, Holmes C, Gallagher K, Feldman EL. Inflammation as a therapeutic target for diabetic neuropathies. Curr Diab Rep. 2016;16(3):29. doi:10.1007/s11892-016-0727-5.
30. Brines M, Dunne AN, van Velzen M, Proto PL, Ostenson CG, Kirk RI, et al. ARA 290, a nonerythropoietic peptide engineered from erythropoietin, improves metabolic control and neuropathic symptoms in patients with type 2 diabetes. Mol Med. 2015;20:658–66.

Chapter 4
Diabetes and Endothelial Dysfunction

Tatsuya Maruhashi, Yasuki Kihara, and Yukihito Higashi

Abstract In patients with diabetes mellitus, endothelial dysfunction is the initial step in the process of atherosclerosis and plays an important role in the development of this condition, leading to diabetic vascular complications. Oxidative stress induced by hyperglycemia and acute glucose fluctuations are associated with endothelial dysfunction through inactivating nitric oxide (NO) by excess production of reactive oxygen species (ROS). Under the condition of insulin resistance, NO production is selectively impaired, whereas endothelin-1 (ET-1) secretion is preferentially activated in endothelial cells, leading to endothelial dysfunction in obese or overweight diabetic patients. On the other hand, endothelial dysfunction might contribute to insulin resistance in skeletal muscle. Reduced NO production through oxidative stress and selective insulin resistance in endothelial cells contributes to decreased glucose uptake by skeletal muscle due to a delayed increase in insulin concentration in the interstitium of the skeletal muscle. Therefore, insulin resistance is further exacerbated through a vicious cycle of endothelial dysfunction and reduced glucose uptake by skeletal muscle. From a clinical perspective, it is important to select an appropriate intervention that is effective in improving endothelial dysfunction for treatment of patients with diabetes mellitus.

In addition to lifestyle modifications, antidiabetic agents that improve insulin sensitivity are anticipated to improve endothelial function and prevent cardiovascular events in patients with diabetes mellitus.

Keywords Endothelial function • Diabetes mellitus • Oxidative stress • Insulin resistance

---

T. Maruhashi, M.D., Ph.D. (✉) • Y. Kihara
Department of Cardiovascular Medicine, Graduate School of Biomedical and Health Sciences, Hiroshima University, Hiroshima, Japan
e-mail: 55maruchin@gmail.com

Y. Higashi, M.D., Ph.D., F.A.H.A. (✉)
Department of Cardiovascular Regeneration and Medicine, Research Institute for Radiation Biology and Medicine, Hiroshima University, Hiroshima, Japan

Division of Regeneration and Medicine, Medical Center for Translational and Clinical Research, Hiroshima University Hospital, Hiroshima, Japan
e-mail: yhigashi@hiroshima-u.ac.jp

S.-i. Yamagishi (ed.), *Diabetes and Aging-related Complications*,
https://doi.org/10.1007/978-981-10-4376-5_4

4.1 Diabetic Vascular Complications

Diabetes mellitus is associated with an increased risk of microvascular and macrovascular complications. A recent study has shown that adults aged 50 years or older with diabetes mellitus die 4.6 years earlier, develop disabilities 6–7 years earlier, and spend 1–2 more years in a disabled state than do those without diabetes mellitus in the USA [1]. Microvascular complications, including retinopathy, nephropathy, and neuropathy, and macrovascular complications, including coronary artery disease, ischemic stroke, and peripheral artery disease, are important causes of morbidity and mortality in patients with diabetes mellitus. Macrovascular complications, namely, cardiovascular diseases (CVDs), are associated with increased mortality in patients with diabetes mellitus. CVD is the most common underlying cause of death, accounting for about 45% of deaths in patients with type 1 diabetes mellitus and about 50% of deaths in patients with type 2 diabetes mellitus [2]. It is therefore important to prevent the onset and progression of CVD for better prognosis in the management of patients with diabetes mellitus.

Endothelial dysfunction is the initial step in the pathogenesis of atherosclerosis and plays a key role in the development of this condition, leading to cardiovascular complications [3]. In addition, it has been demonstrated that endothelial function is an independent predictor of cardiovascular events [4]. Diabetes mellitus has been shown to be associated with endothelial dysfunction [5, 6]. For the prevention of CVD in patients with diabetes mellitus, it is therefore important to understand the causative mechanisms linking diabetes mellitus and endothelial dysfunction and to select an appropriate intervention that will effectively ameliorate endothelial function. In this section, the current understanding of the relationship between diabetes mellitus and endothelial function and treatment options are discussed.

4.2 Endothelial Function

It had been thought that the vascular endothelium was just a structural barrier separating the blood vessel wall and the inside cavity. In the 1980s, it was revealed that the vascular endothelium functions not only as a barrier but also as an endocrine organ secreting various vasoactive agents such as the vasodilators nitric oxide (NO), prostacyclin, and endothelium-derived hyperpolarizing factor (EDHF) and the vasoconstrictors endothelin-1 (ET-1), angiotensin II, and thromboxane A_2 [7]. Thus, the vascular endothelium might be one of the biggest endocrine organs in the human body, with an estimated total weight equal to that of the liver and an estimated total area equal to that of six tennis courts. A healthy endothelium acts as a gatekeeper controlling vascular tone and structure by regulating the balance between vasodilation and vasoconstriction, growth inhibition and growth promotion, anti-thrombosis and pro-thrombosis, anti-inflammation and pro-inflammation, and anti-oxidation and pro-oxidation. Endothelial dysfunction refers to a condition characterized by an inability of the endothelium to maintain vascular homeostasis as a result of an imbalance between endothelium-derived relaxing and contracting factors, leading to the progression of atherosclerosis. Endothelial dysfunction is an early feature of atherosclerosis and is associated with the development of this condition in human [3]. It is expected that improvement or augmentation of endothelial function may prevent the development and progression of atherosclerosis and consequently reduce cardiovascular events. Therefore, endothelial dysfunction has emerged as a therapeutic target in patients with cardiovascular risk factors such as hypertension, dyslipidemia, and diabetes mellitus and in patients with CVD. NO, one of the various vasoactive agents released from the endothelium, has various anti-atherosclerotic effects including vasodilation, inhibition of platelet aggregation and adhesion, inhibition of leucocyte adhesion, and suppression of vascular smooth muscle cell proliferation. Considering the wide range of anti-atherosclerotic effects of NO, reduced NO bioavailability is generally referred to as endothelial dysfunction.

Diabetes mellitus is associated with endothelial dysfunction. Impaired endothelium-dependent vasodilation has been demonstrated in patients with type 1 and type 2 diabetes [8, 9]. Although the definitive pathogenesis remains unclear, several mechanisms underlying the endothelial dysfunction in patients with diabetes mellitus have been proposed.

4.3 Mechanism Underlying the Endothelial Dysfunction in Diabetes

4.3.1 Oxidative Stress

Oxidative stress has been shown to be associated with the pathology of various diseases including diabetes mellitus. Oxidative stress refers to a condition in which the balance of reactive oxygen species (ROS) and the antioxidant system is disturbed in favor of prooxidant ROS. Excessive production of ROS cannot be sufficiently counteracted by the antioxidant defense system, and the deleterious effects of ROS, such as cell proliferation, hypertrophy, apoptosis, and inflammation, become clinically evident. ROS are produced by various oxidase enzymes, including nicotinamide adenine dinucleotide phosphate (NADPH) oxidase, uncoupled endothelial NO synthase (eNOS), mitochondrial electron transport, cyclooxygenase, glucose oxidase, and lipoxygenase. ROS include superoxide anion (O_{2-}), hydrogen peroxide (H_2O_2), hydroxyl radical (OH), hypochlorous acid (HOCl), NO, and peroxynitrite ($ONOO^-$). O_{2-} is produced by the reduction of molecular oxygen through removal of one electron, and it serves as the precursor of other ROS such as H_2O_2 and OH. In addition, O_{2-} reacts directly with NO and reduces NO bioavailability. In this context, O_{2-} is an important source of oxidative stress associated with endothelial dysfunction. Accumulating evidence has revealed an interaction between oxidative stress and endothelial dysfunction. Excessive O_{2-} reacts directly with NO with high affinity, resulting not only in degradation and inactivation of NO but also in formation of $ONOO^-$, a highly potent oxidant causing lipid peroxidation, DNA damage, and cell death (Fig. 4.1). In addition, $ONOO^-$ can oxidize the essential eNOS cofactor tetrahydrobiopterin (BH_4) to the biologically inactive trihydrobiopterin (BH_3), leading to a deficiency of BH_4. In the absence of sufficient concentrations of BH_4, eNOS is converted from an NO-producing enzyme into an O_{2-}-generating enzyme. This process is referred to as eNOS uncoupling (Fig. 4.1) [10]. Under this condition, impaired endothelial function is further exacerbated through a vicious cycle of increased oxidative stress and eNOS uncoupling, leading to a further increase in O_{2-} production and a decrease in NO bioavailability. In diabetes mellitus, chronic hyperglycemia is known to be a major contributor to elevated oxidative stress and endothelial dysfunction. In addition, recent studies have demonstrated that acute glucose fluctuations are involved in the mechanism underlying the increased oxidative stress in diabetes mellitus.

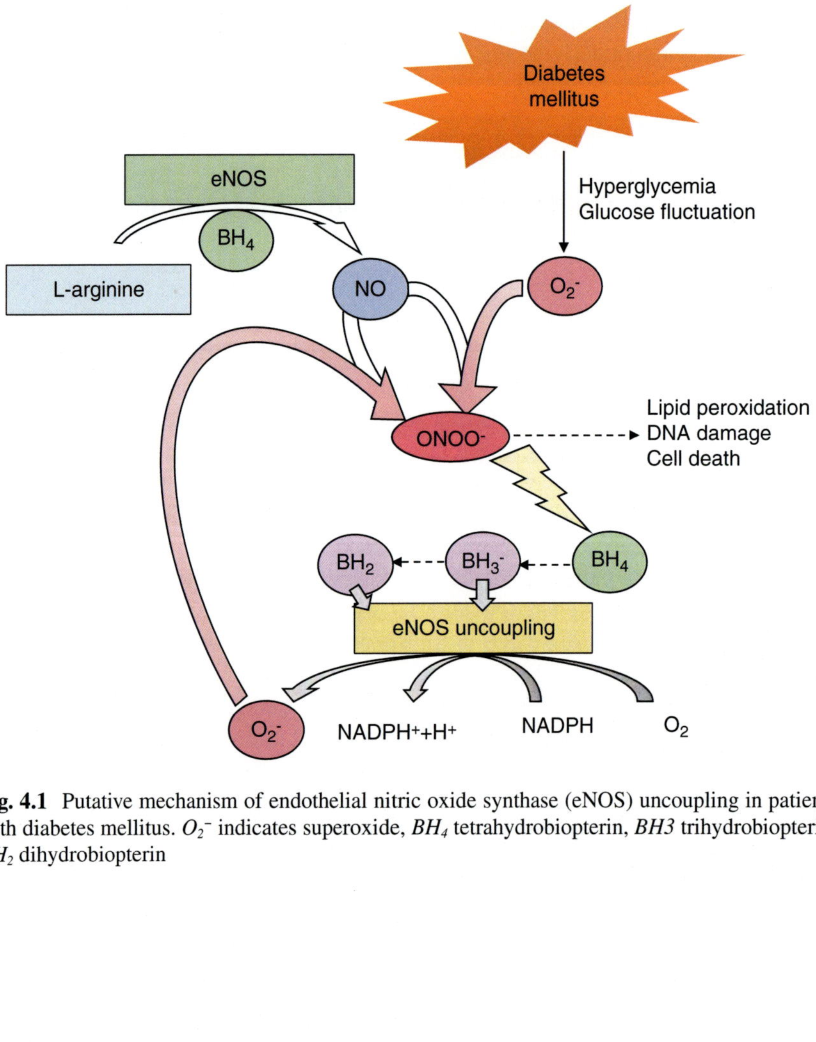

Fig. 4.1 Putative mechanism of endothelial nitric oxide synthase (eNOS) uncoupling in patients with diabetes mellitus. O_2^- indicates superoxide, BH_4 tetrahydrobiopterin, *BH3* trihydrobiopterin, BH_2 dihydrobiopterin

4.3.1.1 Oxidative Stress Induced by Hyperglycemia in Diabetes

Mitochondria are the major intracellular source of O_{2-}. Intracellular glucose oxidation starts with glycolysis, which generates pyruvate for mitochondrial catabolism to form ATP in the cytoplasm. Pyruvate transported into the mitochondria is oxidized to NADH and $FADH_2$ by the tricarboxylic acid (TCA) cycle. NADH and $FADH_2$ serve as donors of electrons used as energy for ATP production through oxidative phosphorylation by the electron transport chain composed of four multiprotein enzyme complexes located in the inner mitochondrial membrane. Electron transfer is coupled with the transfer of protons across the inner mitochondrial membrane. Therefore, electron transfer through the electron transport chain generates a proton gradient by pumping protons across the inner mitochondrial membrane, providing the energy to drive the ATP synthase. Under the condition of hyperglycemia, NADH and $FADH_2$, electron donors, from the TCA cycle are increased, and the proton gradient across the inner mitochondrial membrane is increased due to the enhanced electron transfer through the electron transport chain and a concomitant increase in the proton pumping. An increase in proton gradient above a certain threshold inhibits electron transport through the electron transport chain, resulting in increased electron leak and O_{2-} generation in mitochondria [11].

Hyperglycemia-induced overproduction of mitochondrial O_{2-} inhibits the activity of the glycolytic enzyme glyceraldehyde-3-phosphate, the activity of which is essential for maintenance of glycolytic flux, thereby resulting in the accumulation of upstream glycolysis intermediates and increased flux of these metabolites into glucose overutilization pathways, including the polyol pathway, hexosamine pathway, protein kinase C (PKC) pathway, and advanced glycation end product (AGE) pathway (Fig. 4.2) [11]. Increased glucose flux into the polyol pathway consumes NADPH, which is required for regenerating reduced glutathione (GSH), a main intracellular antioxidant. Therefore, intracellular concentrations of reduced GSH are consequently decreased, leading to an increase in intracellular oxidative stress. Shunting of excess intracellular glucose into the hexosamine pathway increases the modification of transcriptional factor through dysregulated protein glycosylation, resulting in altered protein expression. PKC activation induced by hyperglycemia through increased diacylglycerol has various pathogenic consequences including decreased expression of eNOS, increased expression of ET-1, transforming growth factor-β and plasminogen activator inhibitor-1, and activation of NF-κB and NADPH oxidase, leading to impairment of endothelial function. AGE causes functional alterations of intracellular proteins and modifications of extracellular matrix proteins and plasma proteins. In addition, activation of RAGE, a receptor for AGEs, on endothelial cells mediates the production of ROS and activation of NF-κB. Hyperglycemia causes endothelial dysfunction through overproduction of mitochondrial O_{2-} and diversion of glycolytic flux to alternative metabolic pathways.

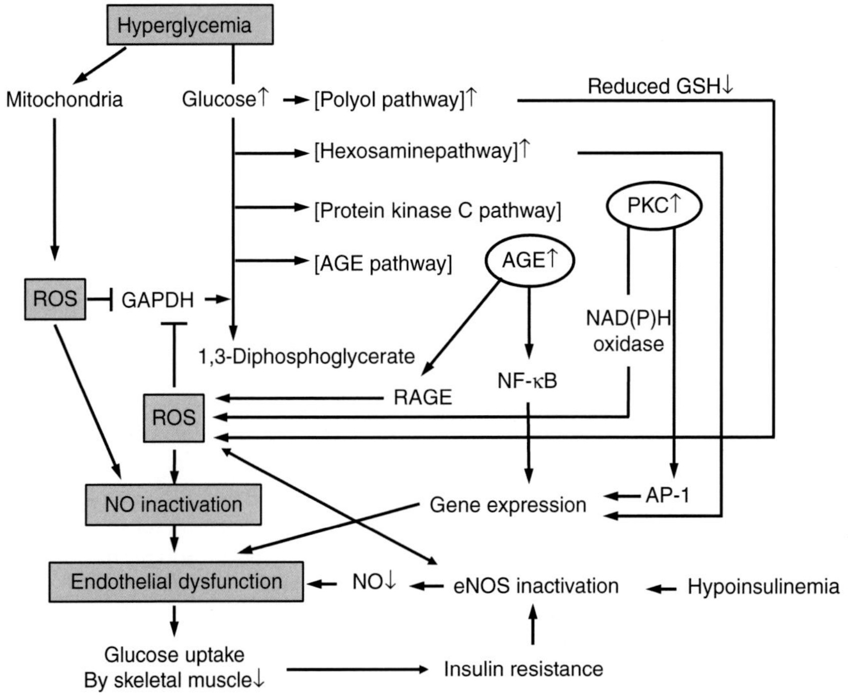

Fig. 4.2 Putative mechanisms of hyperglycemia-induced endothelial dysfunction in patients with diabetes mellitus. *ROS* indicates reactive oxygen species, *GAPDH* glyceraldehyde-3-phosphate, *eNOS* endothelial nitric oxide synthase, *AGE* advanced glycation end product, *RAGE* receptor for AGEs, *AP-1* activator protein-1

4.3.1.2 Oxidative Stress Induced by Acute Glucose Fluctuations in Diabetes

Blood glucose levels are strictly regulated within a narrow range in normal subjects. However, in patients with diabetes mellitus, a rapid and large increase in blood glucose levels in the postprandial phase is observed. Recent studies have demonstrated that the postprandial acute hyperglycemia may play a significant role in the pathogenesis of diabetic vascular complications through increased oxidative stress, reduced NO bioavailability, and consequent endothelial dysfunction [12]. Glucose fluctuations induced by intermittent high glucose might be more deleterious to endothelial cells than a constant high glucose concentration. In in vitro studies, intermittent high glucose has been demonstrated to enhance apoptosis of endothelial cells via the activation of PKC and NADPH oxidase, suggesting the involvement of oxidative stress in endothelial cell injury [13, 14]. In addition, a recent clinical study has demonstrated that glucose fluctuations, obtained from continuous glucose monitoring system data by calculating the mean amplitude of glycemic excursion (MAGE), are associated with increased oxidative stress in patients with type 2 diabetes [15]. Monnier et al. reported that the mean urinary excretion rate of 8-iso

$PGF_{2\alpha}$, an oxidative stress marker, strongly correlated with MAGE, whereas there were no significant correlations between the urinary excretion rates of 8-iso $PGF_{2\alpha}$ and any other glucose control parameters, including HbA_{1c} and fasting plasma glucose [15]. In addition, Torimoto et al. reported that there was a significant association between glucose fluctuations and endothelial dysfunction in patients with type 2 diabetes [16]. MAGE significantly correlated with reactive hyperemia index, a marker of endothelial function, measured by using peripheral arterial tonometry in patients with type 2 diabetes [16]. Although the precise molecular mechanisms for enhanced oxidative stress and consequent endothelial cell injury by glucose fluctuations have not been fully elucidated, a possible explanation is that constant high glucose may facilitate cellular metabolic adaptations against high glucose-induced toxic effects by consistent feedback, whereas such adaptations may be reduced during intermittent exposure to high glucose due to the absence of consistent feedback, resulting in higher glucose toxicity. HbA1c has been used as a clinical marker of glycemic exposure and as a therapeutic marker of glycemic control in treatment of patients with diabetes mellitus. However, HbA1c serves as a time-averaged measure of glycemic exposure without any information regarding glycemic variability and fluctuations. Recent large randomized trials have demonstrated the lack of significant reduction in cardiovascular events with intensive glycemic control using HbA1c as a therapeutic parameter of glucose control. In the treatment of patients with diabetes mellitus, attention should be paid to not only fasting plasma glucose and HbA1c levels but also postprandial hyperglycemia in order to protect the endothelium from oxidative injury for the prevention of vascular complications in patients with diabetes mellitus.

4.3.2 Selective Insulin Resistance in Diabetes

In addition to its essential glucose and lipid metabolic actions, insulin has several important vascular actions including NO production in endothelial cells. Insulin stimulation of endothelial cells through binding to its cognate receptor on the endothelial cell surface phosphorylates insulin receptor substrate (IRS), which stimulates phosphoinositide 3-kinase (PI 3-kinase)/Akt pathway. Akt directly phosphorylates eNOS at Ser^{1177}, resulting in activation of eNOS and increased NO production (Fig. 4.3). Insulin also stimulates the mitogen-activated protein kinase (MAPK)/extracellular signal-regulated kinase (ERK) pathway and downstream release of the vasoconstrictor ET-1 in endothelial cells, which is independent of the PI 3-kinase/Akt pathway (Fig. 4.3). Under the condition of insulin resistance in endothelial cells, insulin-induced activation of the PI 3-kinase/Akt pathway and the downstream phosphorylation of eNOS are selectively impaired due to the decreased endothelial IRS function, whereas the MAPK/ERK pathway is unaffected and preferentially activated due to the compensatory hyperinsulinemia, resulting in decreased NO production and increased ET-1 secretion, a characteristic of endothelial dysfunction. It has been demonstrated that the vasodilatory effect of insulin is

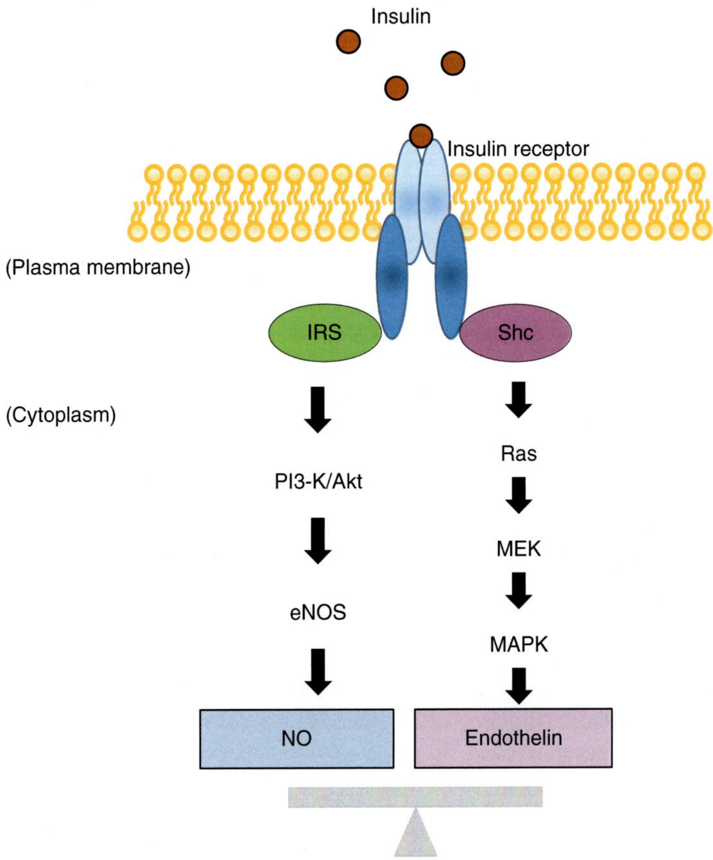

Fig. 4.3 Distinct signaling pathways mediating insulin effects on nitric oxide (NO) and endothelin. *IRS* indicates insulin receptor substrate, *PI* 3-k phosphoinositide 3-kinase, *eNOS* endothelial nitric oxide synthase, *MEK* mitogen-activated protein kinase kinase, *MAPK* mitogen-activated protein kinase

enhanced under the condition of ET-1 blockade in patients with type 2 diabetes but not in healthy control subjects [17]. Insulin resistance causes endothelial dysfunction through the selectively impaired PI 3-kinase/Akt pathway due to impaired IRS function and enhanced stimulation of the MAPK/ERK pathway due to compensatory hyperinsulinemia in endothelial cells.

4.4 Insulin Resistance in Skeletal Muscle Associated with Endothelial Dysfunction

Skeletal muscle plays an important role in glucose homeostasis through insulin-induced glucose uptake. Insulin has to be delivered to the interstitium of skeletal muscle for stimulating glucose uptake by the skeletal muscle. Insulin itself acts in

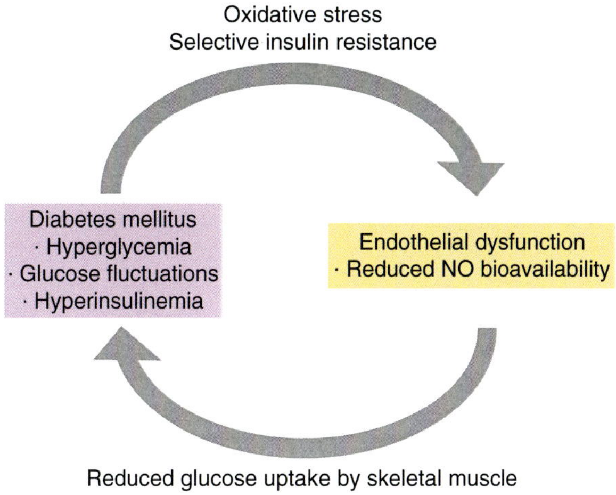

Fig. 4.4 A vicious cycle of endothelial dysfunction and diabetes mellitus

an NO-dependent fashion to increase interstitial insulin concentration by dilating terminal arterioles to increase the number of perfused capillaries and microvascular exchange surface area (microvascular recruitment), dilating larger resistance vessels to increase total limb blood flow, and promoting trans-endothelial transport of insulin to the interstitium of skeletal muscle [18]. Therefore, endothelial dysfunction induced by oxidative stress and selective insulin resistance in endothelial cells causes impairment of vasodilation and insulin transport across the endothelium through reduced NO bioavailability, leading to insulin resistance in skeletal muscle due to a delayed increase in insulin concentration in the interstitium and a consequent decrease in glucose uptake by skeletal muscle. Results of both animal and human studies support the association of insulin resistance with impaired vasodilator action and impaired glucose uptake in skeletal muscle [19, 20]. In clinical studies, skeletal muscle blood flow response to insulin was shown to decrease in diabetic and obese subjects compared with that in lean subjects [19]. In in vivo studies, eNOS knockout mice have been shown to exhibit insulin resistance through decreased muscle blood flow and glucose uptake by skeletal muscle [20]. Therefore, insulin resistance is further exacerbated through a vicious cycle of endothelial dysfunction induced by selective insulin resistance and reduced glucose uptake by skeletal muscle (Fig. 4.4).

4.5 Current Treatment Targeting Endothelial Dysfunction in Diabetes Mellitus

From a clinical perspective, early detection of endothelial dysfunction and early intervention for maintaining endothelial function in a healthy condition are important for the prevention of future cardiovascular events in patients with cardiovascular risk factors. Therefore, in the management of patients with diabetes mellitus, it is important to select an appropriate intervention that effectively improves endothelial function for the prevention of diabetic vascular complications.

Considering the associations of endothelial dysfunction with hyperglycemia, glucose fluctuations, and insulin resistance, lifestyle modifications and pharmacological therapies aiming at lowering glucose level without hypoglycemia, flattening glucose fluctuations, and improving insulin sensitivity may be beneficial for the restoration of endothelial function and prevention of cardiovascular events.

4.5.1 Insulin Therapy

Intensive glycemic control with insulin therapy effectively reduces microvascular complications and cardiovascular events in patients with type 1 diabetes [21]. For patients with type 1 diabetes, in whom insulin resistance does not predominate and a healthy energy balance is achieved, insulin therapy may be safe and beneficial to the endothelium because of the absence of selective insulin resistance in the PI 3-kinase/Akt pathway, leading to increased production of NO in endothelial cells. However, the effect of insulin therapy on endothelial function in patients with type 2 diabetes is still controversial and may be dependent on the achieved metabolic control level [22]. It is possible that high-dose insulin therapy in obese or overweight diabetic patients with insulin resistance who are refractory to its glucose-lowering effect due to excess nutrient supply and positive energy balance may be harmful to the endothelium through an imbalance between impaired PI 3-kinase/Akt pathway and enhanced MAPK/ERK pathway activation caused by selective insulin resistance in endothelial cells, leading to endothelial dysfunction.

4.5.2 Antidiabetic Agents

An antidiabetic agent exerts its glucose-lowering effect by increasing pancreatic insulin secretion and/or ameliorating insulin sensitivity in peripheral tissues. Sulfonylureas, insulin secretagogues, could potentially have an effect similar to that of high-dose insulin therapy and could be harmful to endothelial function in obese or overweight diabetic patients with insulin resistance due to the selective insulin resistance in endothelial cells.

Considering the reciprocal relationship between insulin resistance and endothelial dysfunction, antidiabetic agents that improve insulin sensitivity are anticipated to have beneficial effects on endothelial function through restoration of PI 3-kinase/Akt signaling and downstream NO production. Thiazolidinediones, insulin sensitizers, have been shown to improve endothelium-dependent vasodilation [23, 24]. In addition, thiazolidinediones have been demonstrated to increase the expression and plasma level of adiponectin, which directly stimulates NO production from endothelial cells through activation of the PI 3-kinase/Akt pathway in patients with insulin resistance or type 2 diabetes [25, 26]. Metformin, another insulin-sensitizing agent, has also been shown to improve endothelium-dependent vasodilation with significant association with improvement of insulin resistance assessed by the homeostasis model (HOMA-IR) in patients with type 2 diabetes [27]. Therefore, pharmacological therapies targeting insulin resistance may have beneficial effects on endothelial function through improving insulin sensitivity and increasing NO production in endothelial cells in diabetic patients with insulin resistance.

Antidiabetic agents that decrease the postprandial rise in blood glucose levels are also anticipated to have beneficial effects on endothelial function through decreased oxidative stress and a consequent increase in NO bioavailability. Glinides, dipeptidyl peptidase 4 (DPP-4) inhibitors, and α-glucosidase inhibitors are antidiabetic drugs that improve the control of postprandial glucose levels. These antidiabetic agents have been shown to improve postprandial endothelial function [28–31]. However, there are conflicting reports showing that α-glucosidase inhibitors, glinides, and DPP-4 inhibitors have no significant beneficial effects or even have adverse effects on endothelial function in patients with type 2 diabetes [28, 32, 33]. Although the precise reasons for the discrepancy of the results remain unknown, some explanations, including differences in the vascular beds assessed for endothelial function, subject selection, and treatment period, have been postulated. As for glinides and DPP-4 inhibitors, there is a possibility that increased insulin secretion through their pharmacological actions could be harmful to endothelial function in obese or overweight diabetic patients due to the selective insulin resistance in endothelial cells.

4.5.3 *Other Treatment*

In patients with type 2 diabetes, other cardiovascular risk factors such as hypertension and dyslipidemia are highly prevalent. Therefore, a multiple risk factor intervention approach is important for the prevention of cardiovascular events in patients with type 2 diabetes. The Steno-2 study demonstrated that an intensified and targeted multifactorial intervention including behavior modifications and polypharmacologic therapy aimed at controlling several modifiable risk factors reduced the risk of cardiovascular and microvascular events by about 50% compared with a conventional strategy [34]. In the management of other risk factors in patients with type 2 diabetes, it is also important to select an appropriate intervention that will be expected to improve endothelial function, including administration of antihypertensive agents such as angiotensin-converting enzyme inhibitors and angiotensin II type I receptor blockers [35, 36], administration of statins [37], and lifestyle modifications such as aerobic exercise and body weight reduction [38, 39].

4.6 Conclusions

In patients with diabetes mellitus, endothelial dysfunction is the early feature of atherosclerosis and plays an important role in the development of this condition, leading to diabetic vascular complications. Oxidative stress induced by hyperglycemia and glucose fluctuations causes endothelial dysfunction through inactivating NO by excess production of ROS. Selective insulin resistance in the PI 3-kinase/Akt pathway and impaired downstream NO production in endothelial cells may also contribute to endothelial dysfunction, whereas endothelial dysfunction might contribute to insulin resistance. Insulin potentially regulates its own delivery to skeletal muscle in an NO-dependent fashion at multiple steps. Reduced NO production through oxidative stress and selective insulin resistance in endothelial cells causes insulin resistance in skeletal muscle due to a delayed increase in insulin concentration in the interstitium of skeletal muscle. It is clinically important to break out of the cycle of endothelial dysfunction and insulin resistance in obese or overweight diabetic patients for the prevention of cardiovascular events. In addition to lifestyle modifications such as aerobic exercise and body weight reduction, antidiabetic agents that improve insulin sensitivity are expected to ameliorate endothelial function. Although an intervention targeting the reduction of oxidative stress is theoretically attractive, clinical studies in which the effects of antioxidants on cardiovascular events in patients with diabetes mellitus were investigated have revealed disappointing outcomes. Further studies are needed to develop clinically safe and effective treatment strategies targeting oxidative stress for the prevention of cardiovascular events in patients with diabetes mellitus.

References

1. Bardenheier BH, Lin J, Zhuo X, Ali MK, Thompson TJ, Cheng YJ, et al. Disability-free life-years lost among adults aged >/=50 years with and without diabetes. Diabetes Care. 2016;39(7):1222–9. doi:10.2337/dc15-1095.
2. Morrish NJ, Wang SL, Stevens LK, Fuller JH, Keen H. Mortality and causes of death in the WHO Multinational Study of Vascular Disease in Diabetes. Diabetologia. 2001;44(Suppl 2):S14–21.
3. Higashi Y, Noma K, Yoshizumi M, Kihara Y. Endothelial function and oxidative stress in cardiovascular diseases. Circ J. 2009;73(3):411–8.
4. Lerman A, Zeiher AM. Endothelial function: cardiac events. Circulation. 2005;111(3):363–8. doi:10.1161/01.CIR.0000153339.27064.14.
5. Williams SB, Cusco JA, Roddy MA, Johnstone MT, Creager MA. Impaired nitric oxide-mediated vasodilation in patients with non-insulin-dependent diabetes mellitus. J Am Coll Cardiol. 1996;27(3):567–74.
6. Henry RM, Ferreira I, Kostense PJ, Dekker JM, Nijpels G, Heine RJ, et al. Type 2 diabetes is associated with impaired endothelium-dependent, flow-mediated dilation, but impaired glucose metabolism is not; The Hoorn Study. Atherosclerosis. 2004;174(1):49–56. doi:10.1016/j.atherosclerosis.2004.01.002.

7. Vane JR, Anggard EE, Botting RM. Regulatory functions of the vascular endothelium. N Engl J Med. 1990;323(1):27–36. doi:10.1056/NEJM199007053230106.
8. McVeigh GE, Brennan GM, Johnston GD, McDermott BJ, McGrath LT, Henry WR, et al. Impaired endothelium-dependent and independent vasodilation in patients with type 2 (non-insulin-dependent) diabetes mellitus. Diabetologia. 1992;35(8):771–6.
9. Johnstone MT, Creager SJ, Scales KM, Cusco JA, Lee BK, Creager MA. Impaired endothelium-dependent vasodilation in patients with insulin-dependent diabetes mellitus. Circulation. 1993;88(6):2510–6.
10. Forstermann U, Sessa WC. Nitric oxide synthases: regulation and function. Eur Heart J. 2012;33(7):829–37, 37a–37d. doi:10.1093/eurheartj/ehr304.
11. Brownlee M. Biochemistry and molecular cell biology of diabetic complications. Nature. 2001;414(6865):813–20. doi:10.1038/414813a.
12. Ceriello A. The emerging role of post-prandial hyperglycaemic spikes in the pathogenesis of diabetic complications. Diabet Med. 1998;15(3):188–93. doi:10.1002/(SICI)1096-9136(199803)15:3<188::AID-DIA545>3.0.CO;2-V.
13. Risso A, Mercuri F, Quagliaro L, Damante G, Ceriello A. Intermittent high glucose enhances apoptosis in human umbilical vein endothelial cells in culture. Am J Physiol Endocrinol Metab. 2001;281(5):E924–30.
14. Quagliaro L, Piconi L, Assaloni R, Martinelli L, Motz E, Ceriello A. Intermittent high glucose enhances apoptosis related to oxidative stress in human umbilical vein endothelial cells: the role of protein kinase C and NAD(P)H-oxidase activation. Diabetes. 2003;52(11):2795–804.
15. Monnier L, Mas E, Ginet C, Michel F, Villon L, Cristol JP, et al. Activation of oxidative stress by acute glucose fluctuations compared with sustained chronic hyperglycemia in patients with type 2 diabetes. JAMA. 2006;295(14):1681–7. doi:10.1001/jama.295.14.1681.
16. Torimoto K, Okada Y, Mori H, Tanaka Y. Relationship between fluctuations in glucose levels measured by continuous glucose monitoring and vascular endothelial dysfunction in type 2 diabetes mellitus. Cardiovasc Diabetol. 2013;12:1. doi:10.1186/1475-2840-12-1.
17. Cardillo C, Nambi SS, Kilcoyne CM, Choucair WK, Katz A, Quon MJ, et al. Insulin stimulates both endothelin and nitric oxide activity in the human forearm. Circulation. 1999;100(8):820–5.
18. Barrett EJ, Eggleston EM, Inyard AC, Wang H, Li G, Chai W, et al. The vascular actions of insulin control its delivery to muscle and regulate the rate limiting step in skeletal muscle insulin action. Diabetologia. 2009;52(5):752–64. doi:10.1007/s00125-009-1313-z.
19. Laakso M, Edelman SV, Brechtel G, Baron AD. Impaired insulin-mediated skeletal muscle blood flow in patients with NIDDM. Diabetes. 1992;41(9):1076–83.
20. Duplain H, Burcelin R, Sartori C, Cook S, Egli M, Lepori M, et al. Insulin resistance, hyperlipidemia, and hypertension in mice lacking endothelial nitric oxide synthase. Circulation. 2001;104(3):342–5.
21. Nathan DM, Cleary PA, Backlund JY, Genuth SM, Lachin JM, Orchard TJ, et al. Intensive diabetes treatment and cardiovascular disease in patients with type 1 diabetes. N Engl J Med. 2005;353(25):2643–53. doi:10.1056/NEJMoa052187.
22. Nolan CJ, Ruderman NB, Kahn SE, Pedersen O, Prentki M. Insulin resistance as a physiological defense against metabolic stress: implications for the management of subsets of type 2 diabetes. Diabetes. 2015;64(3):673–86. doi:10.2337/db14-0694.
23. Fujishima S, Ohya Y, Nakamura Y, Onaka U, Abe I, Fujishima M. Troglitazone, an insulin sensitizer, increases forearm blood flow in humans. Am J Hypertens. 1998;11(9):1134–7.
24. Hidaka T, Nakagawa K, Goto C, Soga J, Fujii Y, Hata T, et al. Pioglitazone improves endothelium-dependent vasodilation in hypertensive patients with impaired glucose tolerance in part through a decrease in oxidative stress. Atherosclerosis. 2010;210(2):521–4. doi:10.1016/j.atherosclerosis.2009.12.011.
25. Yu JG, Javorschi S, Hevener AL, Kruszynska YT, Norman RA, Sinha M, et al. The effect of thiazolidinediones on plasma adiponectin levels in normal, obese, and type 2 diabetic subjects. Diabetes. 2002;51(10):2968–74.

26. Maeda N, Takahashi M, Funahashi T, Kihara S, Nishizawa H, Kishida K, et al. PPARgamma ligands increase expression and plasma concentrations of adiponectin, an adipose-derived protein. Diabetes. 2001;50(9):2094–9.
27. Mather KJ, Verma S, Anderson TJ. Improved endothelial function with metformin in type 2 diabetes mellitus. J Am Coll Cardiol. 2001;37(5):1344–50.
28. Kato T, Inoue T, Node K. Postprandial endothelial dysfunction in subjects with new-onset type 2 diabetes: an acarbose and nateglinide comparative study. Cardiovasc Diabetol. 2010;9:12. doi:10.1186/1475-2840-9-12.
29. Matsubara J, Sugiyama S, Akiyama E, Iwashita S, Kurokawa H, Ohba K, et al. Dipeptidyl peptidase-4 inhibitor, sitagliptin, improves endothelial dysfunction in association with its anti-inflammatory effects in patients with coronary artery disease and uncontrolled diabetes. Circ J. 2013;77(5):1337–44.
30. Nakamura K, Oe H, Kihara H, Shimada K, Fukuda S, Watanabe K, et al. DPP-4 inhibitor and alpha-glucosidase inhibitor equally improve endothelial function in patients with type 2 diabetes: EDGE study. Cardiovasc Diabetol. 2014;13:110. doi:10.1186/s12933-014-0110-2.
31. Shimabukuro M, Higa N, Chinen I, Yamakawa K, Takasu N. Effects of a single administration of acarbose on postprandial glucose excursion and endothelial dysfunction in type 2 diabetic patients: a randomized crossover study. J Clin Endocrinol Metab. 2006;91(3):837–42. doi:10.1210/jc.2005-1566.
32. Ayaori M, Iwakami N, Uto-Kondo H, Sato H, Sasaki M, Komatsu T, et al. Dipeptidyl peptidase-4 inhibitors attenuate endothelial function as evaluated by flow-mediated vasodilatation in type 2 diabetic patients. J Am Heart Assoc. 2013;2(1):e003277. doi:10.1161/JAHA.112.003277.
33. Maruhashi T, Higashi Y, Kihara Y, Yamada H, Sata M, Ueda S, et al. Long-term effect of sitagliptin on endothelial function in type 2 diabetes: a sub-analysis of the PROLOGUE study. Cardiovasc Diabetol. 2016;15(1):134. doi:10.1186/s12933-016-0438-x.
34. Gaede P, Vedel P, Larsen N, Jensen GV, Parving HH, Pedersen O. Multifactorial intervention and cardiovascular disease in patients with type 2 diabetes. N Engl J Med. 2003;348(5):383–93. doi:10.1056/NEJMoa021778.
35. Higashi Y, Sasaki S, Nakagawa K, Ueda T, Yoshimizu A, Kurisu S, et al. A comparison of angiotensin-converting enzyme inhibitors, calcium antagonists, beta-blockers and diuretic agents on reactive hyperemia in patients with essential hypertension: a multicenter study. J Am Coll Cardiol. 2000;35(2):284–91.
36. Ghiadoni L, Virdis A, Magagna A, Taddei S, Salvetti A. Effect of the angiotensin II type 1 receptor blocker candesartan on endothelial function in patients with essential hypertension. Hypertension. 2000;35(1 Pt 2):501–6.
37. Wolfrum S, Jensen KS, Liao JK. Endothelium-dependent effects of statins. Arterioscler Thromb Vasc Biol. 2003;23(5):729–36. doi:10.1161/01.ATV.0000063385.12476.A7.
38. Higashi Y, Sasaki S, Kurisu S, Yoshimizu A, Sasaki N, Matsuura H, et al. Regular aerobic exercise augments endothelium-dependent vascular relaxation in normotensive as well as hypertensive subjects: role of endothelium-derived nitric oxide. Circulation. 1999;100(11):1194–202.
39. Sasaki S, Higashi Y, Nakagawa K, Kimura M, Noma K, Sasaki S, et al. A low-calorie diet improves endothelium-dependent vasodilation in obese patients with essential hypertension. Am J Hypertens. 2002;15(4 Pt 1):302–9.

Chapter 5
Diabetes and Vascular Calcification

Katsuhito Mori and Masaaki Inaba

Abstract Vascular calcification had been accepted as a passive, degenerative process, but recent findings suggested that it is actively regulated like osteogenesis. In addition, vascular calcification is roughly classified into two types: intimal arterial calcification (IAC) and medial arterial calcification (MAC). IAC is usually associated with atherosclerosis, whereas MAC is often associated with aging, diabetes, and chronic kidney disease. Although MAC does not directly cause stenotic or occlusive lesions, it may exacerbate arterial stiffness with significant hemodynamic changes, resulting in cardiovascular mortality. Transdifferentiation of vascular smooth muscle cells (VSMCs) and changes in extracellular matrix (ECM), which are mainly due to elastin degradation, are involved in the onset and progression of MAC. In particular, runt-related transcription factor 2 (Runx2) seems to play a critical role in the transformation of VSMCs from a vascular contractile phenotype into an osteoblast-like phenotype. The presence of diabetes accelerates both VSMC transdifferentiation through the upregulation of Runx2 and ECM changes by metalloproteinase-induced elastin degradation. Fetuin-A can act as not only an inducer of insulin resistance but also as an inhibitor of ectopic calcification through the formation of calciprotein particles (CPPs). Recently, it has been hypothesized that overproduction of CPPs could cause vascular damage, including vascular calcification. Since fetuin-A is involved in both diabetes and vascular calcification, precise investigation of CPPs may give new insights in this field.

Keywords Diabetes • Vascular calcification • Medial arterial calcification • Smooth muscle cells • Fetuin-A

K. Mori, M.D. (✉) • M. Inaba
The Department of Metabolism, Endocrinology and Molecular Medicine, Osaka City University Graduate School of Medicine, 1-4-3, Asahi-machi, Abeno-ku, Osaka 545-8585, Japan
e-mail: ktmori@med.osaka-cu.ac.jp

S.-i. Yamagishi (ed.), *Diabetes and Aging-related Complications*,
https://doi.org/10.1007/978-981-10-4376-5_5

5.1 Introduction

Diabetes mellitus is highly prevalent in the world and is, inarguably, one of the representative diseases that cause vascular complications. Appropriate treatment of diabetes, especially if with concomitant cardiovascular disease, is a pressing issue in modern society. Historically, understanding the mechanism of atherosclerosis induced by diabetes was the main issue in this field. For example, the formation of occlusive lesions in an atherosclerotic plaque, such as in acute coronary syndrome (ACS), had been focused on. However, emerging evidence suggested that alteration of arterial stiffness, or arteriosclerosis, which is neither stenotic or thrombogenic, plays a critical role in cardiovascular mortality. Vascular calcification, especially in the media, has provided many clues to the significance of hemodynamic changes due to arteriosclerosis [1, 2].

5.2 Clinical Significance of Vascular Calcification

The presence of calcification seems to be a hallmark of the terminal state of a vascular lesion, such as what happens in aging. Therefore, vascular calcification had been recognized for quite a while as a passive, degenerative process of hydroxyapatite precipitation in the arterial wall. In addition, calcification of the aorta or arteries of the lower extremities has not been known to directly cause vascular occlusion or ischemia. Therefore, clinical doctors seldom minded such seemingly innocuous lesions, although some studies have shown a high prevalence of such calcifications on plain soft tissue radiographs in patients with diabetes or chronic kidney disease (CKD).

However, there have been several scenarios that triggered attention to vascular calcification. For example, the spread of percutaneous coronary intervention has been a breakthrough in the treatment of coronary artery disease (CAD). During its development, it was gradually realized that the existence of calcification disturbed dilatation and rotational atherectomy of target coronary lesions. Angiorrhaphy during coronary artery bypass also becomes difficult in the presence of calcifications. Nowadays, vascular calcification has been an evitable matter to solve in intervention-resistant conditions. Recent technical advances have enabled detection and quantification of coronary artery calcification by multidetector coronary computed tomography. Moreover, calcification patterns on intravenous ultrasound have been reported to be associated with ACS. In particular, a calcium burden pattern (i.e., spotty or granular microcalcification) was prone to rupture, whereas a homogenous pattern or sheetlike macrocalcification seemed to be resistant to plaque rupture [1, 3]. Therefore, the diagnosis and treatment of CAD should not leave out vascular calcification.

5.3 Types of Vascular Calcification

Vascular calcification roughly falls into two types: intimal arterial calcification (IAC) and medial arterial calcification (MAC) (Fig. 5.1) [1–3]. IAC is strongly associated with atherosclerosis, which involves inflammatory cell infiltration and formation of a lipid-rich core in the arterial wall. It is exacerbated by classic cardiovascular risk factors, such as dyslipidemia. The presence of IAC usually represents advanced atherosclerosis. However, whether calcification in itself can promote or protect plaque rupture and subsequent formation of an occlusive lesion is still controversial. As described above, it may depend on the calcification pattern (spotty calcification vs. diffuse calcification) [1, 3].

On the other hand, MAC is more often detected in patients with diabetes and CKD, including those on hemodialysis. MAC occurs independent of atherosclerosis and IAC [1, 3, 4]. It is characterized by the deposition of hydroxyapatite crystals in the extracellular matrix (ECM) of the medial interspace of arterial vascular smooth muscle cells (VSMCs) and usually does not contain inflammatory cells. The characteristic conversion of VSMCs and the compositional changes in medial wall ECM seem to play crucial roles in the development of MAC, as discussed below. Clinically, progression of MAC could increase arterial stiffness and cause systolic hypertension with pressure

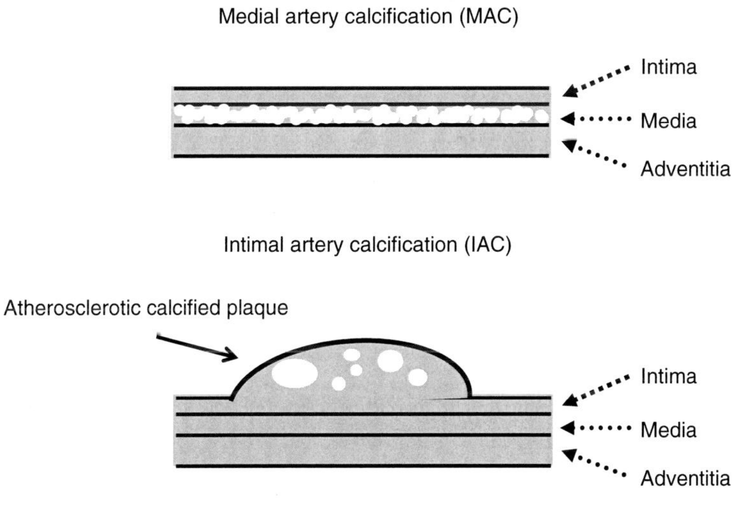

Fig. 5.1 Types of vascular calcification. IAC is strongly associated with atherosclerosis, which involves inflammatory cell infiltration with lipid-rich core in the arterial wall. The presence of IAC is correlated with stenotic, thrombotic lesions with a risk of plaque rupture. MAC is often detected in patients with diabetes, independent of atherosclerosis. MAC influences arterial stiffness and leads to significant hemodynamic changes, although it does not directly cause occlusive lesions. *IAC* intima medial calcification, *MAC* medial arterial calcification

afterload, left ventricular hypertrophy, and heart failure [5]. On the other hand, MAC reduces diastolic hypotension, resulting in a decrease in myocardial perfusion pressure and subsequent myocardial ischemia [5]. Therefore, MAC is associated with higher cardiovascular mortality through profound hemodynamic changes [3, 4].

5.3.1 Mechanism of Vascular Calcification

As mentioned above, MAC is commonly found in patients with diabetes, independent of atherosclerosis. Therefore, we focused on the mechanism of MAC, as follows. The necessity of VSMC transdifferentiation into osteoblast-like cells in the formation of MAC has gained broad acceptance. VSMCs gradually lose their original contractile phenotypes and alternatively express bone-related genes. Simultaneously, medial matrix proteins, such as elastin, undergo drastic changes and lead to altered arterial elasticity, which subsequently provides a scaffold for precipitation of hydroxyapatites. Degradation of elastin by metalloproteinases is a prominent feature in the media. Transdifferentiation of VSMCs and ECM changes may interact during development of MAC (Fig. 5.2), although the predominating mechanism is unknown [6].

5.3.2 Central Role of VSMC Transdifferentiation and ECM Alteration in MAC Formation

Bone morphogenetic protein-2 (BMP-2), which belongs to the transforming growth factor (TGF) superfamily, plays a major role in osteoblastic differentiation. Demer et al. first demonstrated BMP-2 expression in calcified lesions in human arterial

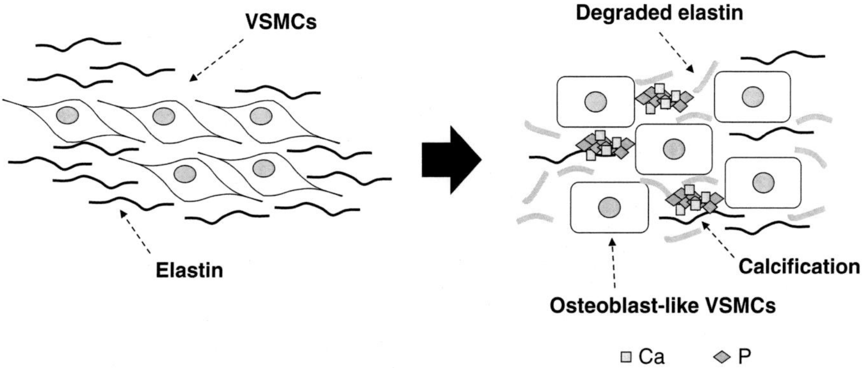

Fig. 5.2 Mechanism of vascular calcification. Two factors may be critical for the onset and progression of MAC: (1) transdifferentiation of VSMCs into osteoblast-like cells and (2) changes in ECM, which are mainly due to elastin degradation by matrix metalloproteinase. Transdifferentiation of VSMCs and ECM changes may interact and accelerate MAC. *MAC* medial arterial calcification, *VSMCs* vascular smooth muscle cells, *ECM* extracellular matrix, *Ca* calcium, *P* phosphate

walls and identified a clonal population of arterial cells with calcifying capability and osteoblastic features; these were named calcifying vascular cells (CVCs) [7]. These findings first shed light on the fact that vascular calcification shares similar pathways with osteogenesis. Another important milestone in the field of vascular calcification was discovered in the study of the phenotype of matrix Gla protein (MGP)-deficient mice [8]. These mice spontaneously showed extensive MAC, suggesting the inhibitory role of MGP in vascular calcification, apart from atherosclerosis-based calcification. However, the critical question on the origin of cells with calcifying capability remains. One possibility is transdifferentiation of VSMCs, which are original components of the medial wall. Another is differentiation from immature, multipotent mesenchymal progenitor cells that reside in the arterial wall or migrate from the circulation.

To answer this question, Giachelli et al. prepared MGP-deficient mice, SM22a-Cre recombinase transgenic mice, and Rosa26-LacZ Cre reporter transgenic mice [9]. After breeding, the VSMCs in these mice were genetically marked by LacZ. Using these mice, the authors clarified that VSMCs were the origin of the cells in the calcified media of MGP-deficient mice. Based on the additional observation that green fluorescent protein (GFP)-positive cells were rare in the arterial wall after engraftment of GFP-expressing bone marrow cells into MGP-deficient mice, they concluded that calcifying cells in the media were unlikely to be derived from multipotent progenitors. Of course, this theory is limited in the mechanism of MAC. In the case of IAC formation, circulating cells may contribute to vascular calcification [1], but this will not be discussed in this manuscript.

The link between hyperphosphatemia and MAC, especially in end-stage renal disease (ESRD), has been predicted. Therefore, addition of inorganic phosphate into cultured SMC was tried in an in vitro model; in this experiment, phosphate calcification in VSMCs was confirmed by upregulation of bone-related genes, probably mediated by Pit-1, which is a sodium-dependent phosphate cotransporter [10].

In contrast to extracellular factors, such as BMP-2, MGP, and phosphate, runt-related transcription factor 2 (Runx2), or Cbfa1/Osf2, is an essential transcriptional factor in osteogenesis [11]. Runx2 expression in mesenchymal stem cells induces some osteogenesis-related genes, such as osteocalcin, osteopontin, and osterix. Although Runx2 is involved in the early stages of osteogenesis, its expression decreases in the late stage, which may be necessary for maturation of osteoblasts and maintenance of bone mass [11]. Fine regulation of Runx2 expression is required during osteogenesis. With regard to vascular calcification, Runx2 may be involved in repression of the primary VSMs phenotype, in addition to acceleration of the osteogenic phenotype. Tanaka et al. precisely investigated the function of Runx2 as a key regulator in transdifferentiation of VSMCs [12].

To maintain the contractile phenotype of VSMCs, a set of regulatory factors is necessary. Among these, serum response factor (SRF), which binds to CArG box [CC(AT)$_6$GG] in the promoter regions of SMC-specific genes, is known to be a key transcriptional factor. In contrast to the ubiquitously expressed SRF, myocardin, which is a coactivator of SRF, is expressed in cardiac myocytes and VSMCs [13]. Therefore, disruption of myocardin affects SRF binding on CArG box and leads to the formation of a synthetic, proliferative phenotype of VSMC. Interestingly, Tanaka et al. demonstrated that Runx2 could interfere with coactivation of SRF and myocardin, resulting in inactivation of SMC-specific genes, such as SM22α and SM-MHC (Fig. 5.3) [12]. Simultaneously, Runx2 could upregulate osteogenic genes, including alkaline phosphatase (ALP), osteopontin, and osterix, in VSMCs (Fig. 5.3) [12].

Similar to Runx2, Msx, which is another critical transcriptional factor in osteogenesis, is considered to be associated with vascular calcification. The Notch signaling pathway is involved in the induction of Msx in VSMCs (Fig. 5.3). Notch ligands on the cell surface bind to Notch receptors on the adjacent VSMCs, and, subsequently, Notch intracellular domains (NICDs) are cleaved [11]. NICDs that are translocated into the nucleus bind to cognate DNA binding sites and interact with RBP-Jk, which is a major mediator of Notch signaling, resulting in the activation of target genes, including Msx (Fig. 5.3) [11]. Although the role of Notch in the promotion or inhibition of osteogenesis is still controversial, Notch-induced Msx upregulation, at the least, stimulates vascular calcification independent of BMP-2 [14]. In this case, cell–cell interaction between infiltrated macrophages, which

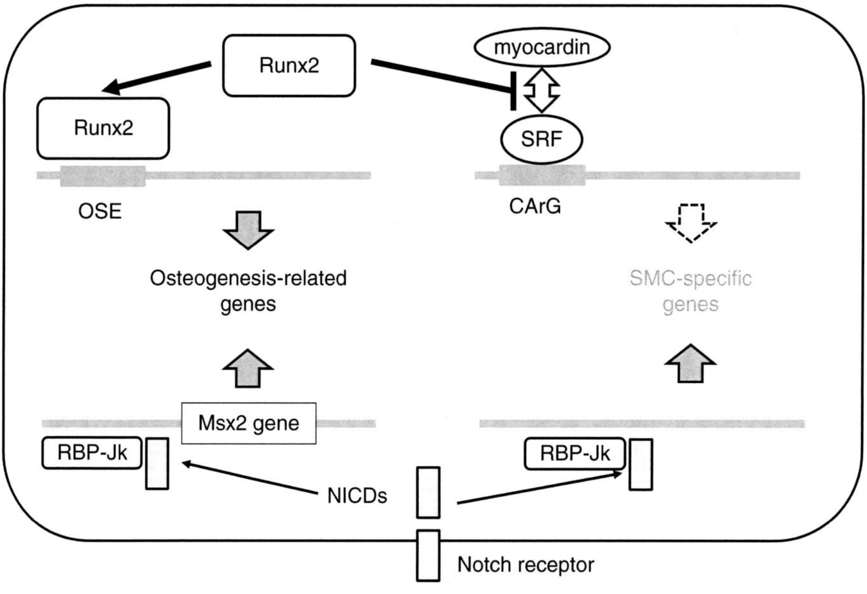

Fig. 5.3 Intracellular pathway of VSMC transdifferentiation from a contractile phenotype to a synthetic, osteoblast-like phenotype. Runx2, an essential transcriptional factor in osteogenesis, plays a critical role in vascular calcification by promoting the osteogenic phenotype of VSMCs. At the same time, Runx2 disrupts myocardin and SRF interaction, which can maintain an intact vascular phenotype of VSMCs. Therefore, Runx2 acts as both promoter of the osteogenic phenotype and repressor of the vascular phenotype of VSMCs. In addition, activation of Notch signaling accelerates the osteogenic phenotype of VSMCs through Msx2 gene upregulation. *Runx2* runt-related transcription factor 2, *VSMCs* vascular smooth muscle cells, *SRF* serum response factor, *OSE* osteocyte-specific element, *NICDs* Notch intracellular domains. Adapted and revised from [12, 14]

express various Notch ligands, and VSMCs, which have Notch receptors, is speculated to cause vascular calcification; however, the significance of macrophages in MAC formation is unknown.

5.3.3 VSMC Transdifferentiation in MAC Under Diabetic Conditions

The existence of diabetes is recognized as one of the major predisposing factors for the development of vascular calcification [1–3]. Although long-standing diabetes can lead to various metabolic disorders, a simple factor may be hyperglycemia. To test this hypothesis, VSMCs were incubated in normal (5 mM) and high-glucose (25 mM) conditions [15]. As expected, high glucose promoted SMC calcification, enhanced Runx2 and osteocalcin expressions, and increased ALP activity and BMP-2 secretion [15]. Addition of a protein kinase C (PKC) inhibitor inhibited the high-glucose condition-induced Runx2 and osteocalcin expressions, suggesting the involvement of PKC in hyperglycemia-induced vascular calcification [15]. On histopathologic examination, diabetic patients with ESRD showed a greater degree of MAC, with increased staining of osteopontin and ALP, compared with nondiabetic patients with ESRD [15].

Glucose in high levels nonenzymatically reacts with various proteins to subsequently form advanced glycation end products (AGEs), which can accelerate calcification of VSMCs via increased Runx2 expression, ALP activation, and increased secretion of osteocalcin [16]. AGE-induced calcification appeared to be mediated by receptors for AGE (RAGE) because the addition of anti-RAGE blocking antibody inhibited calcium deposition in VSMCs [16]. Although RAGE, which is a pattern recognition receptor, has been initially identified with AGEs, other RAGE ligands, including S100, high mobility group box 1, and amyloid fibrils, have been identified as important inflammatory regulators. Therefore, under diabetic conditions, RAGE had been speculated to affect vascular calcification independent of AGEs. RAGE activation suppressed SMC marker genes, such as SM22α and SM-MHC, through the reduction of myocardin [17]. At the same time, Notch–Msx-mediated osteogenic differentiation was promoted by RAGE activation, suggesting another role of the RAGE axis in osteogenic conversion of VSMCs [17].

5.3.4 ECM Changes in MAC Under Diabetic Conditions

High-glucose conditions could also accelerate MAC through elastin degradation by matrix metalloproteinases (MMPs). Compared to subjects without diabetes, patients with diabetes have upregulated MMPs in the arterial wall and higher plasma levels of MMPs. Therefore, diabetic conditions are predicted to enhance the degradation of elastic fibers. Elastin-derived peptides (EDPs), which are products of elastin degradation, can be measured in the serum of diabetic patients. Interestingly, EDPs could induce VSMC expression of osteogenic genes, such as Runx2, osteocalcin, and ALP, possibly through the elastin–laminin receptor (ELR) [18]. Elastin fiber degradation is associated with concomitant degradation of TGFβ binding protein, resulting in the release of TGFβ and increase in the level of free TGFβ. This synergistic effect of TGFβ and EDPs on the osteogenic phenotype of VSMCs had been confirmed [18]. Furthermore, under high-glucose conditions, EDPs and TGFβ have been shown to amplify the osteogenic phenotypes, possibly by activating ELR [19]. These findings suggest that a diabetic state, which causes considerable ECM changes, could promote MAC.

5.4 Fetuin-A and Calciprotein Particles in Diabetes and Vascular Calcification

Fetuin-A is also known as a circulating α2-Heremans–Schmid glycoprotein that is involved in insulin resistance, type 2 diabetes, and atherosclerosis [20, 21]. One of its prominent functions is the potent capability to inhibit ectopic calcification by forming colloidal, water-soluble mineral complexes, termed calciprotein particles (CPPs) or fetuin-A mineral complexes (Fig. 5.4). CPPs do not precipitate

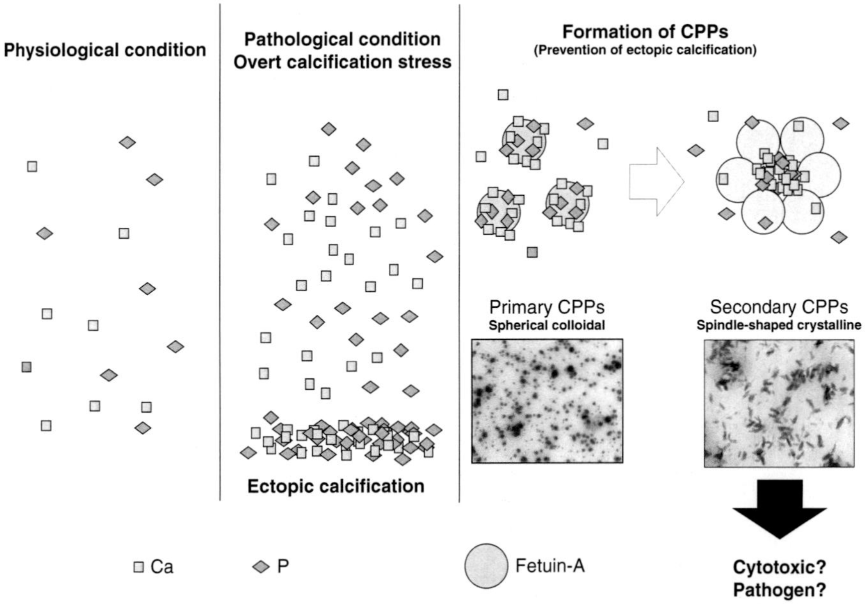

Fig. 5.4 Fetuin-A and calciprotein particles. Fetuin-A forms CPPs to prevent calcification under stress. At the early phase, spherical colloidal CPPs (primary CPPs) are formed. Further calcification stress, including hyperphosphatemia, promotes the transformation of primary CPPs into larger spindle-shaped secondary CPPs. *CPPs* calciprotein particles

spontaneously and are thought to be cleared mainly by macrophages in the liver and spleen [22]. In fact, low fetuin-A levels have already been established to be associated with mortality in patients with ESRD, possibly through accelerated vascular calcification [20, 21]. Therefore, fetuin-A has been recognized to play a protective role against vascular calcification, especially in patients with CKD and ESRD.

However, the fate of overproduced CPPs under conditions of phosphate overload, such as ESRD, has not been considered in detail. Recently, serum CPPs levels have been reported to increase with CKD progression [23]. Moreover, CPPs were found to induce expression and secretion of pro-inflammatory cytokines from macrophages [24]. Therefore, Kuro-o has hypothesized CPPs as endogenous "pathogens" even in subclinical hyperphosphatemia [25]. In the early phase of calcification stress, calcium phosphate crystals bind to fetuin-A to form colloidal nanoparticles (primary CPPs), which measure 50–100 nm in diameter (Fig. 5.4). To prevent further crystal growth and precipitation, primary CPPs form a stable mineral core that is covered by a densely packed fetuin-A monolayer. These particles are termed as secondary CPPs, which are spindle-shaped and measure 100–200 nm in diameter (Fig. 5.4). It was hypothesized that CPPs, especially secondary CPPs, could trigger vascular damage, including VSMC transdifferentiation and vascular calcification [25, 26]. Since fetuin-A is involved in both diabetes and vascular calcification, precise investigation of CPPs may give new insights in this field. This hypothesis will have to be confirmed in future studies.

References

1. Avogaro A, Fadini GP. Mechanisms of ectopic calcification: implications for diabetic vasculopathy. Cardiovasc Diagn Ther. 2015;5:343–52. doi:10.3978/j.issn.2223-3652.2015.06.05.
2. Virmani R, Joner M, Sakakura K. Recent highlights of ATVB: calcification. Arterioscler Thromb Vasc Biol. 2014;34:1329–32. doi:10.1161/ATVBAHA.114.304000.
3. Demer LL, Tintut Y. Vascular calcification: pathobiology of a multifaceted disease. Circulation. 2008;117:2938–48. doi:10.1161/CIRCULATIONAHA.107.743161.
4. London GM, Guerin AP, Marchais SJ, Metivier F, Pannier B, Adda H. Arterial media calcification in end-stage renal disease: impact on all-cause and cardiovascular mortality. Nephrol Dial Transplant. 2003;18:1731–40.
5. Taddei S, Nami R, Bruno RM, Quatrini I, Nuti R. Hypertension, left ventricular hypertrophy and chronic kidney disease. Heart Fail Rev. 2011;16:615–20. doi:10.1007/s10741-010-9197-z.
6. Lei Y, Sinha A, Nosoudi N, Grover A, Vyavahare N. Hydroxyapatite and calcified elastin induce osteoblast-like differentiation in rat aortic smooth muscle cells. Exp Cell Res. 2014;323:198–208. doi:10.1016/j.yexcr.2014.01.011.
7. Bostrom K, Watson KE, Horn S, Wortham C, Herman IM, Demer LL. Bone morphogenetic protein expression in human atherosclerotic lesions. J Clin Invest. 1993;91:1800–9. doi:10.1172/JCI116391.
8. Luo G, Ducy P, McKee MD, Pinero GJ, Loyer E, Behringer RR, et al. Spontaneous calcification of arteries and cartilage in mice lacking matrix GLA protein. Nature. 1997;386(6620):78–81. doi:10.1038/386078a0.
9. Speer MY, Yang HY, Brabb T, Leaf E, Look A, Lin WL, et al. Smooth muscle cells give rise to osteochondrogenic precursors and chondrocytes in calcifying arteries. Circ Res. 2009;104:733–41. doi:10.1161/CIRCRESAHA.108.183053.

10. Jono S, McKee MD, Murry CE, Shioi A, Nishizawa Y, Mori K, et al. Phosphate regulation of vascular smooth muscle cell calcification. Circ Res. 2000;87:E10–7.
11. Xu J, Li Z, Hou Y, Fang W. Potential mechanisms underlying the Runx2 induced osteogenesis of bone marrow mesenchymal stem cells. Am J Transl Res. 2015;7:2527–35.
12. Tanaka T, Sato H, Doi H, Yoshida CA, Shimizu T, Matsui H, et al. Runx2 represses myocardin-mediated differentiation and facilitates osteogenic conversion of vascular smooth muscle cells. Mol Cell Biol. 2008;28:1147–60. doi:10.1128/MCB.01771-07.
13. Xia XD, Zhou Z, Yu XH, Zheng XL, Tang CK. Myocardin: a novel player in atherosclerosis. Atherosclerosis. 2016. doi:10.1016/j.atherosclerosis.2016.12.002.
14. Shimizu T, Tanaka T, Iso T, Doi H, Sato H, Kawai-Kowase K, et al. Notch signaling induces osteogenic differentiation and mineralization of vascular smooth muscle cells: role of Msx2 gene induction via Notch-RBP-Jk signaling. Arterioscler Thromb Vasc Biol. 2009;29:1104–11. doi:10.1161/ATVBAHA.109.187856.
15. Cheng DW, Jiang Y, Shalev A, Kowluru R, Crook ED, Singh LP. An analysis of high glucose and glucosamine-induced gene expression and oxidative stress in renal mesangial cells. Arch Physiol Biochem. 2006;112:189–218. doi:10.1080/13813450601093518.
16. Tanikawa T, Okada Y, Tanikawa R, Tanaka Y. Advanced glycation end products induce calcification of vascular smooth muscle cells through RAGE/p38 MAPK. J Vasc Res. 2009;46:572–80. doi:10.1159/000226225.
17. Suga T, Iso T, Shimizu T, Tanaka T, Yamagishi S, Takeuchi M, et al. Activation of receptor for advanced glycation end products induces osteogenic differentiation of vascular smooth muscle cells. J Atheroscler Thromb. 2011;18:670–83.
18. Simionescu A, Philips K, Vyavahare N. Elastin-derived peptides and TGF-beta1 induce osteogenic responses in smooth muscle cells. Biochem Biophys Res Commun. 2005;334:524–32. doi:10.1016/j.bbrc.2005.06.119.
19. Sinha A, Vyavahare NR. High-glucose levels and elastin degradation products accelerate osteogenesis in vascular smooth muscle cells. Diab Vasc Dis Res. 2013;10:410–9. doi:10.1177/1479164113485101.
20. Mori K, Emoto M, Inaba M. Fetuin-A: a multifunctional protein. Recent Pat Endocr Metab Immune Drug Discov. 2011;5:124–46.
21. Mori K, Emoto M, Inaba M. Fetuin-A and the cardiovascular system. Adv Clin Chem. 2012;56:175–95.
22. Herrmann M, Schafer C, Heiss A, Graber S, Kinkeldey A, Buscher A, et al. Clearance of fetuin-A—containing calciprotein particles is mediated by scavenger receptor-A. Circ Res. 2012;111:575–84. doi:10.1161/CIRCRESAHA.111.261479.
23. Hamano T, Matsui I, Mikami S, Tomida K, Fujii N, Imai E, et al. Fetuin-mineral complex reflects extraosseous calcification stress in CKD. J Am Soc Nephrol. 2010;21:1998–2007. doi:10.1681/ASN.2009090944.
24. Smith ER, Hanssen E, McMahon LP, Holt SG. Fetuin-A-containing calciprotein particles reduce mineral stress in the macrophage. PLoS One. 2013;8:e60904. doi:10.1371/journal.pone.0060904.
25. Kuro-o M. Klotho, phosphate and FGF-23 in ageing and disturbed mineral metabolism. Nat Rev Nephrol. 2013;9:650–60. doi:10.1038/nrneph.2013.111.
26. Kuro-o M. Calciprotein particle (CPP): a true culprit of phosphorus woes? Nefrologia. 2014;34:1–4. doi:10.3265/Nefrologia.pre2013.Dec.12385.

Chapter 6
Diabetes and Adipocyte Dysfunction

Yohko Yoshida†**, Ippei Shimizu**†**, and Tohru Minamino**

Abstract The global burden of obesity/diabetes and comorbidities continues to rise in many societies. Obesity predisposes to the development of diabetes and increases the mortality rate, particularly deaths from cardiovascular disease. Chronic sterile inflammation develops in visceral white adipose tissue (WAT) upon metabolic stress and promotes the production of pro-inflammatory adipokines and systemic insulin resistance (hyperinsulinemia). Systemic insulin resistance develops with metabolically unhealthy obesity and diabetes and promotes pathologies in these disorders. Studies indicate that cellular senescence is critically involved in the development of sterile adipose inflammation in obesity. In vitro studies showed that senescent cells have bystander effects to promote aging in surrounding younger cells, and depletion of senescent cells by the genetic manipulation or senolytic agents led to the inhibition of age-related organ dysfunction in rodents. Brown adipose tissue (BAT) is another type of fat initially identified and characterized as a tissue involved in thermogenesis. BAT is nowadays well accepted as an active metabolic organ, which has a potential to contribute for the maintenance of systemic metabolic health. In humans and rodents, obesity linked with reduced BAT function and, recently, capillary rarefaction was shown to have causal role for the functional decline of this organ, which led to systemic metabolic disorders in murine obese model. Metabolically healthy obesity (MHO) is characterized with less visceral adiposity associated with nonsignificant metabolic phenotypes. MHO individuals are enriched in subcutaneous WAT, and this specific fat pad is known to include beige cells that share functional similarities with brown adipocytes. The activation of

---

†Yohko Yoshida and Ippei Shimizu contributed equally to this work.

Y. Yoshida • I. Shimizu, M.D., Ph.D. (✉)
Department of Cardiovascular Biology and Medicine, Niigata University Graduate School of Medical and Dental Sciences, Niigata 951-8510, Japan

Division of Molecular Aging and Cell Biology, Niigata University Graduate School of Medical and Dental Sciences, 1-757 Asahimachidori, Chuo-ku, Niigata 951-8510, Japan
e-mail: ippeishimizu@yahoo.co.jp

T. Minamino, M.D., Ph.D. (✉)
Department of Cardiovascular Biology and Medicine, Niigata University Graduate School of Medical and Dental Sciences, Niigata 951-8510, Japan
e-mail: t_minamino@yahoo.co.jp

S.-i. Yamagishi (ed.), *Diabetes and Aging-related Complications*,
https://doi.org/10.1007/978-981-10-4376-5_6

beige cells contributes for systemic metabolic health in rodents, suggesting that in addition to classical brown adipocytes, targeting beige cells would become next-generation therapies for obesity and diabetes. Accumulating evidence indicates that maintenance of homeostasis in adipose tissues is critically important for systemic metabolic health.

Keywords Cellular senescence • Inflammation • Adipose tissue • Insulin resistance

6.1 Introduction

Obese and/or diabetic population is increasing and continues to be the top health-care problems in many societies. Systemic metabolic dysfunction develops with unhealthy obesity and promotes pathologies in cardiovascular disorders. Several types of fats are known to distribute in our body. White adipose tissue is initially characterized as an organ involved in energy storage, and nowadays it is well appreciated to be an active endocrinal organ involved in the secretion of biologically active molecules described as adipokines. Chronic sterile inflammation in visceral as well as subcutaneous fat develops under metabolic stress and has causal role for the development of systemic metabolic disorders. Brown adipose tissue is another type of fat known to have roles for systemic metabolic health. Brown adipocytes are enriched in mitochondria and consume huge amounts of energy by producing heat. For this reason, BAT was initially thought to be an organ involved in thermogenesis. Recently, studies indicate that BAT is an active metabolic organ involved in the regulation of systemic metabolisms in humans and rodents. It has become clear that several specific fat pads are involved in the maintenance of systemic metabolic homeostasis. In this chapter, we delineate the roles of white and brown adipose tissues in obesity and diabetes.

6.2 The Pathological Role of Systemic Insulin Resistance in Cardiometabolic Disorders

Aging is characterized with a progressive regression of physiological function, leading to an increase in vulnerability and eventually to death. Insulin signaling is the most extensively studied signaling pathway involved in aging processes. It is well known that the mild suppression of this pathway would inhibit the progression of aging in diverse species. Systemic insulin resistance (hyperinsulinemia) develops with metabolically unhealthy obesity, diabetes, and/or heart failure, and studies suggest that it promotes pathologies in these age-related disorders [1, 2]. In vascular cells, such as endothelial cells and vascular smooth muscle cells, insulin/insulin receptor(IR)/insulin receptor substrate(IRS)/phosphoinositide 3-kinase(PI3K)/Akt signaling activates endothelial nitric oxide synthase (eNOS), heme oxygenase-1

(HO-1), and vascular endothelial growth factor (VEGF) production and suppresses vascular cell adhesion molecule-1 (VCAM-1) expression. Thereby, this signaling pathway is well accepted to mediate anti-atherosclerotic responses. In contrast, insulin/IR/Son of sevenless (SOS)/growth factor receptor-bound protein (GRB)/mitogen-activated protein kinase (MAPK) signaling upregulates the expression of plasminogen activator inhibitor-1 (PAI-1) and endothelin-1 (ET-1), and these molecules are well known to promote pro-atherosclerotic actions. In this context, insulin signaling has bidirectional roles for the maintenance of vascular health. In obesity and diabetes, IR/IRS/PI3K/Akt signaling downregulates; conversely, IR/SOS/GRB/MAPK signaling is enhanced in vascular cells. This is described as "selective insulin resistance," and this pathological condition is known to promote pro-atherosclerotic responses by the activation of MAPK signaling that mediates vasoconstriction, proliferation, and migration of vascular cells, thereby promoting vascular remodeling [3].

Evidence suggests that systemic insulin resistance develops with heart failure. Systemic insulin resistance predicted the subsequent onset of heart failure independently of established risk factors. Another study showed that patients who subsequently developed heart failure had higher level of proinsulin, the marker of insulin resistance. In a murine left ventricular (LV) pressure-overload model, heart failure induced systemic insulin resistance (hyperinsulinemia), and this promoted pathologies by mediating the excessive activation of insulin signaling pathway that resulted in cardiac hypertrophy, tissue hypoxia, and systolic cardiac dysfunction. In the chronic phase of LV pressure overload, insulin resistance developed in the visceral fat and liver but was constitutively activated in cardiac tissue, possibly because cardiomyocytes have a unique system to activate insulin signaling mediated by the mechanical stretch of these cells [4].

In addition to obese and diabetic conditions, several lines of evidence indicate that the inhibition of systemic insulin resistance, as well as the modulation of insulin signaling, is critically important to suppress pathologies in heart failure. Among several oral diabetic drugs, sodium glucose cotransporter-2 (SGLT-2) inhibitor and biguanide, drugs that improve systemic insulin resistance, have evidence to inhibit cardiac events including heart failure [5, 6]. Nowadays it is well accepted that adipose tissues are critically involved in systemic glucose metabolism and insulin sensitivity, and these would be discussed in the following sections.

6.3 The Contribution of White Adipose Tissue in Systemic Metabolic Health

In addition to its initially identified roles for energy storage, white adipose tissue is now well described as an active endocrine organ secreting various types of "adipokines." Adiponectin is the best described anti-inflammatory and antidiabetic adipokine that contributes to enhance insulin sensitivity and promote oxidation of free fatty acids (FFA) in metabolic organs. Adiponectin contributes to the clearance of FFA, glucose, and triacylglycerol from the blood, and evidence suggests that it contributes to suppress pathologies in several disease models. Leptin is a satiety hormone secreted from adipocytes, and circulating leptin level tightly links with fat mass. Leptin has biological effects for central nervous system and suppresses hunger and reduces food intake. Obesity links with high leptin level; however, under obese condition, selective leptin resistance is known to develop in arcuate nucleus (ARC) of the hypothalamus, contributing to promote pathologies in obesity [7]. White adipose tissue is also known to secrete series of pro-inflammatory adipokines. Adipocytes including mature lipids are thought to make up 20–40% of total cell components in fat pad, occupying more than 90% of fat pad volume. In obesity, 1 g of adipose tissue includes approximately 2–5 million stromal vascular fraction cells, and around 65% of these cells are shown to be leukocytes. Among several leukocytes, macrophages are the extensively studied and characterized cells contributing for the development of non-sterile inflammation in adipose tissue [2]. There is a broad spectrum of markers for macrophages, and a simplified model favors to classify them into two types according to their roles for inflammation. M1 (classically activated) macrophages express cell surface marker such as CD11c and pro-inflammatory cytokines like tumor necrosis factor (TNF)-α and interleukin 6 (IL-6), thereby categorized into pro-inflammatory macrophages. M2 (alternatively activated) macrophages express cell surface markers such as CD206 and CD301, and anti-inflammatory cytokines like IL-10, and characterized to be anti-inflammatory macrophages. M2 macrophages predominantly exist in adipose tissue of lean animals, and M1 macrophages become dominant under obese conditions. The balance between anti- and pro-inflammatory adipokine production is critically important to maintain metabolic homeostasis. An increase in circulating pro-inflammatory cytokines and FFA released from inflamed adipose tissue suppress insulin signaling pathways in key metabolic organs, including skeletal muscles and the liver, and this results in systemic metabolic disorder and diabetes [8]. In addition to inflammatory macrophage infiltration, chronic sterile inflammation is characterized with the infiltration of other immune cells including neutrophils, B lymphocytes, mast cells, and effector memory T cells, associated with reduction in anti-inflammatory macrophages, eosinophils, and regulatory T cells. Macrophages and other immune cells generate a complex cell-cell interaction to modulate immune responses in adipose tissue, and they are elegantly reviewed by others [9, 10]. Accumulating evidence indicates that cellular senescence is critically involved in these processes leading to the development of systemic metabolic dysfunction, and these would be discussed next.

6.4 The Role of Cellular Senescence in White Adipose Tissue Dysfunction

In somatic cells, telomere attrition develops with cell division, and after reaching a critical threshold, DNA damage response becomes activated and induces cells to enter a state of irreversible growth arrest described as "replicative senescence" [11]. Oxidative stress, oncogenic activation, constitutive activation of mitogenic stimuli, or inflammatory cytokines also induce cellular senescence, and this is described as "stress-induced premature senescence." Cellular senescence is defined as a state of irreversible growth arrest accompanied by changes of both cell morphology and gene expression. Senescent cells secrete pro-inflammatory cytokines leading to tissue remodeling, and this is described as senescence-associated secretory phenotype (SASP) [12]. It is well accepted that the p53/p21 and p16/Rb signaling pathways have central roles for regulating cellular senescence. The p53 protein has roles for broad range of biological processes including DNA repair, cellular senescence, apoptosis, cell metabolism, autophagy, and cell-cycle regulation [13–15]. It now became clear that p53-induced cellular senescence is critically involved in the progression of pathologies in age-related disorders such as heart failure, atherosclerotic diseases, and diabetes [1, 16–18]. In diabetic humans and mice, p53 level was significantly increased in the visceral fat. This was associated with the elevation of senescence-associated β-galactosidase, a marker for cellular senescence, and production of pro-inflammatory cytokines. Studies with transgenic mice models showed that adipose tissue-specific p53 depletion ameliorates adipose inflammation and systemic insulin resistance. In contrast, adipose tissue-specific p53 gain of function induced adipose inflammation and systemic insulin resistance under chow diet. Recently, p53 was reported to increase the expression of semaphorin3E, and this secreted-type protein was shown to have a chemoattractant activity for inflammatory macrophages that express plexinD1, the specific receptor for semaphorin3E. The suppression of p53/semaphorin 3E/plexinD1 axis would become the next-generation therapy for diabetes [16].

The p53-induced cellular senescence was also shown to induce adipose inflammation in visceral fat in murine heart failure models and has causal roles for reducing systolic cardiac function. Studies suggest that systemic insulin resistance links with heart failure in nondiabetic individuals; however, the underlying mechanisms and their pathological implications were not known for a while [19]. Murine left ventricular pressure-overload model showed that constitutive activation of adrenergic signaling would induce excessive lipolysis in visceral fat associated with high reactive oxygen species level. This pathological condition contributed to increase p53 in visceral fat and was causal for inducing adipose inflammation and systemic insulin resistance (hyperinsulinemia). Suppression of adipose p53 and systemic insulin resistance ameliorated cardiac dysfunction upon left ventricular pressure overload. These results suggested that the inhibition of systemic metabolic disorders through the modulation of aging signaling in adipose tissue is crucial for the suppression of pathologies in heart failure [1].

Interestingly, senescent cells are known to damage their local environment. In vitro studies showed that exposure to senescent cells promotes cellular senescence in initially intact bystander fibroblasts via gap junction-mediated processes [20]. Murine genetic models suggested that the elimination of p16-positive senescent cells contributes to suppress age-related pathological changes in several organs including epididymal/inguinal WAT, cardiac tissue, and kidney [21]. Importantly, some pharmacological agents are recently shown to selectively kill senescent cells; thereby these compounds are described as "senolytic agents." In one study,

ABT263, an inhibitor of the anti-apoptotic proteins, was shown to effectively deplete senescent bone marrow hematopoietic stem cells and senescent muscle cells, and this led to the rejuvenation of these cells in chronological aging model [22]. Another study demonstrated that the elimination of senescent cells in aged mice contributes to preserve adipogenesis and increase insulin sensitivity [23]. Taken together, these results indicate that the suppression of cellular senescence and/or elimination of senescent cells would become next-generation therapies for obesity and diabetes.

6.5 The Contribution of Brown Adipose Tissue in Systemic Metabolic Health

Several types of fats are known to distribute in our body in specific locations. Brown adipose tissue (BAT) exists at several locations such as interscapular, supraclavicular, para-aortic, pericardial, paravertebral, and suprarenal areas and is morphologically and functionally different from WAT. BAT is a highly vascularized organ abundant in mitochondria, and initially it was characterized as a thermogenic organ involved in heat production. Now it is well described as a metabolically active organ that has a potential to regulate systemic metabolism. Humans are believed to possess 50–80 g of active brown adipose tissue. Studies with healthy volunteers showed that chronic cold exposure (17 °C for 2 h daily for 6 weeks) recruits BAT, and this led to the reduction in body fat mass [24]. Another study investigating obese humans showed that short-term cold acclimation also recruits BAT in this population [25]. BAT is reported to weigh approximately 5% of the whole-body weight in mice; however, when they get maximally activated, their contribution for triglyceride and glucose clearance is enormous. Mitochondria in brown adipocytes are enriched in uncoupling protein 1 (UCP-1), and this specific protein enables BAT to consume huge amounts of energy as heat by uncoupling respiratory chain in mitochondria. BAT was once thought to exist only in infants and small rodents and disappear in adults. The landmark study by Cypess et al. showed that adult humans also have functional BAT, and in addition to aging, obesity led to reduce their function [26]. The underlying mechanisms were not clearly defined for a while. Recently, metabolic stress was shown to promote the whitened phenotype of BAT, associated with functional decline of this organ, and this was causal for promoting systemic glucose intolerance. Vascular endothelial growth factor-A (VEGF-A) is an angiogenic molecule critically involved in the morphogenesis and maintenance of tissue homeostasis [27]. Metabolic stress led to the significant reduction of VEGF-A, thereby capillary rarefaction and tissue hypoxia developed in BAT. Hypoxic condition in BAT promoted autophagic responses and excessive mitochondria clearance in BAT, and this led to the whitened and dysfunctional phenotype of BAT. Genetic model of adipose tissue-specific *Vegfa* depletion led to capillary rarefaction, tissue hypoxia, and BAT whitening and developed systemic metabolic disorder when fed chow diet. In this genetic model, *Vegfa* was also depleted in white adipose tissue; however, they showed mild phenotype compared with BAT possibly because BAT is more dependent on vasculature and oxygen to maintain high-energy consumption [28]. An important and unanswered question is whether positive regulatory mechanisms for VEGF-A exist in BAT under stressed condition. Under physiological condition, β-adrenergic receptor-protein kinase A (PKA) signaling positively regulates VEGF-A expression in BAT, and excessive fatty acid influx into brown adipocytes suppressed this by the downregulation of phospho-PKA level. Dietary obesity induces hypoxia in BAT, and this is associated with high expression level of hypoxia-inducible factor-1α (HIF-1α) in this tissue. HIF-1α is among the extensively studied angiogenic molecules contributing to upregulate VEGF expression in several organs including cardiac tissue. Interestingly, in white and brown adipose tissues, studies suggest that HIF-1α do not promote angiogenesis. Genetic model of HIF-1α overexpression induced fibrosis in WAT [29]. In BAT, activation of HIF-1α resulted in the induction of HIF-1α target genes involved in autophagy and fibrosis but did not increase VEGF-A. Studies indicate that the maintenance of capillary network formation is important for preserving adipocyte function in BAT as well as WAT [28, 30]. Further studies are needed to find systems contributing for the promotion of capillary network formation in adipose tissues under stressed conditions. We also note that the role of cellular senescence in BAT homeostasis remains as an open question to be explored. Considering their potential contributions for systemic metabolism, maintenance of BAT homeostasis continues to be an important topic to be studied.

6.6 Subcutaneous White Adipose Tissue and the Role of Beige Cells in Systemic Metabolic Health

The expansion of visceral fat associates with obesity-related cardiometabolic disorders. In contrast, subcutaneous fats are thought to contribute more to systemic metabolic health than visceral fat [31]. Previous study showed that transplanting subcutaneous fat to visceral cavity would lead to reduced adiposity associated with systemic metabolic health [32]. Subcutaneous fat is enriched in mitochondrial brown fat uncoupling protein 1 (UCP-1)-positive and myogenic factor 5 (Myf-5)-negative cells, described as beige cells. Beige and brown adipocytes share some functional similarities including high UCP-1 expression; therefore, both cells are well accepted to be highly energy-consuming. In the Myf-5-positive classical brown adipocytes, baseline UCP-1 expression is high; in contrast, this is low in beige adipocytes without stimulation. The activation of adrenergic signaling in beige cells contributes to increase UCP-1 expression in these cells similar to the level of brown adipocytes. Nowadays, it is well accepted that beige cells promote the browning of subcutaneous fat leading to the suppression of systemic metabolic disorder [33, 34]. Several mechanisms including adrenergic signaling, fibroblast growth factor 21 (FGF21), irisin, cold stimulation, thiazolidinediones, and natriuretic peptide-mediated signaling are reported to promote beige cell differentiation and activation. Recently, cold stimulus was shown to activate the eosinophils and type 2 cytokine signaling in alternatively activated macrophages. These synergistically promoted the development of functional beige cells in subcutaneous fat and contributed for an increase in systemic oxygen consumption and metabolic health [35]. In dietary obese model, beige cell deletion resulted in increased susceptibility to weight gain, and this is associated with metabolically unhealthy phenotype [33]. In contrast, activation of beige cells was shown to suppress obesity in mice [36]. Interestingly, selective depletion of classical brown adipocyte (Myf5Cre;Bmpr1a$^{flox/flox}$) led to the induction of beige cells both in subcutaneous and epididymal WAT, and this contributed to restore thermogenesis and suppress systemic metabolic dysfunction [37]. This evidence indicates the existence of the complex compensatory network between classical brown adipocytes and beige cells. In humans, obesity led to a marked reduction in the incidence of brown/beige adipose tissue [38, 39]. Beige adipocytes derived from lean individuals have higher expression profile for UCP-1 compared to those from obese individuals [40]. Further studies are needed to clearly define the contribution of beige cells in systemic metabolic health in humans, and studying the browning processes of fat continues to be interesting research topics.

Chronic sterile inflammation in subcutaneous fat also develops with obesity, and this is also reported to promote systemic metabolic dysfunction. Suppression of subcutaneous fat inflammation contributed for systemic metabolic health even when the visceral fats were inflamed [41]. An interesting report by Lakowa et al. showed that telomere attrition develops more significantly in subcutaneous fat compared to visceral fat in humans, and this was due to shorter telomere length in stromal vascular fraction rather than adipose rich fraction [42]. The role of cellular senescence in subcutaneous fat is yet to be defined; however, studies suggest that the maintenance of subcutaneous fat health is an important concept to combat obesity and diabetes.

6.7 Fat Distribution Defines Metabolically Healthy and Unhealthy Obesity

Some obese individuals with high body mass index (BMI) show less visceral adiposity and mild metabolic phenotypes, and this condition is described as metabolically healthy obesity (MHO) or uncomplicated obesity. MHO condition fits for approximately 10–45% of adult obese populations, and it is prevalent among younger obese individuals and obese women. MHO individuals are generally thought not to develop systemic insulin resistance and do not match the criteria for metabolic syndrome [43]. Levels of circulating pro-inflammatory cytokines were lower, and adiponectin levels were higher in MHO compared to metabolically unhealthy obesity (MUO) [44]. MHO individuals also demonstrate low fasting plasma glucose and insulin, low plasma triglyceride, and higher high-density lipoprotein cholesterol [45]. MHO population shows lower risks for all-cause mortality and cardiovascular events compared to individuals with MUO [46]. Studies indicate that the distribution and quality of fat are among the critical factors contributing for this relative healthier condition. MHO associates with low visceral fat and high peripheral fat distribution compared to MUO. Systemic insulin resistance associates with smaller subcutaneous adipose tissue depots, indicating that inadequate lipid storage has pathological implications for metabolic health [47]. Adiponectin transgenic mice on an *ob/ob* background became obese under chow diet, but they were metabolically healthy [48]. Systemic insulin resistance is also known to develop in individuals with normal weight (BMI less than 25 kg/m^2), and this is described as metabolically unhealthy normal weight (MUHNW). The prevalence of MUHNW is reported to be as high as 23.5% in one study [49]. This group has higher risks for metabolic/cardiovascular disorders compared to MHO subjects, and it is thought that central adiposity promotes pathologies in MUHNW individuals [50, 51]. Nowadays, it is generally accepted that MHO is a transient condition that shifts toward MUO that associates with cardiovascular events. Two-thirds of individuals with MHO developed metabolic syndrome during 10-year observation [52]. One report showed that MHO does not increase the risk for myocardial infarction but increase the risk of heart failure compared to metabolically healthy nonobese individuals [53]. Further studies are needed to generate criteria that can clearly define MHO, and whether this relatively healthier condition become therapeutic target remains an open question to be explored.

6.8 Drugs, Compound, or Treatment Targeting Fats to Combat Obesity and Diabetes

6.8.1 Brown Adipose Tissue

Anti-obesity drugs mediating their biological effects through the promotion of energy consumption have been developed and tested in clinical trials. Activation of adrenergic signaling would promote BAT function and may lead to weight loss; however, clinical trials targeting this signaling were discouraging. Activation of adrenergic signaling led to weight loss as expected; however, clinical usefulness of these compounds were diminished due to serious side effects mediated by nonselective catecholamine signaling [54, 55]. Accumulating evidence indicates that noncanonical activation of BAT may become next-generation therapies for obesity and diabetes. Fibroblast growth factor 21 (FGF21) is predominantly secreted from the liver, and it binds to the FGF receptor/β-klotho complex in BAT, resulting in the uncoupled respiration associated with glucose oxidation [56]. In addition to the activation of BAT, FGF21 promotes the browning of WAT depots in adults; however, bone loss is reported as potential side effects related with this molecule [57, 58]. Bile acids were shown to bind to G-protein-coupled bile acid receptor and upregulate BAT function through the induction of *Ucp-1* gene expression and/or modulation of glucagon-like peptide-1 (GLP1) signaling [59–61]. Heart-derived ANP and BNP bind to NP receptors (NPRs) on the surface of brown adipocytes. NPR-mediated signalings activate cGMP-dependent protein kinase and promote the expression of thermogenic genes [62]. BAT secretes bone morphogenetic protein-8b (BMP8b) that acts in an autocrine fashion to sensitize BAT to adrenergic stimulation [63]. These results indicate that modulation of noncanonical pathways targeting BAT would become therapies for obesity and diabetes (reviewed in [10, 34, 64, 65]). Therapeutic potential of sirtuin1 (SIRT1) is extensively studied. SIRT1 regulates cellular energy homeostasis and mitochondrial biogenesis, and the activation of SIRT1 signaling is reported to extend life span in rodents. Resveratrol, a SIRT1 inducer, was shown to increase mitochondrial size and mitochondrial DNA content in the BAT of dietary obese mice, and this led to the suppression of BAT whitening, associated with higher energy expenditure. These biological effects of SIRT1 are thought to be mediated via SIRT1-peroxisome proliferator-activated receptor gamma coactivator 1-alpha (PGC1α) signaling. We also note that cold exposure, per se, may become therapy to combat obesity, as demonstrated in humans [24, 25].

6.8.2 *White Adipose Tissue*

Thiazolidinediones (TZDs) are antidiabetic drugs known to have beneficial biological effects through the activation of PPARγ signaling pathways. PPARγ is predominantly expressed in adipose tissue, and TZDs were shown to suppress inflammation and induce browning and energy expenditure in WAT, contributing to increase systemic insulin sensitivity. PPARγ is also reported to exist in monocytes, and TZDs are shown to promote alternative M2 polarization [66]. Unfortunately some issues related with side effects were raised with these compounds, including fluid retention, and currently moods exist to refrain from using these drugs in clinical practice. However, considerations for PPARγ signaling pathways as therapies for diabetes are reviving recently. Findings from Choi et al. indicated that phosphorylation at Ser273 of PPARγ changes the pattern of gene expression driven by this protein. Cdk5 was the critical regulator to mediate this response, and Cdk5-induced Ser273 phosphorylation reduced adiponectin expression without affecting some other PPARγ target genes. Inhibition of this Cdk5-mediated phosphorylation by a compound, SR1664, showed antidiabetic function in insulin-resistant mice, and importantly, this was mediated without the development of fluid retention [67]. This evidence indicates that selective activation of specific PPARγ signaling is possible, which enables to generate drugs with reduced side effects. Another paper showed that PPARγ ligands would induce the browning of inguinal white adipose tissue, and this was mediated by PRDM16, a transcriptional co-regulator known to promote the development of classical brown adipocytes [68].

TZDs contribute to increase the synthesis and secretion of adiponectin. Considering that biological effects of adiponectin are broadly beneficial, enhancement of this molecule would be the promising approach to combat obesity. The half-life of adiponectin is very short; therefore, Iwabu et al. generated small molecule activators of adiponectin receptors described as "AdipoRon" and tested their biological effects. AdipoRon reduced adipose inflammation, increased metabolism in skeletal muscle, and increased insulin sensitivity and glucose tolerance in genetic model of obesity. Importantly, AdipoRon was shown to extend the life span of these murine obese models fed under a high fat diet [69].

6.9 Conclusions

Studies suggest that WAT and BAT dysfunction develops upon metabolic stress and promotes pathologies in obesity and diabetes. The distribution of WAT is among the critical factors for metabolic phenotypes, and now it is well accepted that central adiposity is the determining factor for unhealthy obesity associated with high morbidity for cardiometabolic disorders. Chronic visceral fat inflammation and systemic metabolic disorders develop with unhealthy obesity, and it has become clear that the accumulation of senescent cells has causal roles for adipose inflammation and dysfunction. Inhibition of cellular senescence or elimination of senescent cells suppresses adipose dysfunction and contributes for systemic metabolic health. BAT is morphologically and functionally distinct from WAT. BAT is involved in thermogenesis, consuming huge amounts of energy as heat, and nowadays it is well accepted as a metabolically active organ involved in the maintenance of systemic metabolic health. Chronological aging and obesity linked with functional decline of this organ, and recently, metabolic stress-mediated hypoxic signaling was shown to induce BAT dysfunction leading to the development of systemic metabolic disorder. The role of cellular senescence in BAT remains an unanswered topic to be studied. Evidence indicates that subcutaneous fats contribute more for metabolic health compared to visceral fat. One of the possible underlying mechanisms would be that subcutaneous fats are enriched in UCP-1-positive beige cells. Beige cells become metabolically active upon stimulations, like classical brown adipocytes, and suppress pathologies in obesity and diabetes. Accumulation of evidence indicates that the maintenance of adipose tissue homeostasis is crucial for preserving systemic metabolic health. Therapies targeting white as well as brown adipose tissues would become next-generation therapies for obesity and diabetes (Fig. 6.1).

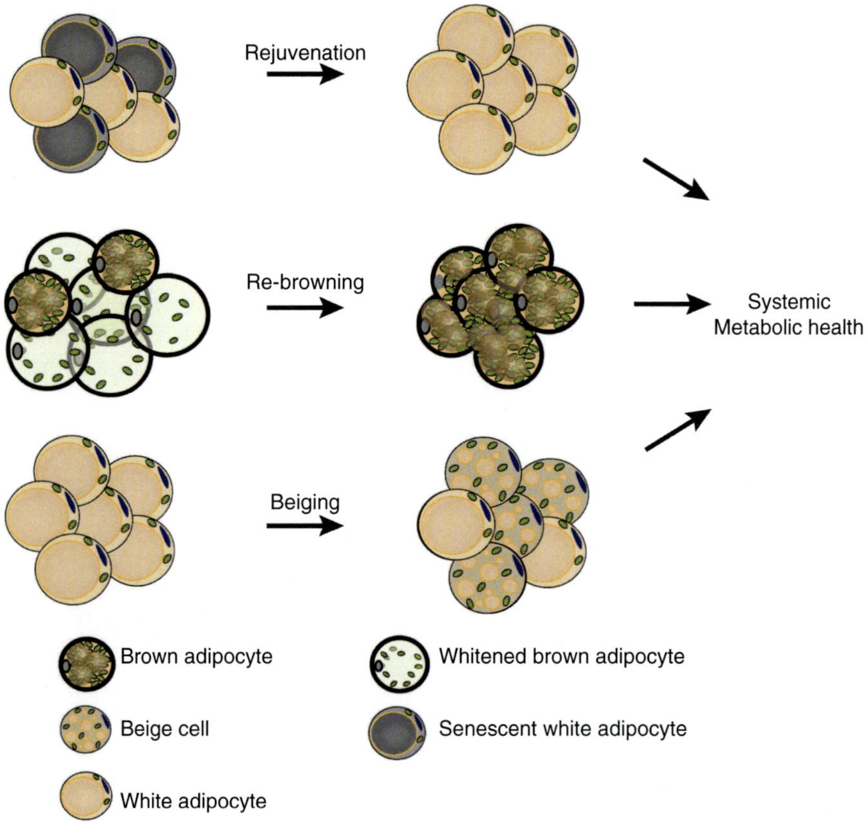

Fig. 6.1 Elimination of senescent white adipocytes, re-browning of whitened brown adipocytes, and beiging would contribute for systemic metabolic health

Acknowledgments This work was supported by a Grant-in-Aid for Scientific Research, a Grant-in-Aid for Scientific Research on Innovative Areas (Stem Cell Aging and Disease, Grant number 26115008), and a Grant-in-Aid for Exploratory Research from the Ministry of Education, Culture, Sports, Science, and Technology (MEXT, Grant number 15K15306) of Japan and grants from the Ono Medical Research Foundation, the Japan Diabetes Foundation, the Takeda Science Foundation, and the Takeda Medical Research Foundation (to T.M.) as well as by a Grants-in-Aid for Young Scientists (Start-up) (JSPS KAKENHI, Grant Number 26893080) and grants from the Uehara Memorial Foundation, Takeda Science Foundation, Kowa Life Science Foundation, Manpei Suzuki Diabetes Foundation, Kanae Foundation, Japan Heart Foundation Research Grant, The Senri Life Science Foundation, SENSHIN Medical Research Foundation, ONO Medical Research Foundation, Tsukada Grant for Niigata University Medical Research, The Nakajima Foundation, SUZUKEN memorial foundation, HOKUTO Corporation, Inamori Foundation, Mochida Memorial Foundation for Medical & Pharmaceutical Research, Banyu Foundation Research Grant, Grant for Basic Science Research Projects from The Sumitomo Foundation, Grants-in-Aid for Encouragement of Young Scientists (A) (JSPS KAKENHI Grant Number 16H06244), The Bayer Scholarship for Cardiovascular Research, and Japan Diabetes Foundation (to I.S.), by a Grants-in-Aid for Encouragement of Young Scientists (B) (JSPS KAKENHI Grant Number 16K19531), a Japan Heart Foundation Dr. Hiroshi Irisawa & Dr. Aya Irisawa Memorial Research

Grant, Senshin Medical Research Foundation grant, SUZUKEN memorial foundation, Takeda Science Foundation, ONO Medical Research Foundation, Uehara Memorial Foundation, Research Foundation for Community Medicine, Kanae Foundation, Banyu Foundation Research Grant, and HOKUTO Corporation (to Y.Y.) and by a grant from Bourbon (to T.M., I.S., and Y.Y.).

Disclosures: Y.Y., I.S., and T.M. disclose no conflict of interest.

References

1. Shimizu I, Yoshida Y, Katsuno T, Tateno K, Okada S, Moriya J, et al. p53-induced adipose tissue inflammation is critically involved in the development of insulin resistance in heart failure. Cell Metab. 2012;15(1):51–64.
2. Hotamisligil GS, Shargill NS, Spiegelman BM. Adipose expression of tumor necrosis factor-alpha: direct role in obesity-linked insulin resistance. Science. 1993;259(5091):87–91.
3. King GL, Park K, Li Q. Selective insulin resistance and the development of cardiovascular diseases in diabetes: the 2015 Edwin Bierman Award Lecture. Diabetes. 2016;65(6):1462–71.
4. Shimizu I, Minamino T, Toko H, Okada S, Ikeda H, Yasuda N, et al. Excessive cardiac insulin signaling exacerbates systolic dysfunction induced by pressure overload in rodents. J Clin Invest. 2010;120(5):1506–14.
5. Zinman B, Wanner C, Lachin JM, Fitchett D, Bluhmki E, Hantel S, et al. Empagliflozin, cardiovascular outcomes, and mortality in type 2 diabetes. N Engl J Med. 2015;373(22):2117–28.
6. Eurich DT, Weir DL, Majumdar SR, Tsuyuki RT, Johnson JA, Tjosvold L, et al. Comparative safety and effectiveness of metformin in patients with diabetes mellitus and heart failure systematic review of observational studies involving 34,000 patients. Circ Heart Fail. 2013;6(3):395–402.
7. Konner AC, Bruning JC. Selective insulin and leptin resistance in metabolic disorders. Cell Metab. 2012;16(2):144–52.
8. Hotamisligil GS. Inflammation and metabolic disorders. Nature. 2006;444(7121):860–7.
9. Kanneganti TD, Dixit VD. Immunological complications of obesity. Nat Immunol. 2012;13(8):707–12.
10. Rosen ED, Spiegelman BM. What we talk about when we talk about fat. Cell. 2014;156(1–2):20–44.
11. Hayflick L, Moorhead PS. The serial cultivation of human diploid cell strains. Exp Cell Res. 1961;25:585–621.
12. Tchkonia T, Zhu Y, van Deursen J, Campisi J, Kirkland JL. Cellular senescence and the senescent secretory phenotype: therapeutic opportunities. J Clin Invest. 2013;123(3):966–72.
13. Berkers CR, Maddocks OD, Cheung EC, Mor I, Vousden KH. Metabolic regulation by p53 family members. Cell Metab. 2013;18(5):617–33.
14. Green DR, Chipuk JE. p53 and metabolism: inside the TIGAR. Cell. 2006;126(1):30–2.
15. Vousden KH, Lane DP. p53 in health and disease. Nat Rev Mol Cell Biol. 2007;8(4):275–83.
16. Shimizu I, Yoshida Y, Moriya J, Nojima A, Uemura A, Kobayashi Y, et al. Semaphorin3E-induced inflammation contributes to insulin resistance in dietary obesity. Cell Metab. 2013;18(4):491–504.
17. Minamino T, Orimo M, Shimizu I, Kunieda T, Yokoyama M, Ito T, et al. A crucial role for adipose tissue p53 in the regulation of insulin resistance. Nat Med. 2009;15(9):1082–7.
18. Minamino T, Komuro I. Vascular cell senescence: contribution to atherosclerosis. Circ Res. 2007;100(1):15–26.
19. Arnlov J, Lind L, Zethelius B, Andren B, Hales CN, Vessby B, et al. Several factors associated with the insulin resistance syndrome are predictors of left ventricular systolic dysfunction in a male population after 20 years of follow-up. Am Heart J. 2001;142(4):720–4.
20. Nelson G, Wordsworth J, Wang C, Jurk D, Lawless C, Martin-Ruiz C, et al. A senescent cell bystander effect: senescence-induced senescence. Aging Cell. 2012;11(2):345–9.

21. Baker DJ, Childs BG, Durik M, Wijers ME, Sieben CJ, Zhong J, et al. Naturally occurring p16(Ink4a)-positive cells shorten healthy lifespan. Nature. 2016;530(7589):184–9.
22. Chang J, Wang Y, Shao L, Laberge RM, Demaria M, Campisi J, et al. Clearance of senescent cells by ABT263 rejuvenates aged hematopoietic stem cells in mice. Nat Med. 2016;22(1):78–83.
23. Xu M, Palmer AK, Ding H, Weivoda MM, Pirtskhalava T, White TA, et al. Targeting senescent cells enhances adipogenesis and metabolic function in old age. Elife. 2015;4:e12997.
24. Yoneshiro T, Aita S, Matsushita M, Kayahara T, Kameya T, Kawai Y, et al. Recruited brown adipose tissue as an antiobesity agent in humans. J Clin Invest. 2013;123(8):3404–8.
25. Hanssen MJ, van der Lans AA, Brans B, Hoeks J, Jardon KM, Schaart G, et al. Short-term cold acclimation recruits brown adipose tissue in obese humans. Diabetes. 2016;65(5):1179–89.
26. Cypess AM, Lehman S, Williams G, Tal I, Rodman D, Goldfine AB, et al. Identification and importance of brown adipose tissue in adult humans. N Engl J Med. 2009;360(15):1509–17.
27. Sano M, Minamino T, Toko H, Miyauchi H, Orimo M, Qin Y, et al. p53-induced inhibition of Hif-1 causes cardiac dysfunction during pressure overload. Nature. 2007;446(7134):444–8.
28. Shimizu I, Aprahamian T, Kikuchi R, Shimizu A, Papanicolaou KN, MacLauchlan S, et al. Vascular rarefaction mediates whitening of brown fat in obesity. J Clin Invest. 2014;124(5):2099–112.
29. Halberg N, Khan T, Trujillo ME, Wernstedt-Asterholm I, Attie AD, Sherwani S, et al. Hypoxia-inducible factor 1alpha induces fibrosis and insulin resistance in white adipose tissue. Mol Cell Biol. 2009;29(16):4467–83.
30. Elias I, Franckhauser S, Ferre T, Vila L, Tafuro S, Munoz S, et al. Adipose tissue overexpression of vascular endothelial growth factor protects against diet-induced obesity and insulin resistance. Diabetes. 2012;61(7):1801–13.
31. Tran TT, Yamamoto Y, Gesta S, Kahn CR. Beneficial effects of subcutaneous fat transplantation on metabolism. Cell Metab. 2008;7(5):410–20.
32. Tran TT, Kahn CR. Transplantation of adipose tissue and stem cells: role in metabolism and disease. Nat Rev Endocrinol. 2010;6(4):195–213.
33. Cohen P, Levy JD, Zhang Y, Frontini A, Kolodin DP, Svensson KJ, et al. Ablation of PRDM16 and beige adipose causes metabolic dysfunction and a subcutaneous to visceral fat switch. Cell. 2014;156(1–2):304–16.
34. Harms M, Seale P. Brown and beige fat: development, function and therapeutic potential. Nat Med. 2013;19(10):1252–63.
35. Qiu Y, Nguyen KD, Odegaard JI, Cui X, Tian X, Locksley RM, et al. Eosinophils and type 2 cytokine signaling in macrophages orchestrate development of functional beige fat. Cell. 2014;157(6):1292–308.
36. Wang J, Liu R, Wang F, Hong J, Li X, Chen M, et al. Ablation of LGR4 promotes energy expenditure by driving white-to-brown fat switch. Nat Cell Biol. 2013;15(12):1455–63.
37. Schulz TJ, Huang P, Huang TL, Xue RD, McDougall LE, Townsend KL, et al. Brown-fat paucity due to impaired BMP signalling induces compensatory browning of white fat. Nature. 2013;495(7441):379–83.
38. Sharp LZ, Shinoda K, Ohno H, Scheel DW, Tomoda E, Ruiz L, et al. Human BAT possesses molecular signatures that resemble beige/brite cells. PLoS One. 2012;7(11):e49452.
39. Saito M, Okamatsu-Ogura Y, Matsushita M, Watanabe K, Yoneshiro T, Nio-Kobayashi J, et al. High incidence of metabolically active brown adipose tissue in healthy adult humans effects of cold exposure and adiposity. Diabetes. 2009;58(7):1526–31.
40. Carey AL, Vorlander C, Reddy-Luthmoodoo M, Natoli AK, Formosa MF, Bertovic DA, et al. Reduced UCP-1 content in in vitro differentiated beige/brite adipocytes derived from preadipocytes of human subcutaneous white adipose tissues in obesity. PLoS One. 2014;9(3):e91997.
41. Liu Y, Ge X, Dou X, Guo L, Liu Y, Zhou SR, et al. Protein inhibitor of activated STAT 1 (PIAS1) protects against obesity-induced insulin resistance by inhibiting inflammation cascade in adipose tissue. Diabetes. 2015;64(12):4061–74.

42. Lakowa N, Trieu N, Flehmig G, Lohmann T, Schon MR, Dietrich A, et al. Telomere length differences between subcutaneous and visceral adipose tissue in humans. Biochem Biophys Res Commun. 2015;457(3):426–32.
43. Goncalves CG, Glade MJ, Meguid MM. Metabolically healthy obese individuals: key protective factors. Nutrition. 2016;32(1):14–20.
44. Ahl S, Guenther M, Zhao S, James R, Marks J, Szabo A, et al. Adiponectin levels differentiate metabolically healthy vs unhealthy among obese and nonobese white individuals. J Clin Endocr Metab. 2015;100(11):4172–80.
45. Kramer CK, Zinman B, Retnakaran R. Are metabolically healthy overweight and obesity benign conditions?: a systematic review and meta-analysis. Ann Intern Med. 2013;159(11):758–69.
46. Ortega FB, Lee DC, Katzmarzyk PT, Ruiz JR, Sui X, Church TS, et al. The intriguing metabolically healthy but obese phenotype: cardiovascular prognosis and role of fitness. Eur Heart J. 2013;34(5):389–97.
47. Scott RA, Fall T, Pasko D, Barker A, Sharp SJ, Arriola L, et al. Common genetic variants highlight the role of insulin resistance and body fat distribution in type 2 diabetes, independent of obesity. Diabetes. 2014;63(12):4378–87.
48. Kim JY, De Wall EV, Laplante M, Azzara A, Trujillo ME, Hofmann SM, et al. Obesity-associated improvements in metabolic profile through expansion of adipose tissue. J Clin Investig. 2007;117(9):2621–37.
49. Wildman RP, Muntner P, Reynolds K, McGinn AP, Rajpathak S, Wylie-Rosett J, et al. The obese without cardiometabolic risk factor clustering and the normal weight with cardiometabolic risk factor clustering: prevalence and correlates of 2 phenotypes among the US population (NHANES 1999-2004). Arch Intern Med. 2008;168(15):1617–24.
50. Yang HK, Han K, Kwon HS, Park YM, Cho JH, Yoon KH, et al. Obesity, metabolic health, and mortality in adults: a nationwide population-based study in Korea. Sci Rep. 2016;6:30329.
51. Ruderman N, Chisholm D, Pi-Sunyer X, Schneider S. The metabolically obese, normal-weight individual revisited. Diabetes. 1998;47(5):699–713.
52. Hwang YC, Hayashi T, Fujimoto WY, Kahn SE, Leonetti DL, McNeely MJ, et al. Visceral abdominal fat accumulation predicts the conversion of metabolically healthy obese subjects to an unhealthy phenotype. Int J Obes. 2015;39(9):1365–70.
53. Morkedal B, Vatten LJ, Romundstad PR, Laugsand LE, Janszky I. Risk of myocardial infarction and heart failure among metabolically healthy but obese individuals. J Am Coll Cardiol. 2014;63(11):1071–8.
54. Arch JR. beta(3)-Adrenoceptor agonists: potential, pitfalls and progress. Eur J Pharmacol. 2002;440(2–3):99–107.
55. Buemann B, Toubro S, Astrup A. Effects of the two beta3-agonists, ZD7114 and ZD2079 on 24 hour energy expenditure and respiratory quotient in obese subjects. Int J Obes Relat Metab Disord. 2000;24(12):1553–60.
56. Hondares E, Rosell M, Gonzalez FJ, Giralt M, Iglesias R, Villarroya F. Hepatic FGF21 expression is induced at birth via PPARalpha in response to milk intake and contributes to thermogenic activation of neonatal brown fat. Cell Metab. 2010;11(3):206–12.
57. Fisher FM, Kleiner S, Douris N, Fox EC, Mepani RJ, Verdeguer F, et al. FGF21 regulates PGC-1alpha and browning of white adipose tissues in adaptive thermogenesis. Genes Dev. 2012;26(3):271–81.
58. Wei W, Dutchak PA, Wang X, Ding X, Bookout AL, Goetz R, et al. Fibroblast growth factor 21 promotes bone loss by potentiating the effects of peroxisome proliferator-activated receptor gamma. Proc Natl Acad Sci U S A. 2012;109(8):3143–8.
59. Watanabe M, Houten SM, Mataki C, Christoffolete MA, Kim BW, Sato H, et al. Bile acids induce energy expenditure by promoting intracellular thyroid hormone activation. Nature. 2006;439(7075):484–9.
60. Thomas C, Gioiello A, Noriega L, Strehle A, Oury J, Rizzo G, et al. TGR5-mediated bile acid sensing controls glucose homeostasis. Cell Metab. 2009;10(3):167–77.

61. Lockie SH, Heppner KM, Chaudhary N, Chabenne JR, Morgan DA, Veyrat-Durebex C, et al. Direct control of brown adipose tissue thermogenesis by central nervous system glucagon-like peptide-1 receptor signaling. Diabetes. 2012;61(11):2753–62.
62. Bordicchia M, Liu D, Amri EZ, Ailhaud G, Dessi-Fulgheri P, Zhang C, et al. Cardiac natriuretic peptides act via p38 MAPK to induce the brown fat thermogenic program in mouse and human adipocytes. J Clin Invest. 2012;122(3):1022–36.
63. Whittle AJ, Carobbio S, Martins L, Slawik M, Hondares E, Vazquez MJ, et al. BMP8B increases brown adipose tissue thermogenesis through both central and peripheral actions. Cell. 2012;149(4):871–85.
64. Villarroya F, Vidal-Puig A. Beyond the sympathetic tone: the new brown fat activators. Cell Metab. 2013;17(5):638–43.
65. Peirce V, Carobbio S, Vidal-Puig A. The different shades of fat. Nature. 2014;510(7503):76–83.
66. Bouhlel MA, Derudas B, Rigamonti E, Dievart R, Brozek J, Haulon S, et al. PPAR gamma activation primes human monocytes into alternative M2 macrophages with anti-inflammatory properties. Cell Metab. 2007;6(2):137–43.
67. Choi JH, Banks AS, Kamenecka TM, Busby SA, Chalmers MJ, Kumar N, et al. Antidiabetic actions of a non-agonist PPAR gamma ligand blocking Cdk5-mediated phosphorylation. Nature. 2011;477(7365):477–U131.
68. Ohno H, Shinoda K, Spiegelman BM, Kajimura S. PPAR gamma agonists induce a white-to-brown fat conversion through stabilization of PRDM16 protein. Cell Metab. 2012;15(3):395–404.
69. Okada-Iwabu M, Yamauchi T, Iwabu M, Honma T, Hamagami K, Matsuda K, et al. A small-molecule AdipoR agonist for type 2 diabetes and short life in obesity. Nature. 2013;503(7477):493–9.

Chapter 7
Diabetes and Liver Disorders

Tsuguhito Ota

Abstract In the last decade, nonalcoholic fatty liver disease (NAFLD) has emerged as the most common cause of the chronic liver disease in the developed countries. The prevalence of NAFLD is as high as 90% in obese individuals, and up to 70% of patients with type 2 diabetes mellitus (T2DM) develop NAFLD. NAFLD is characterized by a wide range of liver changes, from simple steatosis to nonalcoholic steatohepatitis (NASH), cirrhosis, and hepatocellular carcinoma. The pathogenesis of NAFLD is complicated and involves lipid accumulation, insulin resistance, inflammation, and fibrogenesis. During the progression of NAFLD, reactive oxygen species (ROS) are activated and induce oxidative stress. Recent attempts at establishing effective NAFLD therapy have identified potential micronutrient antioxidants that may reduce the accumulation of ROS and finally ameliorate the disease. Overall, the clinical spectrum, pathophysiology, and therapeutic options of NAFLD share many things in common with T2DM and diabetes or aging-related complications. Therefore, this chapter is to highlight NAFLD as a common diabetes-associated liver disease from a diabetologist's perspective. In particular, we present the molecular mechanisms involved in the pathogenesis of NAFLD and introduce some nutraceutical antioxidants that may be used to prevent or cure NAFLD.

Keywords Nonalcoholic fatty liver disease (NAFLD) • Nonalcoholic steatohepatitis (NASH) • Type 2 diabetes mellitus (T2DM) • Macrophage/Kupffer cell • Carotenoid

7.1 Introduction

In recent years, nonalcoholic fatty liver disease (NAFLD) has emerged as the most common cause of the chronic liver disease in the developed countries. The global epidemic of obesity and diabetes accounts for the alarming rise in NAFLD. NAFLD affects 20–30% of the general population and 70–80% of obese and diabetic

---

T. Ota, M.D., Ph.D.
Department of Cell Metabolism and Nutrition, Brain/Liver Interface Medicine Research Center, Kanazawa University, Kanazawa, Ishikawa 920-8640, Japan
e-mail: tota@staff.kanazawa-u.ac.jp

S.-i. Yamagishi (ed.), *Diabetes and Aging-related Complications*,
https://doi.org/10.1007/978-981-10-4376-5_7

subjects [1]. Both NAFLD and type 2 diabetes mellitus (T2DM) share many similarities in their risk factors, pathogenic mechanisms, and complications. T2DM is further complicated by NAFLD, while coexistence of T2DM accelerates the progression of NAFLD to nonalcoholic steatohepatitis (NASH) and cirrhosis. Insulin resistance is an underlying basis for the pathogenesis of T2DM and NAFLD. Indeed, NAFLD and insulin resistance coexist frequently in subjects with obesity and T2DM [1, 2]. As in T2DM, the most important preventive or therapeutic approach is lifestyle modifications targeted at weight reduction. Other treatment options include insulin sensitizers, antioxidant nutrients such as vitamin E, incretin mimetics, lipid-lowering agents, and bariatric surgery. The clinical spectrum, pathophysiology, and therapeutic options of NAFLD share many things in common with T2DM. Therefore, this chapter is to highlight NAFLD as a common diabetes-associated chronic liver disease from a diabetologist's perspective.

7.2 Pathogenesis of NAFLD

NAFLD is characterized by a wide histologic spectrum of liver damage, including, simple steatosis, NASH, hepatic fibrosis, and cirrhosis [1]. NASH, an advanced form of NAFLD, was originally used by Ludwig et al. [3] in 1980, to define histological features of the liver resembling alcoholic hepatitis in patients without a history of significant alcohol consumption. NASH is described as steatosis combined with inflammation and ballooning and has become the second leading hepatic disease resulting in liver transplantation in the US [4]. Approximately one third of adults in the US who have NAFLD also have NASH, and 30% of these individuals have the potential to progress to advanced cirrhosis, hepatocellular carcinoma, and liver-related mortality [1, 2].

The mainstream concept of NAFLD is the "multiple parallel hits" hypothesis [5], which developed from the two-hit theory proposed by Day et al. [6] in 1998. The two-hit theory states that a high-fat diet or diabetes-induced steatosis (the first hit) will make the liver more sensitive to other risk factors related to oxidative stress and induce severe lipid peroxidation (the second hit) [6]. In our previous studies, we found that insulin resistance promoted the progression of NASH from simple fatty liver [7] (Fig. 7.1). The overload of liver lipids and/or hyperinsulinemia-driven de novo lipogenesis enhances lipid peroxidation, which induces the production of reactive oxygen species (ROS) and steatohepatitis (Fig. 7.1). Currently, this traditional view has been developed within a more complex "multiple parallel-hit hypothesis," which comprises a wide spectrum of parallel hits (Fig. 7.2), including insulin resistance, oxidative stress, genetic and epigenetic mechanisms, environmental elements, cytokines, and microbiota changes [5] (Fig. 7.2). The multiple parallel hits theory states that NAFLD is a more comprehensive effect of diverse factors than a simple effect of one or two factors, which may explain why NAFLD is also observed in lean or aged people [5].

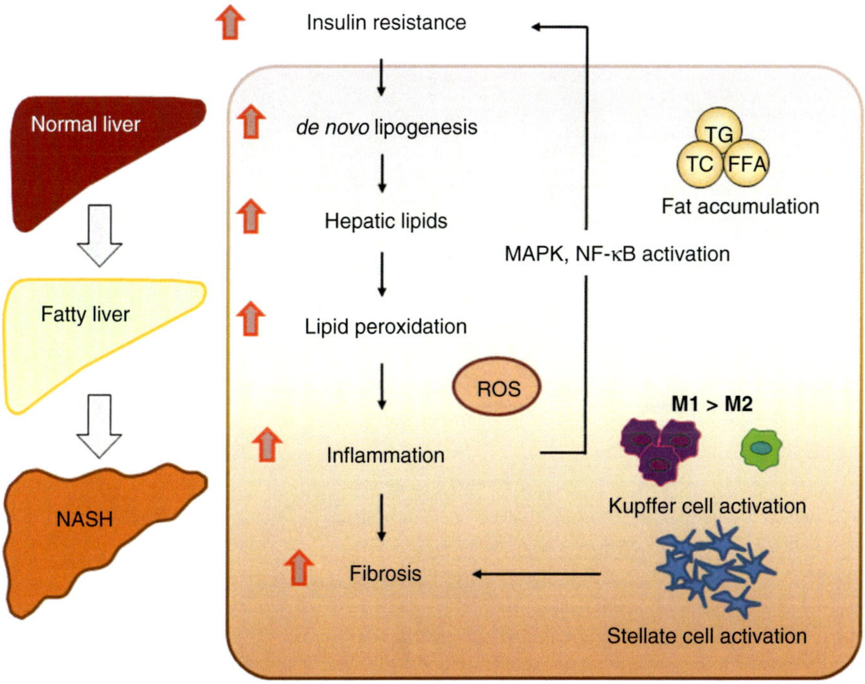

Fig. 7.1 Hypothetic mechanism of nonalcoholic fatty liver disease/nonalcoholic steatohepatitis (NAFLD/NASH) progression. Excessive intake of calories and fat results in accumulation of triglycerides, total cholesterol, and free fatty acids, inducing hepatic steatosis. The overload of liver lipids enhances lipid peroxidation, which induces the production of reactive oxygen species (ROS) and steatohepatitis. Hepatic inflammation activates the mitogen-activated protein kinase pathway and nuclear factor-κB, resulting in insulin resistance. Insulin resistance also promotes de novo lipogenesis, forcing the healthy liver to develop NASH. The inflammation also recruits Kupffer cells and polarizes M1 macrophages, activating hepatic stellate cells and finally leading to liver fibrosis. *TG* triglycerides, *TC* total cholesterol, *FFA* free fatty acids, *MAPK* mitogen-activated protein kinase, *NF-κB* nuclear factor-κB

7.2.1 Obesity

Adipocytes, as important mediators of systemic lipid storage and adipokine release, gather the excessive fatty acids as TGs in tissues, which then influence processes including lipid metabolism, glucose regulation, and inflammation [8]. The free fatty acids (FFAs) obtained from TG lipolysis are the central source of fat in patients with NAFLD. These FFAs contribute to the development of insulin resistance as a common complication of NAFLD [9, 10]. The activity of lipolysis in visceral adipose tissue is higher than that in subcutaneous adipose tissue, which causes patients with visceral fat accumulation-induced central obesity to be universally insulin resistant and more likely to develop NAFLD secondary to their increasing FFA content [11].

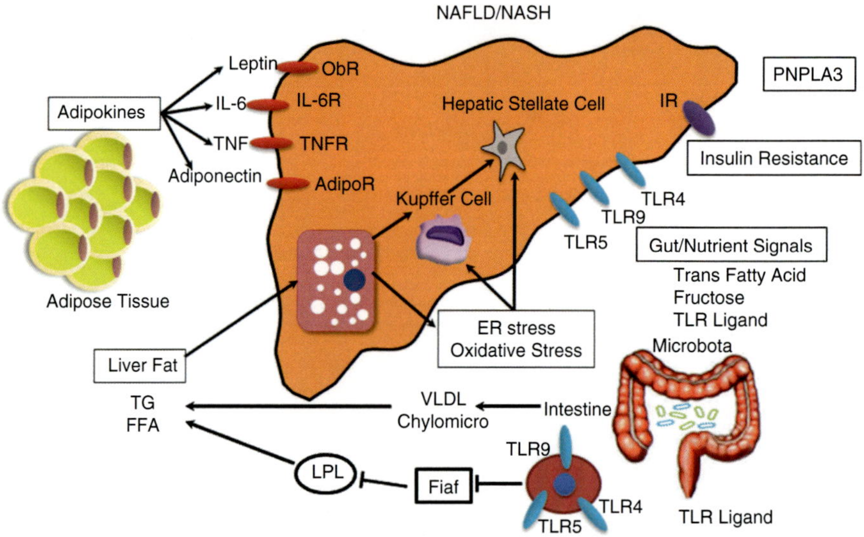

Fig. 7.2 Multiple parallel-hit hypothesis of the progression of NAFLD/NASH. Overloading of lipids consisting primarily of triglycerides (TGs) and free fatty acids (FFAs) induces hepatic steatosis. Adipokines, such as interleukin (IL)-6 and tumor necrosis factor (TNF)-α, produced by adipocytes lead to hepatocyte fat accumulation and liver inflammation. The microbiota decreases epithelial expression of fasting-induced adipocyte factor (Fiaf), which functions as a circulating lipoprotein lipase (LPL) inhibitor and, therefore, is an important regulator of peripheral fat storage. Gut-derived signals can be affected by ingested trans-fatty acids, fructose, or Toll-like receptor (TLR) ligands. Ingested FFAs and free cholesterol induce endoplasmic reticulum (ER) stress and oxidative stress, leading to hepatic inflammation and fibrogenesis. The presence of single nucleotide polymorphisms (SNPs) in the patatin-like phospholipase 3 (PNPLA3) gene increases the risk for NAFLD and NASH development across ethnicities

Adiponectin is an adipose-specific secretory adipokine that can induce FFA oxidation and lipid transfer to inhibit FFA accumulation with its corresponding receptor in the liver [11]. Adiponectin is a link between adipose tissue and whole-body glucose metabolism, which can affect hepatic insulin sensitivity [12]. Hypoadiponectinemia, a typical trait of NAFLD, suggests that adiponectin, as an antagonist of tumor necrosis factor α (TNF-α), has anti-lipogenic and anti-inflammatory effects that can protect the liver from damage by maintaining the balance between pro-inflammatory and anti-inflammatory cytokines in hepatocytes [13]. Furthermore, the serum adiponectin concentration coupled with the waist-to-hip ratio and AST/ALT ratio could serve as a novel tool with which to diagnose advanced fibrosis of NAFLD, suggesting that increasing adiponectin levels may be a new therapeutic method for inflammation and fibrosis in patients with NAFLD [14]. Interestingly, because adiponectin is secreted mostly by subcutaneous fat rather than visceral fat, hypoadiponectinemia may also help to explain why patients with central obesity more commonly develop insulin resistance among patients with NAFLD [11] (Table 7.1).

Table 7.1 Major adipokines involved in nonalcoholic fatty liver disease (NAFLD) pathogenesis

Adipokines	Function
Adiponectin	Anti-inflammatory, improve insulin sensitivity, prevent lipid accumulation, attenuate fibrosis, inhibit tumor necrosis factor (TNF-α) synthesis and/or release
Leptin	Prevent lipid accumulation, amplify inflammation, induce fibrosis, increase TNF-α concentration
TNF-α	Promote inflammation, induce lipid accumulation and insulin resistance, pro-fibrotic effect
Resistin	Cause insulin resistance, reduce *interleukin 6 (*IL-6) secretion, participate in liver fibrogenesis
IL-6	Suppress oxidative stress and prevent mitochondrial dysfunction

7.2.2 Diabetes to NAFLD

As a consequence of obesity and low adiponectin production induced by long-term oversupply of calories, hyperlipidemia and insulin resistance are frequently found in patients with NAFLD, considerably strengthening the association between this metabolic syndrome and diabetes. A few studies have found a strong link between insulin-dependent diabetes mellitus (also known as type 1 diabetes mellitus) and NASH in adolescents [15]. Many other studies have focused on the relationship between T2DM and NAFLD, which is complex and bidirectional [16]. A clinical study of general health examinations in Japan found that about 29% of middle-aged Japanese adults have NAFLD and that a substantial proportion of them also had metabolic syndrome [17]. With their impaired glucose metabolism and abnormally elevated TG concentration, patients with concurrent T2DM and NAFLD have a greater risk of progression to NASH [18, 19].

7.2.3 Diabetes to NAFLD

Likewise, NAFLD also increases the risk of developing T2DM. Using liver ultrasound technology and hepatic biopsy, a study in the US indicated that the incidence of diabetes is threefold higher in patients with NAFLD than in the general population [20]. Hepatic steatosis causes redundant nonesterified fatty acid as an intrinsic defect and induces peripheral insulin resistance and endocrine overreaction, the typical features of T2DM [21]. Due to the precise relationship between NAFLD and diabetes, the most effective therapy for NAFLD appears to be the indirect method of improving abnormal hepatic lipid metabolism by ameliorating glucose dysregulation and enhancing insulin sensitivity [16].

The prevalence of some other fatal diseases is also heightened in populations with these two complications. In patients with diabetes, for instance, the highest standardized mortality ratio is associated with liver cirrhosis; hepatic cirrhosis also elevates the risk of death from cardiovascular disease in patients with diabetes [22]. More than 34% of patients with diabetes have NAFLD and that the combination of these two diseases enhances the risk of death from malignancy [23]. Frequently, NAFLD also increases the risk of developing microvascular diseases such as chronic kidney disease in patients with T2DM. The increased γ-glutamyltransferase concentrations caused by NAFLD may be associated with some severe subclinical renal disease and the risk of T2DM [24]. A recent study in Italy involving a large number of participants estimated that the prevalence of chronic kidney disease in diabetic patients with NAFLD is 60% higher than that in their counterparts without NAFLD [25].

7.2.4 Role of Immune Cells in the Development of NASH

Efforts have been made to understand the roles of immune cells, such as macrophages, natural killer cells, Th1/Th2 cells, and T regulatory cells (T regs), in the pathogenesis of NASH and their potential therapeutic relevance. Specifically, hepatic macrophages, which consist of resident Kupffer cells and recruited bone marrow-derived macrophages, are the major cells that produce inflammatory mediators, such as tumor necrosis factor (TNF)-α and interleukin (IL)-1β, causing systemic insulin resistance and, ultimately, NASH [26]. In tissues, macrophages mature and acquire specialized functional phenotypes upon activation by different stimuli. In general, classical M1 activation is stimulated by Toll-like receptor (TLR) ligands, such as lipopolysaccharide (LPS) and interferon-gamma (IFN-γ), while alternative M2 activation is stimulated by IL-4/IL-13 [27]. A network of signaling molecules, transcription factors, epigenetic mechanisms, and post-transcriptional regulators underlie the different forms of macrophage activation (Fig. 7.3).

Dysregulation and polarization of M1/M2 macrophages can lead to chronic inflammation, infection, cancer, obesity and its associated disorders, and NAFLD [21]. Recently, the protective effects of M2 macrophages/Kupffer cells were reported against alcoholic fatty liver disease and NAFLD by promoting M1 macrophage/Kupffer cell apoptosis [28]. Therefore, specific macrophage-targeted therapies are now starting to appear in the clinical arena. In particular, the reorienting and reshaping of macrophage polarization is extremely important in macrophage therapeutic targeting [29]. In this chapter, we discuss the involvement of hepatic macrophages/Kupffer cells on the pathogenesis of NASH and the impact of carotenoids on NAFLD prevention and treatment.

7.2.5 Fibrosis

As a crucial response to chronic injury and macrophage activation, fibrosis indisputably plays a key role during the progression of NAFLD to NASH [30]. In the course of hepatic fibrosis, the trans-differentiation of hepatic stellate cells (HSCs) into myofibroblasts (known as activated HSCs) produces extracellular matrix components and causes extensive scarring with the formation of abundant dying necrotic

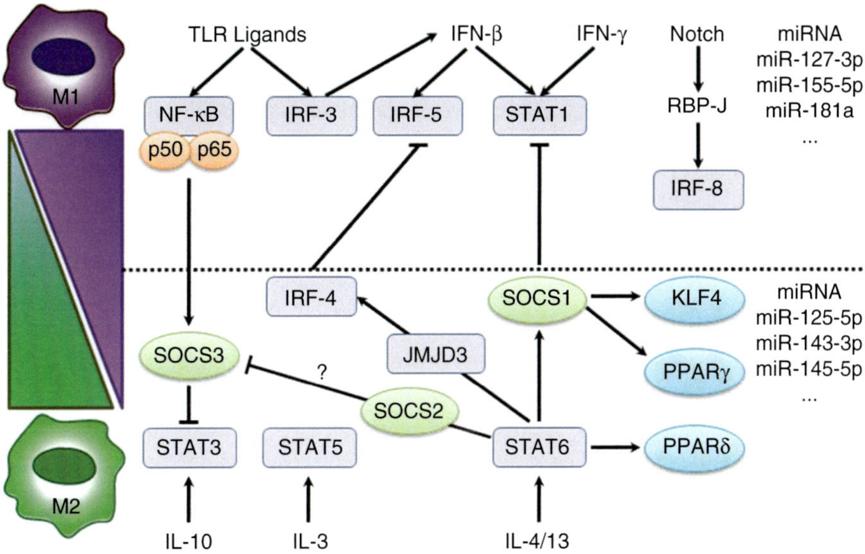

Fig. 7.3 Mechanisms of macrophage polarization. The major pathways of macrophage polarization, which belong to the interferon regulatory factor (IRF)/signal transducer and activator of transcription (STAT)/suppressor of cytokine signaling (SOCS) (IRF-STAT-SOCS) families, are outlined. Cross talk between SOCS/STAT and IRF components in M1 and M2 macrophage polarization is indicated. PPARγ and PPARδ control distinct aspects of M2 macrophage activation and oxidative metabolism. KLF4 participates in the promotion of M2 macrophage functions by cooperating with STAT6. IL-4 also induces the M2-polarizing Jmjd3-IRF4 axis to inhibit IRF5-mediated M1 polarization. IL-10 promotes M2 polarization through the induction of p50 NF-κB homodimers and STAT3 activities. MicroRNAs (miRNAs) have also emerged as critical regulators of macrophage polarization

cells and debris [31, 32]. The Kupffer cells and recruited macrophages then guide phagocytosis of the dying necrotic cells and debris; this can induce the formation of TGF-β which also accelerates fibrosis [33, 34]. Furthermore, monocytes and macrophages expressing chemokine receptors, including CCR2 and CCR5, are thought to be involved in the activation and migration of HSCs through TGF-β to promote liver fibrosis [35, 36].

7.3 Pharmacological Agents for NASH

In addition to the established treatment involving sustained weight loss by increased physical training and diet control, there is no consensus on the most effective pharmacological therapies for NAFLD/NASH. One popular approach involves the use of components for secondary therapy of complications, such as hepatic fat accumulation, insulin resistance, inflammation, and fibrosis. For example, pioglitazone and metformin, common treatments for T2DM, can enhance insulin sensitivity in patients with NAFLD/NASH; however, other histological features, such as fibrosis, are not significantly influenced [37, 38]. In the TONIC trial, both metformin and vitamin E did not lead to a sustained reduction in alanine aminotransferase (ALT) levels in children and adolescents with NAFLD. Although NASH resolution was greater in vitamin E-treated subjects, fibrosis was not improved [38]. In the PIVENS trial, pioglitazone improved steatosis and inflammation but led to significant weight gain. In contrast, compared with placebo, vitamin E improved liver enzyme levels and all histological features of NASH, except fibrosis [37].

7.4 Micronutrients and NAFLD/NASH

There is a clear need for additional therapies for NAFLD/NASH. Thus, most recommendations encourage the consumption of micronutrients such as vitamin E, which have anti-oxidative and anti-inflammatory effects, to prevent and treat NAFLD [39, 40]. So far, it remains unclear whether micronutrient antioxidant supplementation, particularly carotenoids, can be used to prevent and treat NAFLD/NASH.

7.4.1 Vitamin E

As a common antioxidant, vitamin E has been used as a therapeutic component for NAFLD by inhibiting ROS production during the development of steatohepatitis. One study showed that, compared with the control group, 43% of patients with NASH showed clinical improvement with significant reductions in their ALT and AST levels and lobular inflammation after treatment with vitamin E [37]. Similar effects were reported in a clinical study in which vitamin E ameliorated NASH by decreasing the ALT concentration and histological activity and promoted weight control [41]. More generally, vitamin E is often used with other therapeutic methods, such as comprehensive weight reduction programs, leading to weight loss and normalized serum enzyme concentrations in obese children with NASH [42]. A prospective, double-blind, randomized, placebo-controlled trial observed that 6 months of combination treatment with vitamins E and C alleviated fibrosis in patients with NASH without improvement in the necroinflammatory activity or ALT concentration [43]. Nevertheless, some studies have shown that vitamin E is not superior to placebo in ameliorating NAFLD or, even worse, that daily supplementation of vitamin E may increase the risk of prostate cancer [38, 44].

7.4.2 *β-Cryptoxanthin in Nutrients*

β-Cryptoxanthin is a xanthophyll carotenoid specifically found in the Satsuma mandarin (Citrus unshiu Marc.). β-Cryptoxanthin is readily absorbed and relatively abundant in human plasma, together with α-carotene, β-carotene, lycopene, lutein, and zeaxanthin [45–47]. Similar to other carotenoids, β-cryptoxanthin has antioxidant activity [48, 49] and higher bioavailability than those of β-carotene in rodents [50]. Serum β-cryptoxanthin concentrations were found to be inversely associated with indices of oxidative DNA damage and lipid peroxidation [51]. Recent epidemiological studies showed that serum β-cryptoxanthin levels were inversely associated with insulin resistance risk and alcohol-induced increases in serum γ-glutamyltransferase levels in nondiabetic subjects and alcohol drinkers, respectively [45, 46]. In addition, β-cryptoxanthin suppressed LPS-induced osteoclast formation in co-cultures of bone marrow cells and osteoblasts and restored alveolar bone loss induced by LPS in mice [52]. Moreover, β-cryptoxanthin can accumulate in RAW264.7 monocyte cells and induce changes in the intracellular redox status, in turn regulating the immune function of macrophages [53].

In our previous study, we found that β-cryptoxanthin prevented the development of NASH by attenuating fat accumulation, increases in Kupffer cell numbers, activation of stellate cells, and fibrosis in mouse models of lipotoxicity-induced NASH [54, 55]. Comprehensive gene expression studies have shown that β-cryptoxanthin is more effective in inhibiting the inflammatory gene expression changes that accompany NASH [54]. β-Cryptoxanthin downregulated the expression of genes associated with cell death, inflammatory responses, free radical scavenging, and infiltration and activation of macrophages, leukocytes, and T cells [54]. However, it showed little effect on the expression of genes related to the metabolism of cholesterol and other lipids [54]. Moreover, β-cryptoxanthin reversed pre-existing NASH in mice [55]. β-Cryptoxanthin inhibited lipid accumulation and peroxidation in the liver due to its strong anti-oxidative properties. Furthermore, β-cryptoxanthin reduced the accumulation of T cells and macrophages and regulated the M1/M2 status of macrophages/KCs in the liver without affecting the recruitment of monocytes from the bone marrow [55]. Additionally, β-cryptoxanthin directly decreased LPS-induced M1 activation and augmented IL-4-induced M2 macrophage activation in vitro, suggesting macrophages may be directly targeted by β-cryptoxanthin (Fig. 7.4) [55].

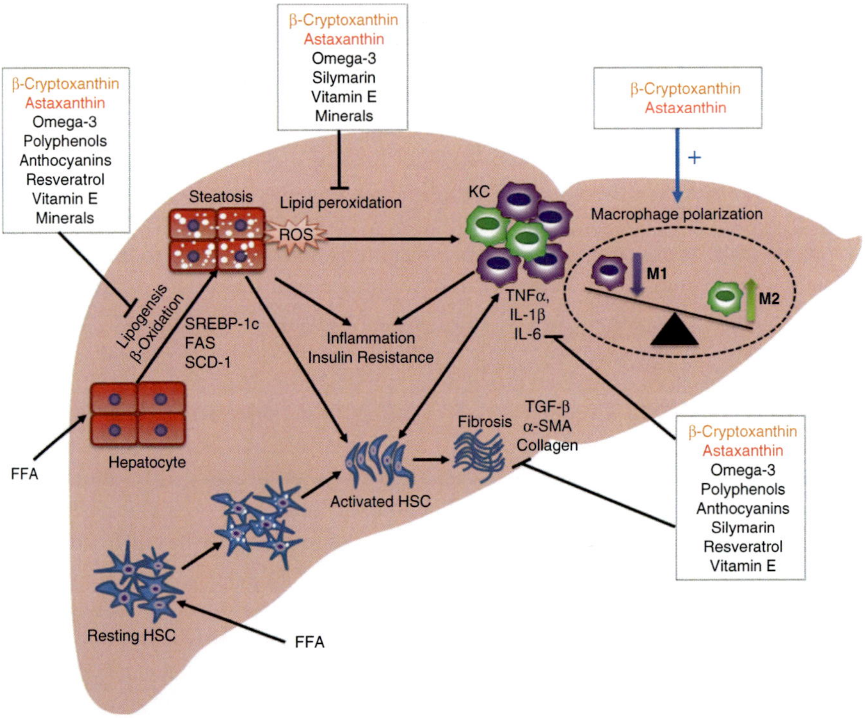

Fig. 7.4 Schematic representation of the hepato-protective effect of carotenoids on the progression of NAFLD/NASH. Carotenoids may improve NAFLD/NASH by inhibiting lipogenesis, β-oxidation of free fatty acids, inflammation, and HSC activation. In addition, apart from their common anti-oxidative and anti-inflammatory properties, carotenoids, such as β-cryptoxanthin and astaxanthin, can contribute to liver homeostasis by regulating the polarization of M1/M2 macrophages/Kupffer cells

7.4.3 Astaxanthin in Nutrients

Astaxanthin is another xanthophyll carotenoid found in various microorganisms and marine animals, including salmon, crabs, and crustaceans [56]. Astaxanthin is well known for its strong antioxidant capacity [56]. It is 100–500-fold more effective than vitamin E at preventing lipid peroxidation. It has hepato-protective effects and can protect against inflammation, ulcers, cancer, neurodegeneration, diabetes, immune system attacks, and cardiovascular disease [56, 57]. Astaxanthin has been reported to inhibit carbon tetrachloride-induced lipid peroxidation and to increase glutathione (GSH) levels and superoxide dismutase (SOD) activity in rat liver [58]. Astaxanthin prevented diet-induced obesity and hepatic lipid accumulation in mice [59]. Moreover, astaxanthin prevented and reversed the activation of mouse primary HSCs and suppressed the upregulation of fibrogenic genes by blocking TGF-β/Smad3 signaling [60, 61]. In addition, astaxanthin ameliorated insulin resistance by protecting cells from oxidative stress [62]. Therefore, the use of astaxanthin as a nutritional supplement has increased significantly in recent years.

We compared the preventative and therapeutic effects of astaxanthin and vitamin E in a lipotoxic NASH mouse model [63]. We found that astaxanthin had significant preventative and therapeutic effects (Fig. 7.4). Astaxanthin attenuated insulin resistance, hepatic lipid accumulation and peroxidation, stellate cell activation, and fibrosis, and it decreased the proportion of pro-inflammatory or M1-type macrophages/Kupffer cells in diet-induced NASH. In addition, astaxanthin ameliorated simple steatosis, the early stage of NAFLD, in both genetically and diet-induced obese mice. Finally, we demonstrated that astaxanthin has the potential to improve NASH in humans [63].

The different mechanisms of action of astaxanthin and vitamin E in NASH mouse models are intriguing, because both of these lipophilic antioxidants suppress hepatic lipid peroxidation to an equivalent extent. Collectively, these results suggest that astaxanthin is more effective at preventing and treating NASH than is vitamin E [63]. First, astaxanthin was superior to vitamin E at improving steatosis by suppressing lipid accumulation. Second, astaxanthin reduced inflammation and insulin resistance more potently than did vitamin E. Of note, these anti-inflammatory and insulin-sensitizing effects were associated with attenuated MAPK (JNK/p38 MAPK) signaling and NF-κB activation, decreased macrophage/Kupffer cell and T cell accumulation, and enhanced alternative M2 macrophage activation in the liver. Finally, astaxanthin prevented and reversed hepatic fibrosis to a greater extent than did vitamin E. Our in vitro study demonstrated that astaxanthin can act directly on hepatocytes by decreasing lipid accumulation, enhancing insulin signaling, and suppressing inflammatory signaling. Additionally, astaxanthin administration decreased M1 macrophage marker activation and increased M2 macrophage marker activation in RAW264.7 macrophages, indicating macrophages are also a direct target of astaxanthin [63]. Therefore, astaxanthin confers its beneficial effects by regulating macrophage homeostasis and may be a potential candidate for the prevention or treatment of insulin resistance and NASH.

References

1. Chalasani N, Younossi Z, Lavine JE, Diehl AM, Brunt EM, Cusi K, et al. The diagnosis and management of non-alcoholic fatty liver disease: practice Guideline by the American Association for the Study of Liver Diseases, American College of Gastroenterology, and the American Gastroenterological Association. Hepatology. 2012;55(6):2005–23. doi:10.1002/hep.25762.
2. Farrell GC, Larter CZ. Nonalcoholic fatty liver disease: from steatosis to cirrhosis. Hepatology. 2006;43(2 Suppl 1):S99–S112. doi:10.1002/hep.20973.
3. Ludwig J, Viggiano TR, McGill DB, Oh BJ. Nonalcoholic steatohepatitis: Mayo Clinic experiences with a hitherto unnamed disease. Mayo Clin Proc. 1980;55(7):434–8.
4. Wong RJ, Aguilar M, Cheung R, Perumpail RB, Harrison SA, Younossi ZM, et al. Nonalcoholic steatohepatitis is the second leading etiology of liver disease among adults awaiting liver

transplantation in the United States. Gastroenterology. 2015;148(3):547–55. doi:10.1053/j.gastro.2014.11.039.
5. Tilg H, Moschen AR. Evolution of inflammation in nonalcoholic fatty liver disease: the multiple parallel hits hypothesis. Hepatology. 2010;52(5):1836–46. doi:10.1002/hep.24001.
6. Day CP, James OF. Steatohepatitis: a tale of two "hits"? Gastroenterology. 1998;114(4):842–5.
7. Ota T, Takamura T, Kurita S, Matsuzawa N, Kita Y, Uno M, et al. Insulin resistance accelerates a dietary rat model of nonalcoholic steatohepatitis. Gastroenterology. 2007;132(1):282–93. doi:10.1053/j.gastro.2006.8.014. S0016-5085(06)02237-2 [pii].
8. Scherer PE. Adipose tissue: from lipid storage compartment to endocrine organ. Diabetes. 2006;55(6):1537–45. doi:10.2337/db06-0263.
9. Marchesini G, Brizi M, Bianchi G, Tomassetti S, Bugianesi E, Lenzi M, et al. Nonalcoholic fatty liver disease: a feature of the metabolic syndrome. Diabetes. 2001;50(8):1844–50.
10. Ota T, Gayet C, Ginsberg HN. Inhibition of apolipoprotein B100 secretion by lipid-induced hepatic endoplasmic reticulum stress in rodents. J Clin Invest. 2008;118(1):316–32. doi:10.1172/JCI32752.
11. Angulo P. GI epidemiology: nonalcoholic fatty liver disease. Aliment Pharmacol Ther. 2007;25(8):883–9. doi:10.1111/j.1365-2036.2007.03246.x.
12. Berg AH, Combs TP, Du X, Brownlee M, Scherer PE. The adipocyte-secreted protein Acrp30 enhances hepatic insulin action. Nat Med. 2001;7(8):947–53. doi:10.1038/90992.
13. Pagano C, Soardo G, Esposito W, Fallo F, Basan L, Donnini D, et al. Plasma adiponectin is decreased in nonalcoholic fatty liver disease. Eur J Endocrinol. 2005;152(1):113–8.
14. Savvidou S, Hytiroglou P, Orfanou-Koumerkeridou H, Panderis A, Frantzoulis P, Goulis J. Low serum adiponectin levels are predictive of advanced hepatic fibrosis in patients with NAFLD. J Clin Gastroenterol. 2009;43(8):765–72. doi:10.1097/MCG.0b013e31819e9048.
15. Rashid M, Roberts EA. Nonalcoholic steatohepatitis in children. J Pediatr Gastroenterol Nutr. 2000;30(1):48–53.
16. Anstee QM, Targher G, Day CP. Progression of NAFLD to diabetes mellitus, cardiovascular disease or cirrhosis. Nat Rev Gastroenterol Hepatol. 2013;10(6):330–44. doi:10.1038/nrgastro.2013.41.
17. Jimba S, Nakagami T, Takahashi M, Wakamatsu T, Hirota Y, Iwamoto Y, et al. Prevalence of non-alcoholic fatty liver disease and its association with impaired glucose metabolism in Japanese adults. Diabet Med. 2005;22(9):1141–5. doi:10.1111/j.1464-5491.2005.01582.x.
18. Ratziu V, Bellentani S, Cortez-Pinto H, Day C, Marchesini G. A position statement on NAFLD/NASH based on the EASL 2009 special conference. J Hepatol. 2010;53(2):372–84. doi:10.1016/j.jhep.2010.04.008.
19. Ryysy L, Hakkinen AM, Goto T, Vehkavaara S, Westerbacka J, Halavaara J, et al. Hepatic fat content and insulin action on free fatty acids and glucose metabolism rather than insulin absorption are associated with insulin requirements during insulin therapy in type 2 diabetic patients. Diabetes. 2000;49(5):749–58.
20. Williams CD, Stengel J, Asike MI, Torres DM, Shaw J, Contreras M, et al. Prevalence of nonalcoholic fatty liver disease and nonalcoholic steatohepatitis among a largely middle-aged population utilizing ultrasound and liver biopsy: a prospective study. Gastroenterology. 2011;140(1):124–31. doi:10.1053/j.gastro.2010.09.038.
21. Bugianesi E, Gastaldelli A, Vanni E, Gambino R, Cassader M, Baldi S, et al. Insulin resistance in non-diabetic patients with non-alcoholic fatty liver disease: sites and mechanisms. Diabetologia. 2005;48(4):634–42. doi:10.1007/s00125-005-1682-x.
22. de Marco R, Locatelli F, Zoppini G, Verlato G, Bonora E, Muggeo M. Cause-specific mortality in type 2 diabetes. The Verona Diabetes Study. Diabetes Care. 1999;22(5):756–61.
23. Adams LA, Harmsen S, St Sauver JL, Charatcharoenwitthaya P, Enders FB, Therneau T, et al. Nonalcoholic fatty liver disease increases risk of death among patients with diabetes: a community-based cohort study. Am J Gastroenterol. 2010;105(7):1567–73. doi:10.1038/ajg.2010.18.

24. Chang Y, Ryu S, Sung E, Woo HY, Oh E, Cha K, et al. Nonalcoholic fatty liver disease predicts chronic kidney disease in nonhypertensive and nondiabetic Korean men. Metabolism. 2008;57(4):569–76. doi:10.1016/j.metabol.2007.11.022.
25. Targher G, Bertolini L, Rodella S, Zoppini G, Lippi G, Day C, et al. Non-alcoholic fatty liver disease is independently associated with an increased prevalence of chronic kidney disease and proliferative/laser-treated retinopathy in type 2 diabetic patients. Diabetologia. 2008;51(3):444–50. doi:10.1007/s00125-007-0897-4.
26. Odegaard JI, Ricardo-Gonzalez RR, Red Eagle A, Vats D, Morel CR, Goforth MH, et al. Alternative M2 activation of Kupffer cells by PPARdelta ameliorates obesity-induced insulin resistance. Cell Metab. 2008;7(6):496–507. doi:10.1016/j.cmet.2008.04.003. S1550-4131(08)00113-7 [pii].
27. Sica A, Mantovani A. Macrophage plasticity and polarization: in vivo veritas. J Clin Invest. 2012;122(3):787–95. doi:10.1172/JCI59643.
28. Wan J, Benkdane M, Teixeira-Clerc F, Bonnafous S, Louvet A, Lafdil F, et al. M2 Kupffer cells promote M1 Kupffer cell apoptosis: a protective mechanism against alcoholic and nonalcoholic fatty liver disease. Hepatology. 2014;59(1):130–42. doi:10.1002/hep.26607.
29. Xue J, Sharma V, Hsieh MH, Chawla A, Murali R, Pandol SJ, et al. Alternatively activated macrophages promote pancreatic fibrosis in chronic pancreatitis. Nat Commun. 2015;6:7158. doi:10.1038/ncomms8158.
30. Wynn TA, Barron L. Macrophages: master regulators of inflammation and fibrosis. Semin Liver Dis. 2010;30(3):245–57. doi:10.1055/s-0030-1255354.
31. Schuppan D, Kim YO. Evolving therapies for liver fibrosis. J Clin Invest. 2013;123(5):1887–901. doi:10.1172/JCI66028.
32. Iredale JP, Benyon RC, Pickering J, McCullen M, Northrop M, Pawley S, et al. Mechanisms of spontaneous resolution of rat liver fibrosis. Hepatic stellate cell apoptosis and reduced hepatic expression of metalloproteinase inhibitors. J Clin Invest. 1998;102(3):538–49. doi:10.1172/JCI1018.
33. Takehara T, Tatsumi T, Suzuki T, Rucker EB III, Hennighausen L, Jinushi M, et al. Hepatocyte-specific disruption of Bcl-xL leads to continuous hepatocyte apoptosis and liver fibrotic responses. Gastroenterology. 2004;127(4):1189–97.
34. Tacke F, Zimmermann HW. Macrophage heterogeneity in liver injury and fibrosis. J Hepatol. 2014;60(5):1090–6. doi:10.1016/j.jhep.2013.12.025.
35. Seki E, de Minicis S, Inokuchi S, Taura K, Miyai K, van Rooijen N, et al. CCR2 promotes hepatic fibrosis in mice. Hepatology. 2009;50(1):185–97. doi:10.1002/hep.22952.
36. Karlmark KR, Weiskirchen R, Zimmermann HW, Gassler N, Ginhoux F, Weber C, et al. Hepatic recruitment of the inflammatory Gr1+ monocyte subset upon liver injury promotes hepatic fibrosis. Hepatology. 2009;50(1):261–74. doi:10.1002/hep.22950.
37. Sanyal AJ, Chalasani N, Kowdley KV, McCullough A, Diehl AM, Bass NM, et al. Pioglitazone, vitamin E, or placebo for nonalcoholic steatohepatitis. N Engl J Med. 2010;362(18):1675–85. doi:10.1056/NEJMoa0907929. NEJMoa0907929 [pii].
38. Lavine JE, Schwimmer JB, Van Natta ML, Molleston JP, Murray KF, Rosenthal P, et al. Effect of vitamin E or metformin for treatment of nonalcoholic fatty liver disease in children and adolescents: the TONIC randomized controlled trial. JAMA. 2011;305(16):1659–68. doi:10.1001/jama.2011.520. 305/16/1659 [pii].
39. McCarthy EM, Rinella ME. The role of diet and nutrient composition in nonalcoholic fatty liver disease. J Acad Nutr Diet. 2012;112(3):401–9. doi:10.1016/j.jada.2011.10.007.
40. Dongiovanni P, Lanti C, Riso P, Valenti L. Nutritional therapy for nonalcoholic fatty liver disease. J Nutr Biochem. 2016;29:1–11. doi:10.1016/j.jnutbio.2015.08.024.
41. Hoofnagle JH, Van Natta ML, Kleiner DE, Clark JM, Kowdley KV, Loomba R, et al. Vitamin E and changes in serum alanine aminotransferase levels in patients with non-alcoholic steatohepatitis. Aliment Pharmacol Ther. 2013;38(2):134–43. doi:10.1111/apt.12352.
42. Lavine JE. Vitamin E treatment of nonalcoholic steatohepatitis in children: a pilot study. J Pediatr. 2000;136(6):734–8.

43. Harrison SA, Torgerson S, Hayashi P, Ward J, Schenker S. Vitamin E and vitamin C treatment improves fibrosis in patients with nonalcoholic steatohepatitis. Am J Gastroenterol. 2003;98(11):2485–90. doi:10.1111/j.1572-0241.2003.08699.x.
44. Klein EA, Thompson IM Jr, Tangen CM, Crowley JJ, Lucia MS, Goodman PJ, et al. Vitamin E and the risk of prostate cancer: the Selenium and Vitamin E Cancer Prevention Trial (SELECT). JAMA. 2011;306(14):1549–56. doi:10.1001/jama.2011.1437.
45. Sugiura M, Nakamura M, Ikoma Y, Yano M, Ogawa K, Matsumoto H, et al. High serum carotenoids are inversely associated with serum gamma-glutamyltransferase in alcohol drinkers within normal liver function. J Epidemiol. 2005;15(5):180–6. JST.JSTAGE/jea/15.180 [pii].
46. Sugiura M, Nakamura M, Ikoma Y, Yano M, Ogawa K, Matsumoto H, et al. The homeostasis model assessment-insulin resistance index is inversely associated with serum carotenoids in non-diabetic subjects. J Epidemiol. 2006;16(2):71–8. JST.JSTAGE/jea/16.71 [pii].
47. Sugiura M, Nakamura M, Ogawa K, Ikoma Y, Matsumoto H, Ando F, et al. Synergistic interaction of cigarette smoking and alcohol drinking with serum carotenoid concentrations: findings from a middle-aged Japanese population. Br J Nutr. 2009;102(8):1211–9. doi:10.1017/S0007114509382124.
48. Lorenzo Y, Azqueta A, Luna L, Bonilla F, Dominguez G, Collins AR. The carotenoid beta-cryptoxanthin stimulates the repair of DNA oxidation damage in addition to acting as an antioxidant in human cells. Carcinogenesis. 2009;30(2):308–14. doi:10.1093/carcin/bgn270. bgn270 [pii].
49. Unno K, Sugiura M, Ogawa K, Takabayashi F, Toda M, Sakuma M, et al. Beta-cryptoxanthin, plentiful in Japanese mandarin orange, prevents age-related cognitive dysfunction and oxidative damage in senescence-accelerated mouse brain. Biol Pharm Bull. 2011;34(3):311–7.
50. Sugiura M, Ogawa K, Yano M. Comparison of bioavailability between beta-cryptoxanthin and beta-carotene and tissue distribution in its intact form in rats. Biosci Biotechnol Biochem. 2014;78(2):307–10. doi:10.1080/09168451.2014.878220.
51. Haegele AD, Gillette C, O'Neill C, Wolfe P, Heimendinger J, Sedlacek S, et al. Plasma xanthophyll carotenoids correlate inversely with indices of oxidative DNA damage and lipid peroxidation. Cancer Epidemiol Biomark Prev. 2000;9(4):421–5.
52. Matsumoto C, Ashida N, Yokoyama S, Tominari T, Hirata M, Ogawa K, et al. The protective effects of beta-cryptoxanthin on inflammatory bone resorption in a mouse experimental model of periodontitis. Biosci Biotechnol Biochem. 2013;77(4):860–2.
53. Katsuura S, Imamura T, Bando N, Yamanishi R. beta-Carotene and beta-cryptoxanthin but not lutein evoke redox and immune changes in RAW264 murine macrophages. Mol Nutr Food Res. 2009;53(11):1396–405. doi:10.1002/mnfr.200800566.
54. Kobori M, Ni Y, Takahashi Y, Watanabe N, Sugiura M, Ogawa K, et al. beta-Cryptoxanthin alleviates diet-induced nonalcoholic steatohepatitis by suppressing inflammatory gene expression in mice. PLoS One. 2014;9(5):e98294. doi:10.1371/journal.pone.0098294.
55. Ni Y, Nagashimada M, Zhan L, Nagata N, Kobori M, Sugiura M, et al. Prevention and reversal of lipotoxicity-induced hepatic insulin resistance and steatohepatitis in mice by an antioxidant carotenoid, beta-cryptoxanthin. Endocrinology. 2015;156(3):987–99. doi:10.1210/en.2014-1776.
56. Ambati RR, Phang SM, Ravi S, Aswathanarayana RG. Astaxanthin: sources, extraction, stability, biological activities and its commercial applications--a review. Mar Drugs. 2014;12(1):128–52. doi:10.3390/md12010128.
57. Yuan JP, Peng J, Yin K, Wang JH. Potential health-promoting effects of astaxanthin: a high-value carotenoid mostly from microalgae. Mol Nutr Food Res. 2011;55(1):150–65. doi:10.1002/mnfr.201000414.
58. Kang JO, Kim SJ, Kim H. Effect of astaxanthin on the hepatotoxicity, lipid peroxidation and antioxidative enzymes in the liver of CCl4-treated rats. Methods Find Exp Clin Pharmacol. 2001;23(2):79–84.
59. Ikeuchi M, Koyama T, Takahashi J, Yazawa K. Effects of astaxanthin in obese mice fed a high-fat diet. Biosci Biotechnol Biochem. 2007;71(4):893–9. doi:10.1271/bbb.60521.

60. Yang Y, Kim B, Park YK, Koo SI, Lee JY. Astaxanthin prevents TGFbeta1-induced profibrogenic gene expression by inhibiting Smad3 activation in hepatic stellate cells. Biochim Biophys Acta. 2015;1850(1):178–85. doi:10.1016/j.bbagen.2014.10.014.
61. Yang Y, Bae M, Kim B, Park YK, Koo SI, Lee JY. Astaxanthin prevents and reverses the activation of mouse primary hepatic stellate cells. J Nutr Biochem. 2016;29:21–6. doi:10.1016/j.jnutbio.2015.11.005.
62. Ishiki M, Nishida Y, Ishibashi H, Wada T, Fujisaka S, Takikawa A, et al. Impact of divergent effects of astaxanthin on insulin signaling in L6 cells. Endocrinology. 2013;154(8):2600–12. doi:10.1210/en.2012-2198.
63. Ni Y, Nagashimada M, Zhuge F, Zhan L, Nagata N, Tsutsui A, et al. Astaxanthin prevents and reverses diet-induced insulin resistance and steatohepatitis in mice: a comparison with vitamin E. Sci Rep. 2015;5:17192. doi:10.1038/srep17192.

Chapter 8
Diabetes and Alzheimer's Disease

Shuko Takeda and Ryuichi Morishita

Abstract It is well documented that diabetes mellitus increases patients' risk of developing cerebrovascular diseases and subsequent vascular dementia. Recent epidemiological studies have provided intriguing evidence that diabetes increases patients' risk of developing Alzheimer's disease, the most common cause of dementia in the elderly population. This might be partly explained by vascular complications in patients with diabetes, which lead to neurodegeneration. The results of the Nun Study, a longitudinal study of aging Catholic sisters that examined the onset of Alzheimer's disease, demonstrated the impact of cerebrovascular alterations on the progression of dementia. However, a growing body of research indicates that diabetes directly affects the pathogenesis of Alzheimer's disease via multiple mechanisms. This chapter will discuss the current knowledge of (1) epidemiological studies supporting the interplay between diabetes and Alzheimer's disease, (2) the role of insulin signaling in the central nervous system, (3) the pathophysiology of Alzheimer's disease, and (4) the molecular mechanisms that link diabetes to Alzheimer's disease in order to provide new therapeutic targets for Alzheimer's disease.

Keywords Alzheimer's disease • Aβ • Tau • Dementia • Brain insulin signaling

8.1 Epidemiology: Diabetes Is Associated with a High Risk of Alzheimer's Disease

The incidence of dementia is increasing at an alarming rate, not only in the developed countries but also in countries with low and middle incomes [1]. More than 35 million people worldwide are affected by dementia, with numbers expected to almost double every 20 years to 115.4 million in 2050 [1]. AD is the most common form of dementia, and it is estimated that currently more than 12 million individuals

S. Takeda (✉) • R. Morishita
Department of Clinical Gene Therapy, Graduate School of Medicine, Osaka University, Yamada-oka 2-2, Suita, Osaka 565-0871, Japan
e-mail: takeda@cgt.med.osaka-u.ac.jp

S.-i. Yamagishi (ed.), *Diabetes and Aging-related Complications*,
https://doi.org/10.1007/978-981-10-4376-5_8

around the world suffer from the devastating disease [2]. The global prevalence of DM also continues to be rising worldwide [3].

Interestingly, epidemiological studies have demonstrated that diabetic individuals have a higher risk of developing AD, independent of the risk for vascular dementia [4, 5]. Ott et al., in a prospective population-based Rotterdam study, found that DM almost double the risk of AD. They reported that patients with DM treated with insulin were at highest risk. Another population-based study reported that hyperinsulinemia was highly associated with a risk of AD and decline in memory-related cognitive scores [6]. A clinicopathological study from Japan, Hisayama study, found a strong association between insulin resistance and a development of AD pathology (senile plaque), giving a direct evidence demonstrating that DM conditions could affect fundamental mechanisms of AD [7]. These imply common cellular and molecular mechanisms underlying AD and DM.

8.2 Pathophysiology of Alzheimer's Disease

AD is the most common form of neurodegenerative dementia and is characterized by progressive cognitive and behavioral deficits. AD is characterized by a typical symmetric pattern of brain atrophy predominantly affecting the medial temporal lobes, including hippocampus, which is associated with typical memory deficit observed in AD.

Microscopically, AD is characterized by two main neuropathological features: senile plaques and neurofibrillary tangles. Amyloid plaque is the abnormal extracellular accumulation and deposition of beta-amyloid (Aβ) in the brain. Aβ is a 38- to 43-amino acid peptide produced by sequential cleavage of amyloid precursor protein (APP) by β- and γ-secretase in neurons [8]. Three genes with a missense mutation that cause familial AD have been identified: APP, presenilin 1, and presenilin 2. All these mutations lead to abnormal accumulation of Aβ, suggesting the significant role of Aβ in AD pathogenesis. The so-called amyloid hypothesis, in which accumulation of neurotoxic Aβ is the initial trigger of a cascade leading to neurodegeneration, has been widely accepted by researchers and the main therapeutic target in drug development against AD [8].

Cerebral accumulation and aggregation of tau protein, as intracellular inclusions known as neurofibrillary tangles (NFTs), is another neuropathological hallmark of AD [9]. Tau is a member of microtubule-associated protein family, enriched in axons of neurons, that contributes to the assembly and stabilization of microtubules. Importantly, cognitive decline in patients of AD are most tightly linked with progression of NFTs in a hierarchical pattern, starting in the medial temporal lobes and marching throughout the brain during disease progression [10]. Pathological accumulation of tau is believed to be more directly linked with a neuronal malfunction and cell death.

Considerable research efforts have been directed toward the development of therapeutic strategies to slow, or even stop, the progression of AD, focusing on Aβ or tau pathology. However, promising therapies targeting Aβ such as γ-secretase inhibitors or immunotherapy tested in clinical trials have been disappointing so far. On the other hand, the therapeutic strategy is shifting to the prevention of AD by management of the risk factors, such as DM and hypertension. It is estimated that delaying the onset of AD by just a few years could substantially decrease the number of patients with AD over the next 50 years [2].

8.3 Insulin Signaling, Cognitive Function, and AD Pathogenesis

8.3.1 Brain Is Insulin-Insensitive?

The brain has been generally considered a so-called "insulin-insensitive" organ; however, it is becoming accepted that insulin plays physiological and pathophysiological roles in the brain, including neuronal development, synapse formation, learning and memory, glucoregulatory function, and feeding behavior [11]. Although the origin of brain insulin remains largely unknown, the presence of high concentration of insulin in the brain has been reported in human and animal models [12], suggesting that insulin is produced locally in the brain or actively transported from peripheral source. Detection of insulin C-peptide and mRNA in the brain strongly suggest that brain has its own insulin producing machinery. Furthermore, experiments using primary neuron culture demonstrated neurons produce and release insulin in vitro [13]. Insulin has been shown to be able to cross the blood-brain barrier (BBB) in animal models (Fig. 8.1). It is assumed that insulin crosses the BBB via specific transporter, which can be regulated by multiple conditions including AD and DM.

Insulin receptors (IRs) are known to be expressed in various regions of the central nervous system. IR is a transmembrane receptor that mediates a cascade of signaling pathways regulating a variety of cellular events, including cell proliferation, protein synthesis, and glucose transport [14]. Notably, IRs are demonstrated in the hippocampus and cerebral cortex, which play a critical role in learning and memory formation [14]. Learning and memory are cognitive domains often impaired in patients with AD in the early stage.

Although the role and significance of IRs in the central nervous system remain largely unknown, IRs are reported to be involved in a variety of neuronal functions (Fig. 8.1). Phosphatidylinositol 3-kinase (PI3K) and extracellular signal-regulated kinase (ERK) are major downstream targets of IR signaling. Binding of insulin to IR initiates activation of Ras-ERK cascade, which is thought to play a role in synaptic plasticity [15]. Activation of cAMP response element binding protein (CREB), a downstream target of ERK, induces structural changes associated with long-term memory formation [16]. Activated PI3K is known to promote GABAergic transmission that plays a vital role in learning and memory [17]. Significance of IR signaling

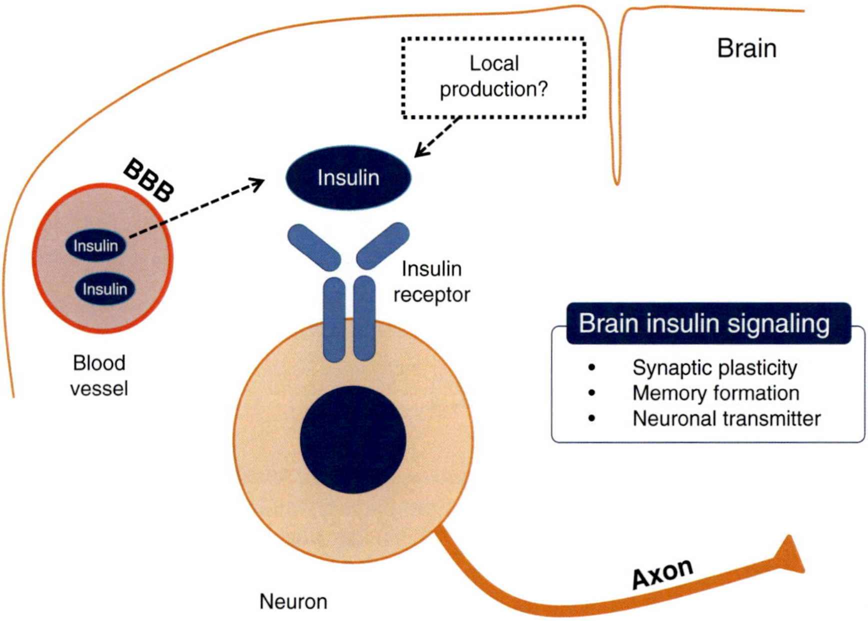

Fig. 8.1 Insulin signaling and neuronal functions. Insulin and insulin receptors exist in the central nervous system. Insulin receptors are involved in a variety of neuronal functions, including synaptic plasticity, memory formation, and the regulation of neuronal transmitters. *BBB* blood-brain barrier

pathway in cognitive function has been demonstrated in animal models as well. Kleinridders et al. reported age-related behavioral impairment in brain-specific knockout of IR mice [18], which was associated with altered dopamine turnover.

8.3.2 Insulin Signaling in Alzheimer's Brain

Aβ itself has been shown to affect the insulin signaling pathway. Xie and coworkers reported that synthetic Aβ peptide could attenuate insulin binding and receptor autophosphorylation, suggesting that Aβ is a direct competitive inhibitor of insulin binding and action [19]. Another report demonstrated that Aβ could induce insulin resistance in cultured cells via downregulation of IRs [20].

Postmortem analyses of brain tissues from patients with AD revealed a downregulated expression of insulin and insulin signaling pathway molecules, including IR, insulin-like growth factor (IGF)-1 receptor, IRS-1, and IRS-2 [21], indicating an attenuation of insulin signaling in the AD brain. Mammalian target of rapamycin (mTOR), which is downstream target of IR signaling, has been also implicated in the pathogenesis of AD [22].

8.4 Diabetes Affects Alzheimer's Amyloid Pathology Via Multiple Mechanisms

Pathological accumulation and aggregation of Aβ, a major component of senile plaque, contribute to the AD pathogenesis. Aβ is a normal product of APP and present in healthy brain. At physiological concentrations, Aβ exists as a soluble, non-toxic form, mainly in the extracellular space of the brain. A physiological role of Aβ (and other APP-related products) is not yet well understood. In the AD brain, rise in Aβ levels leads to pathological aggregation and formation of senile plaques. The steady-state level of Aβ in the brain is determined by the balance between its production and clearance [23]; increased production, decreased clearance, or both can lead to rise in Aβ concentration. Senile plaque, fibrillar form of Aβ, has been believed to cause neuronal dysfunction and cell death; however, recent studies highlight the critical role of soluble, intermediate oligomers in AD pathogenesis [24]. Diabetic conditions have been reported to affect Aβ turnover and aggregation mechanisms (Fig. 8.2).

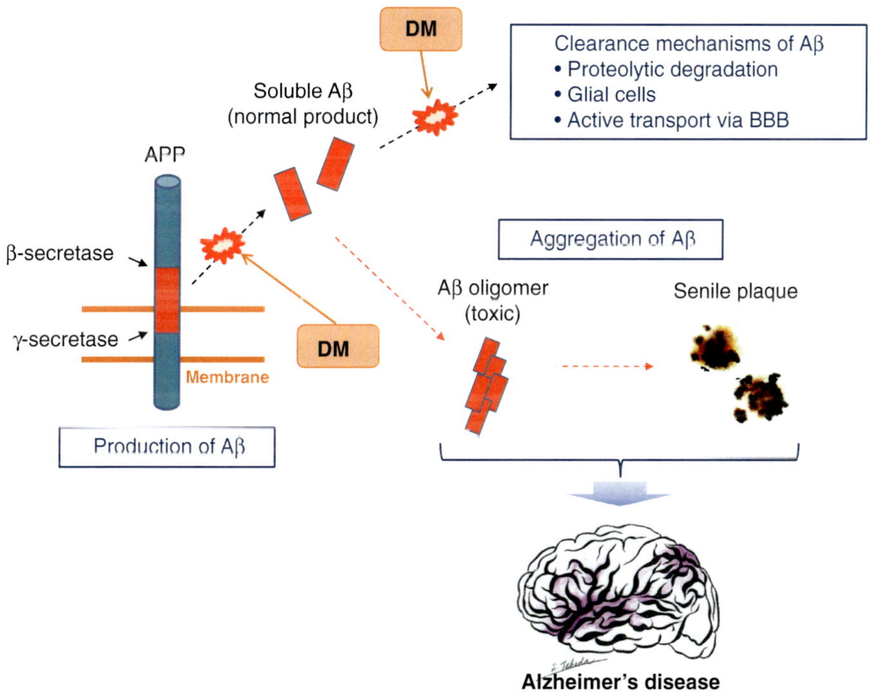

Fig. 8.2 Effect of diabetes on Alzheimer's amyloid pathology via multiple mechanisms. DM increases the brain's Aβ load via multiple mechanisms, which leads to toxic Aβ oligomer and senile plaque formation. *APP* amyloid precursor protein, *BBB* blood-brain barrier, *DM* diabetes mellitus

8.4.1 Effect of DM of Aβ Synthesis

Cellular resistance for insulin/insulin-like growth factor-1 (IGF-1) represents one of the key molecular bases of DM. The role of insulin signaling in the APP processing and Aβ accumulation has been reported by independent research groups using animal models [21, 25]. Stohr et al. generated a unique mouse model by crossing neuron-specific insulin receptor (IR) knockout mice with Alzheimer's APP transgenic mice [25]. The crossed mice had significantly lower levels of Aβ in the brain, suggesting that neuronal IR signaling mediates APP processing and contribute to AD pathogenesis. Along the same line, Ho et al. demonstrated that diet-induced insulin resistance in Alzheimer's APP transgenic mice promoted Aβ synthesis in the brain with increased γ-secretase activities [26]. They also reported a functional decline in IR-mediated signal transduction in the brains. Another group reported that insulin resistance, induced by excessive sucrose intake, increased cerebral Aβ peptide levels and exacerbated learning impairment in Alzheimer's APP transgenic mice [27].

8.4.2 Effect of DM on Aβ Clearance from Brain

The clearance of Aβ from the brain is accomplished by multiple mechanisms, including proteolytic degradation, uptake by glial cells, and active transport via the blood-brain barrier (BBB). Dysregulation of these mechanisms can lead to increase in brain Aβ load.

Proteolytic degradation is a potent determinant of brain Aβ load. Neprilysin (NEP), angiotensin-converting enzyme (ACE), insulin-degrading enzyme (IDE), matrix metalloproteinases (MMPs), and endothelin-converting enzyme (ECE) have been implicated in the degradation of Aβ in the brain [28]. Hyperinsulinemia in DM condition is postulated to increase Aβ levels via insulin's competition with Aβ for IDE [29]. This hypothesis is partly supported by genetic studies reporting that IDE gene variation is associated with a high risk of AD, as well as DM [29].

Enhancing Aβ clearance from the brain, via the BBB, into peripheral circulation is considered to be one of the therapeutic targets for AD. Exchange of Aβ through BBB is tightly regulated and free exchange is not allowed because of the presence of tight junctions between endothelial cells on the cerebrovascular wall. Active transport of Aβ through BBB is believed to be predominantly mediated by two molecules: low-density lipoprotein receptor related protein 1 (LRP) and the receptor for advanced end glycation products (RAGE) [30].

RAGE, implicated in the pathogenesis DM, is postulated to bind Aβ and mediate influx of Aβ into brain from the peripheral circulation. Increased expression of RAGE on the BBB could enhance Aβ influx, leading to the accumulation and aggregation of Aβ in the brain. Takeda et al. generated a unique mouse model by crossing Alzheimer's APP transgenic mice with ob/ob diabetic mice [31]. The diabetic-Alzheimer mice showed increased expression of RAGE on the cerebrovasculature at an early age and severe cerebral amyloid angiopathy (CAA, deposition of Aβ on cerebral blood vessels) at older age. This implies the role of cerebrovascular RAGE and Aβ in the AD pathogenesis. Dysregulated expression/function of RAGE at the BBB might represent a molecular link between DM and AD.

8.5 Diabetes Affects Alzheimer's Tau Pathology

Abnormal accumulation and aggregation of tau protein in the neurons represent one of the fundamental aspects of AD pathogenesis. Tau plays an important role in stabilizing neuronal microtubules under normal physiological conditions. In pathological condition, such as in the AD brain, tau undergoes a change toward a pathological conformation which leads to aggregation and fibrillization. Phosphorylation of tau is known to play a critical role in aggregation process and neuronal toxicity [32].

8.5.1 Insulin Resistance, GSK-3, and Tau Phosphorylation

Glycogen synthase kinase-3 (GSK-3) is a serine/threonine kinase with multiple physiological roles in the regulation of glycogen synthesis, cellular differentiation and proliferation, and apoptosis. Impaired insulin signaling with inactivation of Akt in diabetic condition leads to an activation of GSK-3, a key target for the development of novel treatment for type 2 diabetes.

GSK-3β is known to be one of key regulators of tau phosphorylation. In diabetic condition, activated GSK-3β induces hyper-phosphorylation of tau, which could enhance NFT formation. Experimental study using rat model of obesity and diabetes reported that obesity-induced peripheral insulin resistance was associated with central insulin resistance and tau hyper-phosphorylation [33] (Fig. 8.3). GSK-3 has been also shown to mediate APP processing, leading to increased Aβ synthesis [34]. Activation of GSK-3, in theory, induces abnormal accumulation of Aβ and development of AD pathology. This is also one potential mechanism through which diabetes accelerates progression of AD.

Importantly, GSK-3 expression is reported to be upregulated in the hippocampus of the brain and peripheral lymphocytes of patients with AD [34]. Dysregulation of GSK-3 activity may represent a common molecular mechanism between DM and AD.

8.5.2 Other Effects of Diabetes on Tau Pathology

Protein glycation plays a role in the pathogenesis of diabetic complications. Glycation happens even in the normal physiological conditions; however, excessive glycation due to prolonged hyperglycemia interferes with the protein's normal

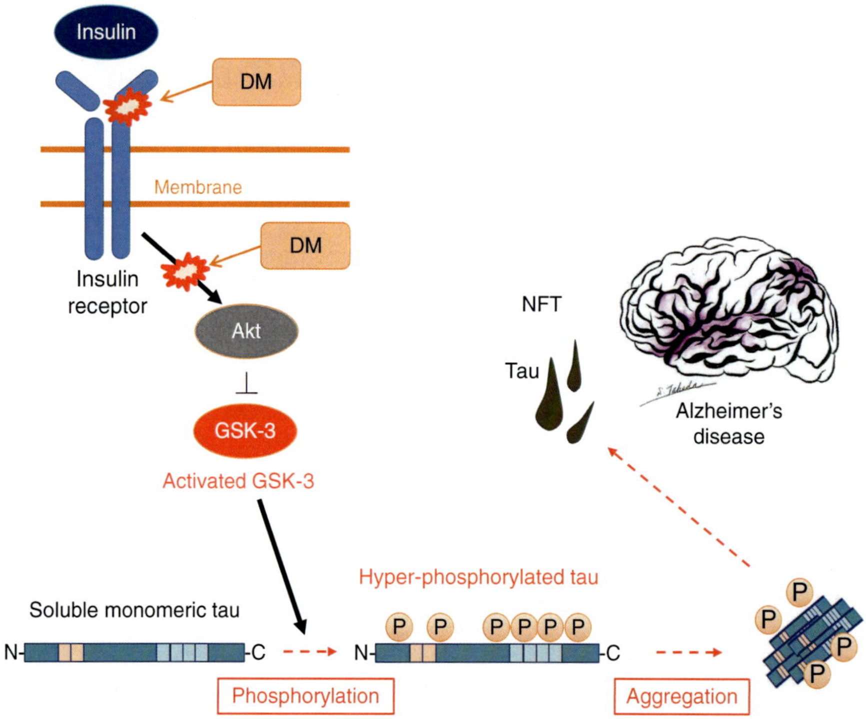

Fig. 8.3 Effect of diabetes on Alzheimer's tau pathology. Insulin resistance caused by DM induces the activation of GSK-3, which enhances the phosphorylation of the tau protein. Phosphorylation plays an important role in the aggregation of tau, leading to Alzheimer's NFT formation. *GSK-3* glycogen synthase kinase-3, *NFT* neurofibrillary tangle, *DM* diabetes mellitus, *P* phosphorylation

function by disrupting molecular conformation. In line with Alzheimer's tau pathology, glycation of tau is reported to mediate NFT formation in AD brain [35].

Tau pathology is known to "spread" in a stereotypical pattern in AD brain during disease progression, likely by transsynaptic mechanism between neurons [10]. So-called "tau propagation" phenomenon has been getting attention among researchers lately since it may provide new therapeutic opportunities for AD. Effects of diabetic conditions on tau propagation remain largely unknown and need to be investigated in future studies.

8.6 Therapeutic Aspects of Diabetes-Alzheimer Interaction

An important question that remains to be answered is whether altered insulin signaling in the brain is a cause or a consequence of neurodegeneration in AD. Lester et al. clearly demonstrated that multiple aspects of AD neuropathology, such as Aβ accumulation and tau hyper-phosphorylation, can be reproduced by selectively impairing insulin/IGF signaling using an intracerebral streptozotocin injection model in rodent [36]. This means that altered brain insulin signaling might be a causative event in the AD pathogenesis. Other reports, however, indicate that reduction in brain insulin signaling could be a compensatory response against AD pathology [21, 37]. The causal relationship issue between altered insulin signaling and AD pathogenesis is critical when considering the therapeutic implications of modulating brain insulin signaling. Although further research is needed to reveal the role and significance of brain insulin signaling in AD pathogenesis, modulating the signaling pathway could be a potentially promising strategy for AD treatment. In line with therapeutic potential, nasal insulin delivery has been widely investigated by researchers, and recent pilot studies have reported promising results in mild AD patients [38].

Takeda et al. reported the possibility that Alzheimer's pathogenesis might exacerbate glucose intolerance in peripheral organs [31]. It has been becoming apparent that the central nervous system plays a role in the regulation of energy metabolism in peripheral organs. There may be a mutual interaction between DM and AD, which establish a vicious cycle (Fig. 8.4). Management of DM in patients with AD may halt the vicious cycle and prevent the progression of both diseases.

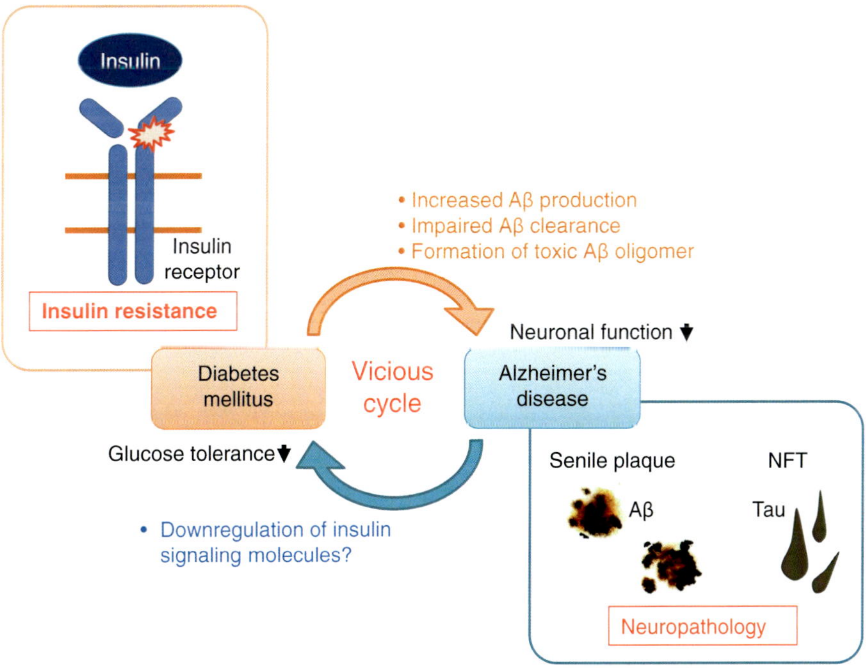

Fig. 8.4 Interaction between diabetes and Alzheimer's disease. Results from animal models suggest an interaction between DM and AD, which establishes a vicious cycle. *NFT* neurofibrillary tangle

References

1. Prince M, et al. The global prevalence of dementia: a systematic review and metaanalysis. Alzheimers Dement. 2013;9(1):63–75.e2.
2. Citron M. Strategies for disease modification in Alzheimer's disease. Nat Rev Neurosci. 2004;5(9):677–85.
3. Adeghate E, Schattner P, Dunn E. An update on the etiology and epidemiology of diabetes mellitus. Ann N Y Acad Sci. 2006;1084:1–29.
4. Maher PA, Schubert DR. Metabolic links between diabetes and Alzheimer's disease. Expert Rev Neurother. 2009;9(5):617–30.
5. Ott A, et al. Diabetes mellitus and the risk of dementia: The Rotterdam Study. Neurology. 1999;53(9):1937–42.
6. Luchsinger JA, et al. Hyperinsulinemia and risk of Alzheimer disease. Neurology. 2004;63(7):1187–92.
7. Matsuzaki T, et al. Insulin resistance is associated with the pathology of Alzheimer disease: the Hisayama study. Neurology. 2010;75(9):764–70.
8. Hardy J, Selkoe DJ. The amyloid hypothesis of Alzheimer's disease: progress and problems on the road to therapeutics. Science. 2002;297(5580):353–6.
9. Hyman BT. Tau propagation, different tau phenotypes, and prion-like properties of tau. Neuron. 2014;82(6):1189–90.
10. Takeda S, et al. Neuronal uptake and propagation of a rare phosphorylated high-molecular-weight tau derived from Alzheimer's disease brain. Nat Commun. 2015;6:8490.
11. Derakhshan F, Toth C. Insulin and the brain. Curr Diabetes Rev. 2013;9(2):102–16.
12. Blazquez E, et al. Insulin in the brain: its pathophysiological implications for States related with central insulin resistance, type 2 diabetes and Alzheimer's disease. Front Endocrinol (Lausanne). 2014;5:161.
13. Goate A, et al. Segregation of a missense mutation in the amyloid precursor protein gene with familial Alzheimer's disease. Nature. 1991;349(6311):704–6.
14. Cole AR, et al. Molecular connexions between dementia and diabetes. Neurosci Biobehav Rev. 2007;31(7):1046–63.
15. Sweatt JD. Mitogen-activated protein kinases in synaptic plasticity and memory. Curr Opin Neurobiol. 2004;14(3):311–7.
16. Tully T, et al. Targeting the CREB pathway for memory enhancers. Nat Rev Drug Discov. 2003;2(4):267–77.
17. Ma XH, et al. Muscarinic potentiation of GABA(A) receptor currents is gated by insulin signaling in the prefrontal cortex. J Neurosci. 2003;23(4):1159–68.
18. Kleinridders A, et al. Insulin resistance in brain alters dopamine turnover and causes behavioral disorders. Proc Natl Acad Sci U S A. 2015;112(11):3463–8.
19. Xie L, et al. Alzheimer's beta-amyloid peptides compete for insulin binding to the insulin receptor. J Neurosci. 2002;22(10):RC221.
20. Zhao WQ, et al. Amyloid beta oligomers induce impairment of neuronal insulin receptors. FASEB J. 2008;22(1):246–60.
21. Freude S, et al. Neuronal IGF-1 resistance reduces Abeta accumulation and protects against premature death in a model of Alzheimer's disease. FASEB J. 2009;23(10):3315–24.
22. Caccamo A, et al. Molecular interplay between mammalian target of rapamycin (mTOR), amyloid-beta, and Tau: effects on cognitive impairments. J Biol Chem. 2010;285(17):13107–20.
23. Bates KA, et al. Clearance mechanisms of Alzheimer's amyloid-beta peptide: implications for therapeutic design and diagnostic tests. Mol Psychiatry. 2009;14(5):469–86.
24. Walsh DM, et al. Naturally secreted oligomers of amyloid beta protein potently inhibit hippocampal long-term potentiation in vivo. Nature. 2002;416(6880):535–9.
25. Stohr O, et al. Insulin receptor signaling mediates APP processing and beta-amyloid accumulation without altering survival in a transgenic mouse model of Alzheimer's disease. Age (Dordr). 2013;35(1):83–101.

26. Ho L, et al. Diet-induced insulin resistance promotes amyloidosis in a transgenic mouse model of Alzheimer's disease. FASEB J. 2004;18(7):902–4.
27. Cao D, et al. Intake of sucrose-sweetened water induces insulin resistance and exacerbates memory deficits and amyloidosis in a transgenic mouse model of Alzheimer disease. J Biol Chem. 2007;282(50):36275–82.
28. Saido T, Leissring MA. Proteolytic degradation of amyloid beta-protein. Cold Spring Harb Perspect Med. 2012;2(6):a006379.
29. Qiu WQ, Folstein MF. Insulin, insulin-degrading enzyme and amyloid-beta peptide in Alzheimer's disease: review and hypothesis. Neurobiol Aging. 2006;27(2):190–8.
30. Deane R, Wu Z, Zlokovic BV. RAGE (yin) versus LRP (yang) balance regulates Alzheimer amyloid beta-peptide clearance through transport across the blood-brain barrier. Stroke. 2004;35(11 Suppl 1):2628–31.
31. Takeda S, et al. Diabetes-accelerated memory dysfunction via cerebrovascular inflammation and Abeta deposition in an Alzheimer mouse model with diabetes. Proc Natl Acad Sci U S A. 2010;107(15):7036–41.
32. Tepper K, et al. Oligomer formation of tau protein hyperphosphorylated in cells. J Biol Chem. 2014;289(49):34389–407.
33. Spolcova A, et al. Deficient hippocampal insulin signaling and augmented Tau phosphorylation is related to obesity- and age-induced peripheral insulin resistance: a study in Zucker rats. BMC Neurosci. 2014;15:111.
34. Hooper C, Killick R, Lovestone S. The GSK3 hypothesis of Alzheimer's disease. J Neurochem. 2008;104(6):1433–9.
35. Yan SD, et al. Glycated tau protein in Alzheimer disease: a mechanism for induction of oxidant stress. Proc Natl Acad Sci U S A. 1994;91(16):7787–91.
36. Lester-Coll N, et al. Intracerebral streptozotocin model of type 3 diabetes: relevance to sporadic Alzheimer's disease. J Alzheimers Dis. 2006;9(1):13–33.
37. Cohen E, et al. Reduced IGF-1 signaling delays age-associated proteotoxicity in mice. Cell. 2009;139(6):1157–69.
38. Reger MA, et al. Intranasal insulin improves cognition and modulates beta-amyloid in early AD. Neurology. 2008;70(6):440–8.

Chapter 9
Diabetes and Cancers

Hiroshi Noto

Abstract A growing body of evidence from observational studies suggests that diabetes mellitus is associated with an increased risk of cancer. Meta-analyses have demonstrated that patients with diabetes have increased risks of total cancer and of site-specific cancers of the breast, endometrium, bladder, liver, colorectum, and pancreas. Insulin resistance with subsequent hyperinsulinemia is the most frequently proposed hypothesis to explain this link although high-quality evidence investigating the association between glycemic control and cancer risk remains lacking. In addition to several facets of lifestyle including obesity, smoking, and lack of exercise, treatment for diabetes potentially affects the risk of cancer. For instance, metformin, an insulin sensitizer, reportedly may have an anticancer effect. In light of the exploding global epidemic of diabetes, even a modest increase in the cancer risk will translate into a substantial socioeconomic burden, which led to a joint committee being formed, enlisting experts from the Japan Diabetes Society and the Japanese Cancer Association to address this issue, along the lines of those from the American Diabetes Association and the American Cancer Society. The current insights underscore the need for clinical attention and better-designed studies of the complex interactions between diabetes and cancer.

Keywords Diabetes • Cancer • Metformin • Insulin • Pioglitazone

9.1 Introduction

Emerging evidence from observational studies and meta-analyses of the data suggest that diabetes mellitus is associated with an increased risk of cancer. Although the mechanisms are not fully elucidated, insulin resistance with secondary hyperinsulinemia is the favored hypothesis, as insulin might have a possible mitogenic effect via binding the insulin-like growth factor-1 receptor [1]. In addition, hyperglycemia itself may promote carcinogenesis by increasing oxidative stress [2–5].

H. Noto
Endocrinology Department, St. Luke's International Hospital,
9-1, Akashi, Chuo, Tokyo 104-8560, Japan
e-mail: noto-tky@umin.net

S.-i. Yamagishi (ed.), *Diabetes and Aging-related Complications*,
https://doi.org/10.1007/978-981-10-4376-5_9

In light of the exploding global epidemic of diabetes, even a modest increase in the cancer risk will translate into a substantial social burden. The American Diabetes Association and the American Cancer Society recently published a consensus statement which reviewed evidence concerning the association between diabetes and cancer incidence or prognosis, risk factors common to both diabetes and cancer, possible biologic links between diabetes and cancer risk, and whether diabetes treatments influence risk of cancer or cancer prognosis [6]. Subsequently, the joint committee consisting of experts from the Japan Diabetes Society (JDS) and the Japanese Cancer Association (JCA) recently published a report [7] to address this issue.

9.2 Epidemiology

Several meta-analyses have demonstrated that diabetes is associated with increased risks of cancer mortality and cancer incidence including site-specific cancers of the liver, endometrium, pancreas, kidney, colorectum, bladder, and breast (Table 9.1). Exceptionally, the risk of prostate cancer in diabetes is significantly decreased. Evidence has been accumulating to suggest that diabetic patients have a higher risk of cancer death than nondiabetic people [8, 17] (Table 9.1). Furthermore, cancer patients with pre-existing diabetes have poorer short-term [18] and long-term [19] prognosis.

The same as in Western countries, the prevalence of diabetes is markedly increasing in Asia. This trend is presumably attributable to the rapid Westernization of people's lifestyle, a trend that is likely shared by the majority of Asian populations [20]. While cardiovascular disease is the main cause of mortality in Western countries and subjects with diabetes have a high risk of such disease, cancer is emerging as a major cause of death in Asian countries [21, 22]. A meta-analysis [23] demonstrated that

Table 9.1 Cancer risk in diabetes: meta-analysis

Site	Risk ratio (95%CI)
Cancer incidence	
Overall [8]	
Men	1.14 (1.06–1.23)
Women	1.18 (1.08–1.28)
Liver [9]	2.50 (1.93–3.24)
Endometrium [10]	2.10 (1.75–2.53)
Pancreas [11]	1.82 (1.66–1.89)
Kidney [12]	1.42 (1.06–1.91)
Colorectum [13]	1.30 (1.20–1.40)
Bladder [14]	1.24 (1.08–1.42)
Breast [15]	1.20 (1.12–1.28)
Prostate [16]	0.84 (0.76–0.93)
Cancer mortality	
Overall [8]	
Men	1.10 (0.98–1.23)
Women	1.24 (1.11–1.40)

Table 9.2 Comparative cancer risk in diabetes: meta-analysis [23]

	Risk ratio (95%CI)	
	Cancer incidence	Cancer mortality
Men		
Asians	1.24 (1.12–1.38)	1.27 (1.22–1.33)
Non-Asians	1.05 (0.96–1.25)	1.13 (0.99–1.29)
Women		
Asians	1.23 (1.07–1.42)	1.45 (1.05–1.99)
Non-Asians	1.16 (1.09–1.23)	1.29 [1.11–1.49)

the risk ratio (RR) of all-cancer mortality was significantly higher than nondiabetic people (RR, 1.32 [CI, 1.20–1.45] for Asians; RR, 1.16 [CI, 1.01–1.34] for non-Asians). Diabetes was also associated with an increased RR of incidence across all cancer types (RR, 1.23 [CI, 1.09–1.39] for Asians; RR, 1.15 [CI, 0.94–1.43] for non-Asians). The RR of incident cancer for Asian men was significantly higher than for non-Asian men ($p = 0.021$) (Table 9.2). Epidemiological data in Japan provides evidence to demonstrate that diabetes is associated with increased risk for overall (RR, 1.10 [CI, 1.04–1.17]) [8], liver (RR, 1.97 [CI, 1.65–2.36]), pancreatic (RR, 1.85 [CI, 1.46–2.34]), and colorectal cancers (RR, 1.40 [CI, 1.19–1.64]) [7].

9.3 Mechanism

9.3.1 Hyperinsulinemia

Type 2 diabetes is characterized by insulin resistance and compensatory hyperinsulinemia, and people with type 2 diabetes are typically obese and lead sedentary lives, both of which also contribute to their hyperinsulinemia. Multiple and complex mechanisms involving these factors are proposed to explain the link between diabetes and cancer. First, insulin may bind and activate its structurally related insulin-like growth factor 1 (IGF-1) receptor, which is the most frequently proposed mechanism to explain the clearly increased risk of cancer in diabetic patients [1, 24]. Secondly, hyperinsulinemia may increase cancer risk by unregulated insulin receptor signaling, leading to proliferative and anti-apoptotic effects [25]. Finally, the mitogenic activity of insulin might be enhanced at the cellular level by post-receptor molecular mechanisms including insulin residence time on the receptor and the intracellular upregulation of the insulin mitogenic pathway [26]. In humans, patients with type 1 diabetes, who are insulin deficient and receive insulin replacement, have a lower risk of cancer than subjects with type 2 diabetes [27], although the evidence of the risk in patients with type 1 diabetes as compared with that in the general population remains inconclusive.

These speculations, however, need to be interpreted with caution since they are derived from retrospective observational studies and may not necessarily demonstrate causality because of possible biases and confounders, such as coexisting obesity and age [28]. In fact, some of the more recent studies demonstrated no or minimal increments in cancer risk [29], and the data from insulin-treated patients with type 2 diabetes are not supporting this hypothesis [30].

Of note, diabetes reportedly protects against the development of prostate cancer which is testosterone dependent. Testosterone levels have been shown to be partially influenced by insulin resistance, and testosterone deficiency is common in men with diabetes because they have low levels of sex hormone-binding globulin. Thus this effect of diabetes on prostate cancer may have contributed to the attenuation of the increase in cancer risk in men [17]. However, those meta-analyses [16, 31] were mainly based on data for Caucasian men, and the reported risks for Asian men have been either significantly elevated in Taiwan [32, 33] or nonsignificant in Japan [34] and Korea [3], which points to the possibility that the effect of diabetes on prostate cancer may not be universal probably due to genetic/cultural/socioeconomic factors.

9.3.2 *Hyperglycemia*

Hyperglycemia has been shown to promote cancer development and cancer metastasis in type 2 diabetes [35]. Indeed, this forms the basis for 18F-fluorodeoxyglucose-positron emission tomography of cancers, which detects tissues with high rates of glucose uptake. In addition, hyperglycemia itself may promote carcinogenesis by generating oxidative stress [2, 36], which is frequently elevated in a variety of cells in diabetes. The increase in oxidative stress would lead to damages to DNA, the initial step in carcinogenesis [5].

Community-based prospective surveys have documented associations between plasma glucose levels and the risk of cancer [2, 3, 37]. The results of our study [23] support this hypothesis, because the results showed that the risk of both cancer incidence and mortality is also generally higher among Japanese [17] and Korean [3] subjects with diabetes, who have been deemed to be insulinopenic [20, 38]. However, these results are not consistent among the observational studies, and published reports on high-quality epidemiological studies are scarce [39]. On the other hand, a meta-analysis of large randomized-controlled trials (RCTs) of intensified glycemic control did not support the hypothesis that hyperglycemia is causally linked to increased cancer risk [40], although no high-quality RCT has been undertaken to estimate cancer risk associated with glycemic control [39].

Given the paucity of high-quality evidence at present, well-designed RCTs and observational studies are required to explore this issue further [39].

9.3.3 *Potential Confounders*

Observational analyses should be interpreted with caution. A recent review suggested only a minority of associations between type 2 diabetes and risk of developing cancer or death from cancer have robust supporting evidence without hints of

Table 9.3 Shared risk factors of diabetes and cancer

Age
Sex
Genetic factors
Obesity
Diets
Lack of exercise
Smoking
Alcohol intake

bias [41]. Potential risk factors to cancer and diabetes in common need to be addressed as potential confounders because it remains to be clarified whether the association between diabetes and the risk of cancer is mainly because of shared risk factors (Table 9.3) or whether diabetes itself increases cancer risk. For example, coexisting obesity and a sedentary lifestyle, which induce hyperinsulinemia, may be the true causes, and diabetes may merely be an innocent bystander. A meta-analysis revealed that obesity is associated with increased risks for pancreas cancer, thyroid cancer, non-Hodgkin's lymphoma, leukemia, and myeloma [42], whereas bariatric surgery resulted in 60% reduction in cancer mortality over the course of 7 years [43]. Exercise is suggestively associated with overall cancer, colon cancer, hepatocellular cancer, pancreas cancer, and gastric cancer [44]. The other possible confounding factors include age, sex, diet, alcoholic intake, smoking, cirrhosis, hepatitis C viral infection [45], and the indication of insulin therapy. Secondly, an alternative explanation is that diabetic subjects might receive medical care more frequently and have more opportunities for cancer detection than nondiabetic subjects. The third is that diabetes might develop as a consequence of cancer, since cancers generally cause insulin resistance and subsequent hyperglycemia by producing cytokines, such as tumor necrosis-α [46]. The fourth is that the previous studies might have left room for confounding by treatment indication: differences between the treatment of cancer according to whether or not they had diabetes may have contributed to the increased mortality of the subjects. Diabetic subjects often have other diabetes-related comorbidities that may influence the treatment decisions and prognosis. For example, diabetes may be accompanied by a higher risk of infection, and the diagnosis of cancer may result in less stringent glucose management.

9.4 Antidiabetic Drugs and Cancers

Current evidence regarding the cancer risk of any particular antidiabetic agents is limited to determine the casual relation between them not only secondary to their inadequate adjustment for confounding factors and therapeutic indications but also because of not accounting for dosage and duration of medications and their short periods of follow-up.

Table 9.4 Metformin and cancer risk in diabetes: meta-analysis [48]

Site	Risk ratio (95%CI)
Cancer incidence	
Overall	0.67 (0.53–0.85)
Liver	0.20 (0.07–0.88)
Lung	0.67 (0.45–0.99)
Colorectum	0.68 (0.53–0.88)
Cancer mortality	
Overall	0.66 (0.49–0.88)

9.4.1 Metformin

Metformin is an insulin sensitizer that is the drug of first choice in the management of type 2 diabetes [47], given its safety profile and lower cost. Our recent meta-analysis including observational studies and RCTs showed that metformin usage is associated with a lower risk of cancer incidence and mortality in diabetes [48] (Table 9.4), and similar effects have been seen across different regions in the world [33, 49–54], although bias could not be entirely eliminated.

Metformin activates activating adenosine 5′-monophosphate-activated protein kinase (AMPK) through LKB-1, a tumor suppressor protein kinase. AMPK, mammalian target of rapamycin (mTOR), and insulin-signaling pathway represent three interrelated components of a complex mechanism controlling cell responses to nutrient availability. AMPK inhibits protein synthesis and gluconeogenesis during cellular stress and inhibits mTOR, a downstream effector of growth factor signaling, which is frequently activated in cancer cells. Metformin also induces cell cycle arrest and apoptosis and reduces growth factor signaling. To support the hypothesis of these direct effects, metformin potentiated the effect of neoadjuvant chemotherapy in early-stage breast cancer [55], decreased the risk of colorectal cancer in a small RCT involving nondiabetic subjects [56], and was reportedly associated with a decreased cancer risk, while another insulin sensitizer, thiazolidinediones, was not [57].

Our research [48] revealed that metformin use is associated with reduced mortality and incidence of cancer at any site, supporting the generalizability of the proposed anticancer mechanisms. On the other hand, the magnitude of the risk reduction varies among site-specific cancers. This variance may result from differences in carcinogenesis at certain sites. For instance, elevated levels of insulin and glucose may exert an important influence in the development or growth of epithelial malignant tumors of the colon [58–60], pancreas [61, 62], and breast [63]. An animal study suggested that metformin prevented smoking-related lung cancer in mice, probably by inducing some hormone from the liver [64]. The fact that one preliminary study suggested a promising effect of metformin on pathologic complete responses to neoadjuvant chemotherapy in diabetic patients with breast cancer [55] may point to the possibility that metformin simply augmented the efficacy of chemotherapy for breast cancer [65, 66]. There are more recent meta-analyses supporting this potential benefit of metformin [67–70], and several prospective clinical trials to evaluate its safety and efficacy are currently ongoing.

9.4.2 *Pioglitazone*

Pioglitazone is an insulin sensitizer that activates PPAR-γ. Recent reports including meta-analyses have suggested that it might significantly increase the risk of bladder cancer in a exposure/dose-response pattern [54, 57, 71–78], while its effect on total cancer or cancers at other sites might be neutral [79]. The carcinogenic effect was also seen in an animal study [80] although the mechanism is not clarified yet. Though recent evidence did not show an elevated risk of bladder cancer, it now hints increased risks of prostate cancer and pancreatic cancer [81]. The oncogenic safety of pioglitazone is still inconclusive. It is currently out of market in some countries because of this potential harm, and it is prudent to follow its warning label.

9.4.3 *Insulin, Sulfonylureas, and Glinides*

As discussed earlier, insulin treatment might theoretically increase the risk of cancer. In fact, several reports initially suggested that insulin glargine usage might be associated with an elevated risk of cancer [82–85]. However, these observational studies were subject to considerable biases: retrospective studies only demonstrate an association and not necessarily causality; it is very difficult to adjust all possible confounders in observational studies; the effects of treatment by indication and informative censoring cannot be excluded. On the other hand, the oncogenic effect of hyperinsulinemia might be offset by the cancer-protective effect through robust amelioration of hyperglycemia. RCTs and more recent cohort studies have not indicated significant associations of insulin with cancer risk [86–88], and the causality is now practically negated.

Sulfonylureas and glinides induce hyperinsulinemia, and there is a concern of increased cancer risks. However, the estimate in a meta-analysis of the cancer risk of sulfonylureas is neutral [89]. Data for glinides are limited and further investigations are needed to evaluate their oncogenic safety.

9.4.4 *α-Glucosidase Inhibitors*

Data on the cancer risk associated with α-glucosidase inhibitors are sparse and highly biased. Cancer risk associated with α-glucosidase inhibitors is still inconclusive [52, 72, 90, 91].

9.4.5 Glucagon-Like Peptide (GLP)-1 Analogues and Dipeptidyl Peptidase (DPP-4) Inhibitors

The risks of pancreas cancer and thyroid cancer were reportedly elevated among exenatide, a GLP-1 analogue, users [92]. An increased risk of thyroid C-cell cancer was seen in rodent studies. The risk of pancreas cancer was possibly increased with a DPP-4 inhibitor [92]. Although a meta-analysis suggested an oncogenic safety of DPP-4 inhibitors [93], the included studies were of short follow-up periods, and the long-term effect remains elusive. More recent RCTs have not demonstrated a significant risk of cancer [94, 95].

9.4.6 Sodium Glucose Co-transporter (SGLT) 2 Inhibitors

No apparent association has been reported between cancer incidence and these novel agents. However, long-term data on the oncogenic risk/safety remain lacking at present.

9.5 Recommendations on Diabetes and Cancer for Physicians and Healthcare Providers

On the basis of the exploding global epidemic of diabetes, even a modest increase in the cancer risk will translate into a substantial socioeconomic burden, which led to a joint committee being formed, enlisting experts from the Japan Diabetes Society and the Japanese Cancer Association to make the following recommendations [7], along the lines of those from the American Diabetes Association and the American Cancer Society [6].

- Generally, it is reported that diabetes (mainly type 2 diabetes) is associated with an increased risk of colorectal, liver, pancreatic, breast, endometrial, and bladder cancers, while it is also associated with a decreased risk of prostate cancer. To focus attention on cancer risks in Japanese diabetic patients, at present, diabetes appears to be associated with an increased risk of colorectal, liver, and pancreatic cancers in these patients. Available reports suggest no increased risk of other cancers associated with diabetes or offer conflicting views.
- Diabetes may be associated with cancer partly because there are common risk factors, such as aging, obesity, and inappropriate diet/exercise.
- Hyperinsulinemia, hyperglycemia, and inflammation are suggested as potential mechanisms through which diabetes contributes to an increased risk of cancer in affected patients.

Table 9.5 Evidence-based cancer screening [96]

Screening for	Candidates	Screening frequency	Screening procedure
Gastric cancer	Men/women, 40 years of age or older	Once a year	History taking, stomach x-ray
Uterine cancer	Women, 20 years of age or older	Once every 2 years	History taking, inspection, cervical cytology, internal examination
Lung cancer	Men/women, 40 years of age or older	Once a year	History taking, chest x-ray, sputum cytology
Breast cancer	Women, 40 years of age or older	Once every 2 years	History taking, inspection, palpation, breast x-ray (mammography)
Colorectal cancer	Men/women, 40 years of age or older	Once a year	History taking, stool testing for occult blood

- Healthy diet, exercise, body weight control, smoking cessation, and alcohol moderation should be encouraged to reduce the risk for diabetes and cancer.
- Given that inappropriate diets, lack of exercise, smoking, and excessive alcohol drinking represent risk factors for cancer morbidity, diet/exercise therapy, smoking cessation, and alcohol moderation may lead to a decreased risk of cancer in diabetic patients.
- Diabetic patients are encouraged to undergo evidence-based cancer screening as required depending on their sex and age (Table 9.5). Diabetic patients are encouraged to undergo screening for liver cancer if they are hepatitis virus positive.
- Given the insufficient evidence available for determining whether or not a particular antidiabetic drug may be associated with cancer risk, in selecting drug therapy, priority should be given to maximizing the benefits of the drug(s) being used to achieve favorable glycemic control in individual patients, following the labeling.

9.6 Future Directions

The review in this chapter underscores the need for diabetes prevention and for investigation of effective cancer prevention, screening policies, and implementation of diabetes treatment with potentially protective effects against cancer. More attention should be directed to elucidating the association between diabetes and cancer, which is pivotal for making timely, rational, and informed decisions, not only in the areas of public health and economy but also in clinical practice.

For the time being, patients with diabetes should be strongly encouraged by their healthcare professionals to undergo appropriate cancer screenings as recommended for all people in their age and sex, and cancer risk should not be a major factor in choosing between available diabetes therapies for the average patient [6, 7].

References

1. White MF. The insulin signalling system and the IRS proteins. Diabetologia. 1997;40(Suppl 2):S2–17.
2. Barclay AW, Petocz P, McMillan-Price J, Flood VM, Prvan T, Mitchell P, et al. Glycemic index, glycemic load, and chronic disease risk—a meta-analysis of observational studies. Am J Clin Nutr. 2008;87(3):627–37.
3. Jee SH, Ohrr H, Sull JW, Yun JE, Ji M, Samet JM. Fasting serum glucose level and cancer risk in Korean men and women. JAMA. 2005;293(2):194–202.
4. Stocks T, Rapp K, Bjorge T, Manjer J, Ulmer H, Selmer R, et al. Blood glucose and risk of incident and fatal cancer in the metabolic syndrome and cancer project (me-can): analysis of six prospective cohorts. PLoS Med. 2009;6(12):e1000201.
5. Abe R, Yamagishi S. AGE-RAGE system and carcinogenesis. Curr Pharm Des. 2008;14(10):940–5.
6. Giovannucci E, Harlan DM, Archer MC, Bergenstal RM, Gapstur SM, Habel LA et al. Diabetes and cancer: a consensus report. Diabetes Care. 2010;33(7):1674–85. doi:10.2337/dc10-0666. 33/7/1674 [pii].
7. Kasuga M, Ueki K, Tajima N, Noda M, Ohashi K, Noto H, et al. Report of the Japan Diabetes Society/Japanese Cancer Association Joint Committee on Diabetes and Cancer. Cancer Sci. 2013;104(7):965–76. doi:10.1111/cas.12203.
8. Noto H, Tsujimoto T, Sasazuki T, Noda M. Significantly increased risk of cancer in patients with diabetes mellitus. Endocr Pract. 2011;17(4):616–28. doi:10.4158/EP10357.RA.
9. El-Serag HB, Hampel H, Javadi F. The association between diabetes and hepatocellular carcinoma: a systematic review of epidemiologic evidence. Clin Gastroenterol Hepatol. 2006;4(3):369–80.
10. Friberg E, Orsini N, Mantzoros CS, Wolk A. Diabetes mellitus and risk of endometrial cancer: a meta-analysis. Diabetologia. 2007;50(7):1365–74.
11. Huxley R, Ansary-Moghaddam A, Berrington de Gonzalez A, Barzi F, Woodward M. Type-II diabetes and pancreatic cancer: a meta-analysis of 36 studies. Br J Cancer. 2005;92(11):2076–83.
12. Larsson SC, Wolk A. Diabetes mellitus and incidence of kidney cancer: a meta-analysis of cohort studies. Diabetologia. 2011;54(5):1013–8. doi:10.1007/s00125-011-2051-6.
13. Larsson SC, Orsini N, Wolk A. Diabetes mellitus and risk of colorectal cancer: a meta-analysis. J Natl Cancer Inst. 2005;97(22):1679–87.
14. Larsson SC, Andersson SO, Johansson JE, Wolk A. Diabetes mellitus, body size and bladder cancer risk in a prospective study of Swedish men. Eur J Cancer. 2008;44(17):2655–60. doi:10.1016/j.ejca.2008.07.012.
15. Larsson SC, Mantzoros CS, Wolk A. Diabetes mellitus and risk of breast cancer: a meta-analysis. Int J Cancer. 2007;121(4):856–62.
16. Kasper JS, Giovannucci E. A meta-analysis of diabetes mellitus and the risk of prostate cancer. Cancer Epidemiol Biomarkers Prev. 2006;15(11):2056–62.
17. Noto H, Osame K, Sasazuki T, Noda M. Substantially increased risk of cancer in patients with diabetes mellitus: a systematic review and meta-analysis of epidemiologic evidence in Japan. J Diabetes Complications. 2010;24(5):345–53. doi:10.1016/j.jdiacomp.2010.06.004. S1056-8727(10)00069-3 [pii].
18. Barone BB, Yeh HC, Snyder CF, Peairs KS, Stein KB, Derr RL et al. Postoperative mortality in cancer patients with preexisting diabetes: systematic review and meta-analysis. Diabetes Care. 2010;33(4):931–9. doi:10.2337/dc09-1721. dc09-1721 [pii].
19. Barone BB, Yeh HC, Snyder CF, Peairs KS, Stein KB, Derr RL, et al. Long-term all-cause mortality in cancer patients with preexisting diabetes mellitus: a systematic review and meta-analysis. JAMA. 2008;300(23):2754–64.
20. Chan JC, Malik V, Jia W, Kadowaki T, Yajnik CS, Yoon KH, et al. Diabetes in Asia: epidemiology, risk factors, and pathophysiology. JAMA. 2009;301(20):2129–40.

21. Hotta N, Nakamura J, Iwamoto Y, Ohno Y, Kasuga M, Kikkawa R, et al. Causes of death in Japanese diabetics: a questionnaire survey of 18,385 diabetics over a 10-year period. J Diabetes Invest. 2010;1:66–76.
22. Tseng CH. Mortality and causes of death in a national sample of diabetic patients in Taiwan. Diabetes Care. 2004;27(7):1605–9.
23. Noto H, Tsujimoto T, Noda M. Significantly increased risk of cancer in diabetes mellitus patients: a meta-analysis of epidemiologic evidence in Asians and non-Asians. J Diabetes Invest. 2012;3(1):24–33.
24. Biddinger S, Emanuelli B. Insulin resistance in the metabolic syndrome. In: Ahima A, editor. Metabolic basis of obesity. 1st ed. New York: Springer; 2011.
25. Gallagher EJ, Leroith D. Minireview: IGF, insulin, and cancer. Endocrinology. 2011;152(7):2546–51. doi:10.1210/en.2011-0231.
26. Vigneri P, Frasca F, Sciacca L, Pandini G, Vigneri R. Diabetes and cancer. Endocr Relat Cancer. 2009;16(4):1103–23. doi:10.1677/ERC-09-0087.
27. Lindblad P, Chow WH, Chan J, Bergstrom A, Wolk A, Gridley G, et al. The role of diabetes mellitus in the aetiology of renal cell cancer. Diabetologia. 1999;42(1):107–12.
28. Johnson JA, Gale EA. Diabetes, insulin use, and cancer risk: are observational studies part of the solution-or part of the problem? Diabetes. 2010;59(5):1129–31. doi:10.2337/db10-0334. 59/5/1129 [pii].
29. van Staa TP, Patel D, Gallagher AM, de Bruin ML. Glucose-lowering agents and the patterns of risk for cancer: a study with the General Practice Research Database and secondary care data. Diabetologia. 2012;55:654–65. doi:10.1007/s00125-011-2390-3.
30. McFarland MS, Cripps R. Diabetes mellitus and increased risk of cancer: focus on metformin and the insulin analogs. Pharmacotherapy. 2010;30(11):1159–78. doi:10.1592/phco.30.11.1159. 10.1592/phco.30.11.1159 [pii].
31. Bonovas S, Filioussi K, Tsantes A. Diabetes mellitus and risk of prostate cancer: a meta-analysis. Diabetologia. 2004;47(6):1071–8.
32. Tseng CH. Prostate cancer mortality in Taiwanese men: increasing age standardized trend in general population and increased risk in diabetic men. Ann Med. 2011;43(2):142–50. doi:10.3109/07853890.2010.530683.
33. Tseng CH. Diabetes and risk of prostate cancer: a study using the National Health Insurance. Diabetes Care. 2011;34(3):616–21. doi:10.2337/dc10-1640.
34. Inoue M, Iwasaki M, Otani T, Sasazuki S, Noda M, Tsugane S. Diabetes mellitus and the risk of cancer: results from a large-scale population-based cohort study in Japan. Arch Intern Med. 2006;166(17):1871–7.
35. Richardson LC, Pollack LA. Therapy insight: Influence of type 2 diabetes on the development, treatment and outcomes of cancer. Nat Clin Pract Oncol. 2005;2(1):48–53.
36. Gapstur SM, Gann PH, Lowe W, Liu K, Colangelo L, Dyer A. Abnormal glucose metabolism and pancreatic cancer mortality. JAMA. 2000;283(19):2552–8.
37. Seshasai SR, Kaptoge S, Thompson A, Di Angelantonio E, Gao P, Sarwar N, et al. Diabetes mellitus, fasting glucose, and risk of cause-specific death. N Engl J Med. 2011;364(9):829–41. doi:10.1056/NEJMoa1008862.
38. Kadowaki T, Miyake Y, Hagura R, Akanuma Y, Kajinuma H, Kuzuya N, et al. Risk factors for worsening to diabetes in subjects with impaired glucose tolerance. Diabetologia. 1984;26(1):44–9.
39. Goto A, Noto H, Noda M, Ueki K, Kasuga M, Tajima N, et al. Report of the Japan diabetes society/Japanese cancer association joint committee on diabetes and cancer, Second report. Cancer Sci. 2016;107(3):369–71. doi:10.1111/cas.12889.
40. Stefansdottir G, Zoungas S, Chalmers J, Kengne AP, Knol MJ, Leufkens HG, et al. Intensive glucose control and risk of cancer in patients with type 2 diabetes. Diabetologia. 2011;54(7):1608–14. doi:10.1007/s00125-011-2104-x.
41. Tsilidis KK, Kasimis JC, Lopez DS, Ntzani EE, Ioannidis JP. Type 2 diabetes and cancer: umbrella review of meta-analyses of observational studies. BMJ. 2015;350:g7607. doi:10.1136/bmj.g7607.

42. Renehan AG, Tyson M, Egger M, Heller RF, Zwahlen M. Body-mass index and incidence of cancer: a systematic review and meta-analysis of prospective observational studies. Lancet. 2008;371(9612):569–78. doi:10.1016/S0140-6736(08)60269-X.
43. Adams TD, Gress RE, Smith SC, Halverson RC, Simper SC, Rosamond WD, et al. Long-term mortality after gastric bypass surgery. N Engl J Med. 2007;357(8):753–61. doi:10.1056/NEJMoa066603.
44. Inoue M, Yamamoto S, Kurahashi N, Iwasaki M, Sasazuki S, Tsugane S. Daily total physical activity level and total cancer risk in men and women: results from a large-scale population-based cohort study in Japan. Am J Epidemiol. 2008;168(4):391–403. doi:10.1093/aje/kwn146.
45. Noto H, Raskin P. Hepatitis C infection and diabetes. J Diabetes Complications. 2006;20(2):113–20. doi:10.1016/j.jdiacomp.2006.01.001.
46. McCall JL, Tuckey JA, Parry BR. Serum tumour necrosis factor alpha and insulin resistance in gastrointestinal cancer. Br J Surg. 1992;79(12):1361–3.
47. Nathan DM, Buse JB, Davidson MB, Ferrannini E, Holman RR, Sherwin R, et al. Medical management of hyperglycemia in type 2 diabetes: a consensus algorithm for the initiation and adjustment of therapy: a consensus statement of the American Diabetes Association and the European Association for the Study of Diabetes. Diabetes Care. 2009;32(1):193–203. doi:10.2337/dc08-9025.
48. Noto H, Goto A, Tsujimoto T, Noda M. Cancer risk in diabetic patients treated with metformin: a systematic review and meta-analysis. PLoS One. 2012;7(3):e33411. doi:10.1371/journal.pone.0033411.
49. Lee MS, Hsu CC, Wahlqvist ML, Tsai HN, Chang YH, Huang YC. Type 2 diabetes increases and metformin reduces total, colorectal, liver and pancreatic cancer incidences in Taiwanese: a representative population prospective cohort study of 800,000 individuals. BMC Cancer. 2011;11:20. doi:10.1186/1471-2407-11-20.
50. Yang X, So WY, Ma RC, Yu LW, Ko GT, Kong AP, et al. Use of sulphonylurea and cancer in type 2 diabetes—The Hong Kong Diabetes Registry. Diabetes Res Clin Pract. 2010;90(3):343–51. doi:10.1016/j.diabres.2010.08.022.
51. Yang YX, Hennessy S, Lewis JD. Insulin therapy and colorectal cancer risk among type 2 diabetes mellitus patients. Gastroenterology. 2004;127(4):1044–50.
52. Tseng CH. Diabetes and risk of bladder cancer: a study using the National Health Insurance database in Taiwan. Diabetologia. 2011;54(8):2009–15. doi:10.1007/s00125-011-2171-z.
53. Lai SW, Chen PC, Liao KF, Muo CH, Lin CC, Sung FC. Risk of hepatocellular carcinoma in diabetic patients and risk reduction associated with anti-diabetic therapy: a population-based cohort study. Am J Gastroenterol. 2012;107(1):46–52. doi:10.1038/ajg.2011.384.
54. Chang CH, Lin JW, Wu LC, Lai MS, Chuang LM, Chan KA. Association of thiazolidinediones with liver cancer and colorectal cancer in type 2 diabetes mellitus. Hepatology. 2012;55(5):1462–72. doi:10.1002/hep.25509.
55. Jiralerspong S, Palla SL, Giordano SH, Meric-Bernstam F, Liedtke C, Barnett CM, et al. Metformin and pathologic complete responses to neoadjuvant chemotherapy in diabetic patients with breast cancer. J Clin Oncol. 2009;27(20):3297–302. doi:10.1200/JCO.2009.19.6410.
56. Hosono K, Endo H, Takahashi H, Sugiyama M, Uchiyama T, Suzuki K, et al. Metformin suppresses azoxymethane-induced colorectal aberrant crypt foci by activating AMP-activated protein kinase. Mol Carcinog. 2010;49(7):662–71. doi:10.1002/mc.20637.
57. Lewis JD, Ferrara A, Peng T, Hedderson M, Bilker WB, Quesenberry CP Jr, et al. Risk of bladder cancer among diabetic patients treated with pioglitazone: interim report of a longitudinal cohort study. Diabetes Care. 2011;34(4):916–22. doi:10.2337/dc10-1068.
58. Giovannucci E. Metabolic syndrome, hyperinsulinemia, and colon cancer: a review. Am J Clin Nutr. 2007;86(3):s836–42.
59. Zakikhani M, Dowling RJ, Sonenberg N, Pollak MN. The effects of adiponectin and metformin on prostate and colon neoplasia involve activation of AMP-activated protein kinase. Cancer Prev Res (Phila). 2008;1(5):369–75. doi:10.1158/1940-6207.CAPR-08-0081.

60. Algire C, Amrein L, Zakikhani M, Panasci L, Pollak M. Metformin blocks the stimulative effect of a high-energy diet on colon carcinoma growth in vivo and is associated with reduced expression of fatty acid synthase. Endocr Relat Cancer. 2010;17(2):351–60. doi:10.1677/ERC-09-0252.
61. Raimondi S, Maisonneuve P, Lowenfels AB. Epidemiology of pancreatic cancer: an overview. Nat Rev Gastroenterol Hepatol. 2009;6(12):699–708. doi:10.1038/nrgastro.2009.177.
62. Schneider MB, Matsuzaki H, Haorah J, Ulrich A, Standop J, Ding XZ, et al. Prevention of pancreatic cancer induction in hamsters by metformin. Gastroenterology. 2001;120(5):1263–70. doi:10.1053/gast.2001.23258.
63. Xue F, Michels KB. Diabetes, metabolic syndrome, and breast cancer: a review of the current evidence. Am J Clin Nutr. 2007;86(3):s823–35.
64. Memmott RM, Mercado JR, Maier CR, Kawabata S, Fox SD, Dennis PA. Metformin prevents tobacco carcinogen—induced lung tumorigenesis. Cancer Prev Res (Phila). 2010;3(9):1066–76. doi:10.1158/1940-6207.CAPR-10-0055.
65. Decensi A, Puntoni M, Goodwin P, Cazzaniga M, Gennari A, Bonanni B et al. Metformin and cancer risk in diabetic patients: a systematic review and meta-analysis. Cancer Prev Res (Phila). 2010;3(11):1451–61. doi:10.1158/1940-6207.CAPR-10-0157. 1940-6207.CAPR-10-0157 [pii].
66. Jalving M, Gietema JA, Lefrandt JD, de Jong S, Reyners AK, Gans RO, et al. Metformin: taking away the candy for cancer? Eur J Cancer. 2010;46(13):2369–80. doi:10.1016/j.ejca.2010.06.012.
67. Col NF, Ochs L, Springmann V, Aragaki AK, Chlebowski RT. Metformin and breast cancer risk: a meta-analysis and critical literature review. Breast Cancer Res Treat. 2012;135(3):639–46. doi:10.1007/s10549-012-2170-x.
68. Zhang H, Gao C, Fang L, Zhao HC, Yao SK. Metformin and reduced risk of hepatocellular carcinoma in diabetic patients: a meta-analysis. Scand J Gastroenterol. 2013;48(1):78–87. doi:10.3109/00365521.2012.719926.
69. Zhang ZJ, Bi Y, Li S, Zhang Q, Zhao G, Guo Y, et al. Reduced risk of lung cancer with metformin therapy in diabetic patients: a systematic review and meta-analysis. Am J Epidemiol. 2014;180(1):11–4. doi:10.1093/aje/kwu124.
70. Wang Z, Lai ST, Xie L, Zhao JD, Ma NY, Zhu J, et al. Metformin is associated with reduced risk of pancreatic cancer in patients with type 2 diabetes mellitus: a systematic review and meta-analysis. Diabetes Res Clin Pract. 2014;106(1):19–26. doi:10.1016/j.diabres.2014.04.007.
71. Hillaire-Buys D, Faillie JL, Montastruc JL. Pioglitazone and bladder cancer. Lancet. 2011;378(9802):1543–4. doi:10.1016/S0140-6736(11)61662-0. Author reply 4–5.
72. Piccinni C, Motola D, Marchesini G, Poluzzi E. Assessing the association of pioglitazone use and bladder cancer through drug adverse event reporting. Diabetes Care. 2011;34(6):1369–71. doi:10.2337/dc10-2412.
73. Neumann A, Weill A, Ricordeau P, Fagot JP, Alla F, Allemand H. Pioglitazone and risk of bladder cancer among diabetic patients in France: a population-based cohort study. Diabetologia. 2012;55(7):1953–62. doi:10.1007/s00125-012-2538-9.
74. Azoulay L, Yin H, Filion KB, Assayag J, Majdan A, Pollak MN, et al. The use of pioglitazone and the risk of bladder cancer in people with type 2 diabetes: nested case-control study. BMJ. 2012;344:e3645. doi:10.1136/bmj.e3645.
75. Mamtani R, Haynes K, Bilker WB, Vaughn DJ, Strom BL, Glanz K, et al. Association between longer therapy with thiazolidinediones and risk of bladder cancer: a cohort study. J Natl Cancer Inst. 2012;104(18):1411–21. doi:10.1093/jnci/djs328.
76. Actos. Product information as approved by the CHMP on 20 October 2011, pending endorsement by the European Commission (updated 20 Dec 2011). http://www.ema.europa.eu/docs/en_GB/document_library/Other/2011/07/WC500109185.pdf. 2011.
77. Zhu Z, Shen Z, Lu Y, Zhong S, Xu C. Increased risk of bladder cancer with pioglitazone therapy in patients with diabetes: a meta-analysis. Diabetes Res Clin Pract. 2012;98(1):159–63. doi:10.1016/j.diabres.2012.05.006.

78. Colmers IN, Bowker SL, Majumdar SR, Johnson JA. Use of thiazolidinediones and the risk of bladder cancer among people with type 2 diabetes: a meta-analysis. CMAJ. 2012;184(12):E675–83. doi:10.1503/cmaj.112102.
79. Ramos-Nino ME, MacLean CD, Littenberg B. Association between cancer prevalence and use of thiazolidinediones: results from the Vermont Diabetes Information System. BMC Med. 2007;5:17. doi:10.1186/1741-7015-5-17.
80. Suzuki S, Arnold LL, Pennington KL, Kakiuchi-Kiyota S, Wei M, Wanibuchi H, et al. Effects of pioglitazone, a peroxisome proliferator-activated receptor gamma agonist, on the urine and urothelium of the rat. Toxicol Sci. 2010;113(2):349–57. doi:10.1093/toxsci/kfp256.
81. Lewis JD, Habel LA, Quesenberry CP, Strom BL, Peng T, Hedderson MM, et al. Pioglitazone use and risk of bladder cancer and other common cancers in persons with diabetes. JAMA. 2015;314(3):265–77. doi:10.1001/jama.2015.7996.
82. Hemkens LG, Grouven U, Bender R, Gunster C, Gutschmidt S, Selke GW, et al. Risk of malignancies in patients with diabetes treated with human insulin or insulin analogues: a cohort study. Diabetologia. 2009;52(9):1732–44. doi:10.1007/s00125-009-1418-4.
83. Jonasson JM, Ljung R, Talback M, Haglund B, Gudbjornsdottir S, Steineck G. Insulin glargine use and short-term incidence of malignancies-a population-based follow-up study in Sweden. Diabetologia. 2009;52(9):1745–54. doi:10.1007/s00125-009-1444-2.
84. Colhoun HM. Use of insulin glargine and cancer incidence in Scotland: a study from the Scottish Diabetes Research Network Epidemiology Group. Diabetologia. 2009;52(9):1755–65. doi:10.1007/s00125-009-1453-1.
85. Currie CJ, Poole CD, Gale EA. The influence of glucose-lowering therapies on cancer risk in type 2 diabetes. Diabetologia. 2009;52(9):1766–77. doi:10.1007/s00125-009-1440-6.
86. Basal insulin and cardiovascular and other outcomes in dysglycemia. N Engl J Med. 2012;367(4):319–28. doi:10.1056/NEJMoa1203858.
87. Fagot JP, Blotiere PO, Ricordeau P, Weill A, Alla F, Allemand H. Does insulin glargine increase the risk of cancer compared with other basal insulins?: A French nationwide cohort study based on national administrative databases. Diabetes Care. 2013;36(2):294–301. doi:10.2337/dc12-0506.
88. Wu Y, Liu HB, Shi XF, Song Y. Conventional hypoglycaemic agents and the risk of lung cancer in patients with diabetes: a meta-analysis. PLoS One. 2014;9(6):e99577. doi:10.1371/journal.pone.0099577.
89. Soranna D, Scotti L, Zambon A, Bosetti C, Grassi G, Catapano A, et al. Cancer risk associated with use of metformin and sulfonylurea in type 2 diabetes: a meta-analysis. Oncologist. 2012;17(6):813–22. doi:10.1634/theoncologist.2011-0462.
90. Lai SW, Liao KF, Chen PC, Tsai PY, Hsieh DP, Chen CC. Antidiabetes drugs correlate with decreased risk of lung cancer: a population-based observation in Taiwan. Clin Lung Cancer. 2012;13(2):143–8. doi:10.1016/j.cllc.2011.10.002.
91. Lai SW, Liao KF, Lai HC, Tsai PY, Sung FC, Chen PC. Kidney cancer and diabetes mellitus: a population-based case-control study in Taiwan. Ann Acad Med Singapore. 2013;42(3):120–4.
92. Elashoff M, Matveyenko AV, Gier B, Elashoff R, Butler PC. Pancreatitis, pancreatic, and thyroid cancer with glucagon-like peptide-1-based therapies. Gastroenterology. 2011;141(1):150–6. doi:10.1053/j.gastro.2011.02.018.
93. Monami M, Dicembrini I, Martelli D, Mannucci E. Safety of dipeptidyl peptidase-4 inhibitors: a meta-analysis of randomized clinical trials. Curr Med Res Opin. 2011;27(Suppl 3):57–64. doi:10.1185/03007995.2011.602964.
94. Scirica BM, Bhatt DL, Braunwald E, Steg PG, Davidson J, Hirshberg B, et al. Saxagliptin and cardiovascular outcomes in patients with type 2 diabetes mellitus. N Engl J Med. 2013;369(14):1317–26. doi:10.1056/NEJMoa1307684.
95. White WB, Cannon CP, Heller SR, Nissen SE, Bergenstal RM, Bakris GL, et al. Alogliptin after acute coronary syndrome in patients with type 2 diabetes. N Engl J Med. 2013;369(14):1327–35. doi:10.1056/NEJMoa1305889.
96. Ministry of Health LaW, Japan (in Japanese). http://wwwmhlwgojp/bunya/kenkou/dl/ gan_kenshin01pdf. 2013.

Chapter 10
Diabetes and Osteoporosis

Ippei Kanazawa and Toshitsugu Sugimoto

Abstract Accumulating evidence has shown that the risk of osteoporotic fracture is increased in patients with diabetes mellitus independently of bone mineral density. Thus, diabetes-related bone disease is now recognized as one of diabetic complications. Collagen cross-links of advanced glycation end products (AGEs), dysfunction of osteoblasts with low bone turnover, as well as abnormal microstructure of trabecular and cortical bone are involved in bone fragility in diabetes mellitus. Circulating levels of AGEs and homocysteine are increased in patients with diabetes, and AGEs and homocysteine directly inhibited the differentiation of osteoblasts. In addition, these induce the apoptosis and regulate expression levels of sclerostin and RANKL in osteocytes, which play important roles of bone remodeling. Moreover, several antidiabetic drugs affect bone metabolism and fracture risk. Therefore, the underlying mechanism of diabetes-related bone fragility is very complex and not still fully understood. In this review, we described effects of diabetes on bone metabolism and the risk of fracture based on the recent evidence.

Keywords Diabetes-related bone disease • Osteoporosis • Fracture • Bone formation • Advanced glycation end products

10.1 Introduction

Diabetes mellitus is known to cause various complications such as neuropathy, retinopathy, nephropathy, and atherosclerosis, resulting in the deterioration of quality of life and life prognosis. Accumulating evidence has shown that the risk of osteoporotic fractures, such as hip and vertebral fractures, is significantly increased in not only type 1 diabetes mellitus (T1DM) but also type 2 (T2DM). Vestergaard reported a meta-analysis [1] showing that patients with T1DM had slightly decreased bone mineral density (BMD) at the lumbar and hip (z-score −0.22 and −0.37,

I. Kanazawa (✉) • T. Sugimoto
Internal Medicine 1, Shimane University Faculty of Medicine,
89-1 Enya-cho, Izumo, Shimane 693-8501, Japan
e-mail: ippei.k@med.shimane-u.ac.jp

S.-i. Yamagishi (ed.), *Diabetes and Aging-related Complications*,
https://doi.org/10.1007/978-981-10-4376-5_10

respectively) and that T2DM patients had higher BMD at the lumbar and hip (*z*-score +0.41 and +0.27, respectively). Based on these BMD values, the estimated fracture risks were 1.42-fold in T1DM and 0.77-fold in T2DM, respectively. However, the risks of hip fracture compared to nondiabetes controls were 6.94-fold in T1DM and 1.4-fold in T2DM, respectively. Another meta-analysis also showed that hip fracture risks of T1DM and T2DM patients were increased to 6.3-fold and 1.7-fold, respectively, compared to nondiabetes controls [2]. Furthermore, we previously demonstrated that the presence of T2DM was an independent risk factor for prevalent vertebral fractures in Japanese men and women (odds ratio, 4.7 for men and 1.9 for women) after adjusting for age, body mass index, and lumbar BMD [3]. In addition, we tested usefulness of calcaneal quantitative ultrasound (QUS), which is thought to be able to evaluate bone quality of microarchitecture. However, QUS was also not associated with the risk of vertebral fracture in patients with T2DM [4]. These findings suggest that BMD and QUS may not reflect bone fragility in T1DM and T2DM and that measurements of BMD and QUS may lead to underestimate the actual risk of fracture. Therefore, bone mass reduction-independent fracture risk exists in diabetic patients, and impaired bone quality may be a major cause of diabetes-related bone fragility. Estimation of bone mass and microarchitecture by BMD and QUS is not useful in diabetic patients.

10.1.1 Increased Collagen Cross-Links of Advanced Glycation End Products in Diabetes

Advanced glycation end products (AGEs) are generated by sequential nonenzymatic chemical glycoxidation of protein amino groups. AGEs accumulate in various tissues including bone, kidney, brain, and coronary artery atherosclerotic plaques with aging. AGEs have a pivotal role in the development of complications in patients with diabetes, because hyperglycemia and oxidative stress accelerate AGE formation. Among AGEs, pentosidine is a well-characterized compound and is considered a good predictor for the development of micro- and macro-vascular complications in diabetic patients. Previous studies have shown that serum pentosidine levels in patients with diabetes were significantly higher than those in healthy subjects. Saito et al. previously reported that spontaneous diabetic rats displayed significant increases in pentosidine cross-links in bone, which was linked to impaired mechanical properties despite normal bone mass [5]. These findings clearly support the pathophysiology of bone fragility with normal BMD, which is seen in diabetic patients.

Because previous studies have shown that circulating pentosidine levels are significantly correlated with content of pentosidine in cortical bone, serum and urine pentosidine levels could be used as a surrogate marker for its content in bone as well as bone strength. Indeed, our previous study showed that elevated serum pentosidine levels were significantly associated with prevalent vertebral fracture in postmenopausal women with T2DM [6]. Schwartz et al. also reported an observational cohort study showing that higher urine pentosidine was associated with increased clinical fracture incidence in elderly patients with T2DM, but not in those without it [7]. In addition, a recent clinical study using bone biopsy in patients with T1DM showed that pentosidine content in trabecular was significantly and positively associated with HbA1c levels and increased in T1DM patients with fracture [8]. Therefore, accumulation of pentosidine cross-links in bone may be a major cause of impaired bone quality in patients with diabetes.

10.1.2 Dysfunction of Osteoblasts and Osteocytes in Diabetes

Bone tissue is constantly renewed by a balance between osteoblastic bone formation and osteoclastic bone resorption. Several clinical studies and meta-analyses have revealed that bone formation markers, especially serum osteocalcin, which is a marker of bone formation and produced by mature osteoblasts, were significantly decreased in patients with diabetes compared to nondiabetic subjects [9]. We and others previously demonstrated that serum osteocalcin levels were significantly increased after intensive glycemic control in T2DM, while bone specific alkaline phosphatase (BAP), which is a marker of early stage of differentiated osteoblasts, was significantly decreased [10]. Moreover, the ratio of osteocalcin/BAP was significantly associated with prevalent vertebral fracture in T2DM patients [11]. These findings suggest that derangement of osteoblast maturation may be involved in the risk of fracture in diabetic patients. On the other hand, osteocytes account for 90–95% of bone cells, and recent studies have shown that osteocytes play multifunctional roles in orchestrating bone remodeling by regulating both osteoblast and osteoclast functions. Sclerostin is specifically expressed in osteocytes and inhibits osteoblastic function and bone formation by antagonizing canonical Wnt signaling pathway. We previously showed that elevated serum sclerostin levels were associated with an increased risk of vertebral fractures in T2DM patients independently of BMD and bone turnover [12], suggesting that dysfunction of osteocytes also may contribute to the bone fragility in diabetes. In contrast, there are inconsistent results about bone resorption markers. Several studies showed that they are higher in patients with diabetes than those in nondiabetic subjects, while a meta-analysis demonstrated that C-terminal cross-linked telopeptide (CTX) was significantly lower in diabetic patients [9]. It is thus considered that bone resorption may be relatively elevated in patients with diabetes compared to decreased bone formation.

AGEs have a physiological function and act through their receptors. Because receptor for AGEs (RAGE) is expressed in osteoblasts and osteocytes, there is a possibility that AGEs directly affect bone formation and bone remodeling. Our *in vitro* studies have shown that the combination of high glucose and AGEs inhibited the mineralization of osteoblastic cell line, MC3T3-E1 [13], and that AGEs inhibited the osteoblastic differentiation or mineralization of mouse stromal ST2 cells and human mesenchymal stem cells by decreasing osterix expression, increasing transforming growth factor (TGF)-β expression, and suppressing endoplasmic reticulum stress proteins [14, 15] (Fig. 10.1). Moreover, high glucose and AGEs significantly increased the expression of sclerostin in osteocyte-like MLO-Y4 cells [16]. In contrast, AGEs decreased the expression of receptor activator of nuclear factor κB ligand (RANKL)

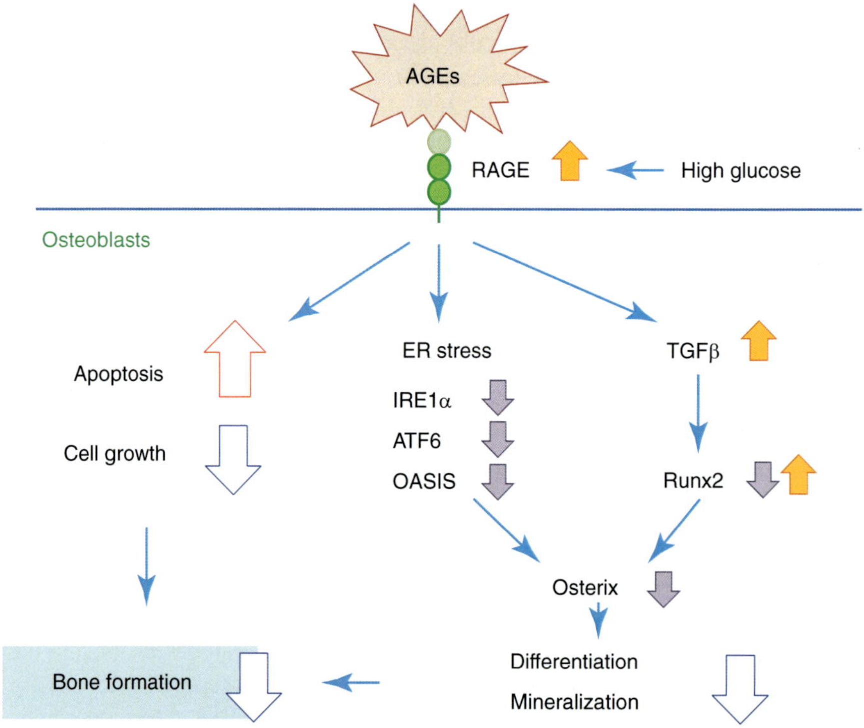

Fig. 10.1 Direct effects of advanced glycation end products (AGEs) on osteoblasts. Receptor for AGEs (RAGE) is expressed in osteoblast, and AGEs act as physiological molecules. AGEs induce apoptosis and suppress cell growth of osteoblasts. AGEs inhibit the differentiation and mineralization of osteoblasts through ER stress and TGFβ expression, resulting in decreased bone formation

in the cells. Furthermore, AGEs induced apoptosis of osteoblasts and osteocytes. Taken together, AGEs directly inhibit osteoblastic differentiation and bone formation and indirectly by increasing sclerostin expression in osteocytes as well as contribute to low turnover of bone remodeling by decreasing RANKL expression.

Homocysteine (Hcy) is a sulfur-containing amino acid formed by the demethylation of methionine, and high plasma Hcy levels are often caused by aging, lifestyle-related diseases such as diabetes, as well as vitamin B12 and folate insufficiency. Hcy has been shown to be an independent risk factor for cardiovascular disease, and several studies have previously shown that hyperhomocysteinemia increases the risk of osteoporotic fracture independently of BMD, suggesting that the deterioration of bone quality may be a dominant cause of Hcy-induced bone fragility. Li et al. previously showed that plasma Hcy levels were significantly increased in patients with T2DM than those in nondiabetes subjects and that higher plasma Hcy levels were associated with the incidence of vertebral fractures and hip fractures in patients with T2DM [17]. Although the mechanism underlying Hcy-related bone fragility in diabetes is still unclear, there are several studies including ours on effects of Hcy on osteoblastic function and collagen cross-links [18, 19]. Diet-induced

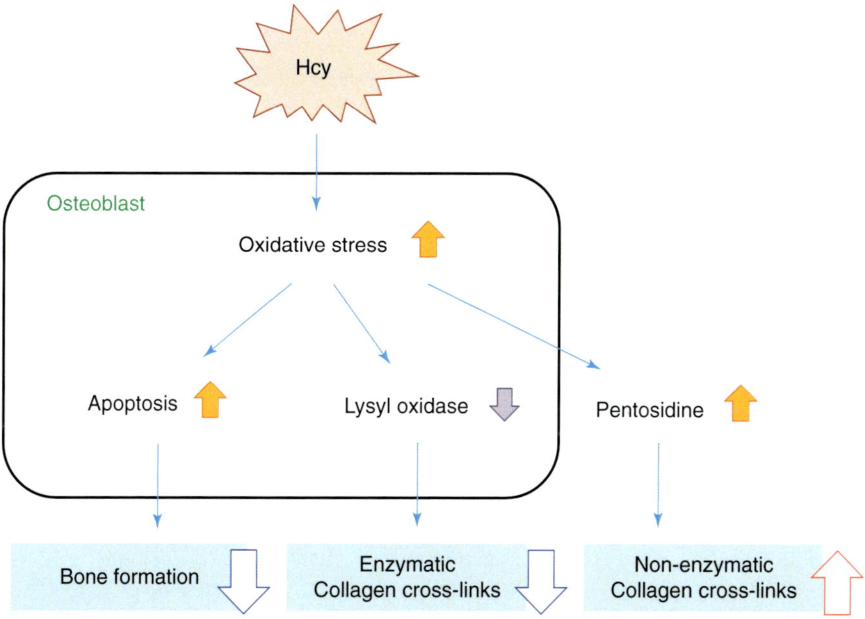

Fig. 10.2 Effects of homocysteine (Hcy) on osteoblasts. Hcy increases intracellular oxidative stress in osteoblasts and induces apoptosis. Hcy suppresses the expression of lysyl oxidase, which is the most important enzyme for collagen cross-links, and increases the extracellular pentosidine accumulation

hyperhomocysteinemia decreased bone quality *in vivo*, and Hcy directly affected osteoblastic lineage cells such as bone marrow stromal cells and osteoblasts. It has been shown that Hcy induces the apoptosis of osteoblastic cells by increasing oxidative stress. In addition, Hcy suppresses the expression of the collagen cross-linker lysyl oxidase and increases the accumulation of extracellular pentosidine in osteoblasts. These findings suggest that Hcy may impair viability and function of osteoblasts as well as deteriorate bone stiffness by inhibiting formation of enzymatic collagen cross-links and increasing nonenzymatic pentosidine cross-links in bone matrix (Fig. 10.2). Moreover, we previously showed that Hcy increased oxidative stress and induced apoptosis of osteocytes by increasing NADPH oxidase 1 (Nox1) and Nox2 expressions although detail of the mechanism is still unclear [20]. Thus, the dysfunction of osteocytes by Hcy may be involved in the bone fragility in diabetes.

Insulin action is important for osteoblastic differentiation, collagen synthesis, and bone formation. Osteoblast-specific insulin receptor gene knockout mice displayed a remarkable reduction in bone volume due to decreased bone formation and deficient numbers of osteoblasts [21]. Blocking insulin signaling suppresses osteoblastic proliferation, induces its apoptosis, and inhibits the differentiation and mineralization of osteoblasts by decreasing a Runx2 inhibitor, Twist2. These results are supported by the clinical finding that patients with T1DM have lower BMD and an increased risk of fragility fracture and can develop early-onset osteoporosis as well as poor bone healing and regeneration after injury. Insulin-like growth factor (IGF)-I is also known to have an anabolic effect on bone. IGF-I is expressed in osteoblasts and promotes osteoblastic differentiation and bone remodeling by autocrine and paracrine pathways in the microenvironment. Circulating IGF-I is mainly produced in the liver via regulation by growth hormone and diet and acts in an endocrine manner on bone as well. Significant reduction in bone mass and deficient mineralization were observed in osteoblast-specific knockout mice of IGF-I receptor, and liver-specific IGF-I gene-null mice showed a marked reduction in bone volume, periosteal circumference, and medial lateral width [22]. Moreover, several laboratory studies have shown that the stimulatory actions of IGF-I on osteoblasts are blunted by high glucose or AGEs and that high glucose significantly impairs the proliferative and functional responses of osteoblastic cells to IGF-I. AGEs also significantly decreased IGF-I secretion in osteoblasts. Thus, high glucose concentrations or AGEs may cause the resistance of osteoblasts to IGF-I actions in local environment. Therefore, IGF-I signaling is important for maintaining bone mass and strength in diabetic patients, and decreased IGF-I levels may be involved in the diabetes-related bone fragility. Indeed, we have previously shown that serum IGF-I level was positively associated with serum osteocalcin levels and inversely with the number of prevalent vertebral fractures in postmenopausal women with T2DM [23].

10.1.3 Abnormal Microstructure of Bone

Previous clinical studies using high-resolution peripheral quantitative computed tomography (HR-pQCT) have shown that cortical porosity is associated with the independent risk of fracture in T2DM patients. Burghardt et al. showed that T2DM patients had 10% higher trabecular volumetric BMD and higher trabecular thickness in the tibia compared to nondiabetic subjects, whereas cortical porosity in the distal radius was significantly 50% higher in T2DM than controls [24]. Furthermore, pore volume of the tibia showed similar trend, but not significant. In addition, HR-pQCT images of the distal radius and tibia showed that T2DM patients with fracture had severe intracortical porosity as well as extremely dense trabecular bone in the peripheral region adjacent to the cortex. Recently, several studies demonstrated consistent results. Therefore, increased cortical porosity may be involved in the fragility fracture in T2DM. However, the underlying mechanism is unknown. Osteocytes exist in the cortex, and it is considered that apoptosis of osteocytes may lead to increased pore volume of cortical bone. As described above, AGEs and Hcy induce the apoptosis of osteocytes. Thus, further studies are necessary to examine the association of AGEs and Hcy levels with cortical porosity.

Trabecular bone score (TBS) is a texture parameter that quantifies local variation in the gray level distribution of dual-energy X-ray absorptiometry images. Although TBS is not a direct physical measurement of bone microarchitecture, it is associated with bone microarchitecture of trabecular and stiffness of vertebra independently of BMD. Because of no need of further invasive examinations, TBS attracts widespread attention to physicians. Several studies showed that TBS was significantly decreased in patient with T2DM, while BMD was increased [25]. Thus, abnormal distribution

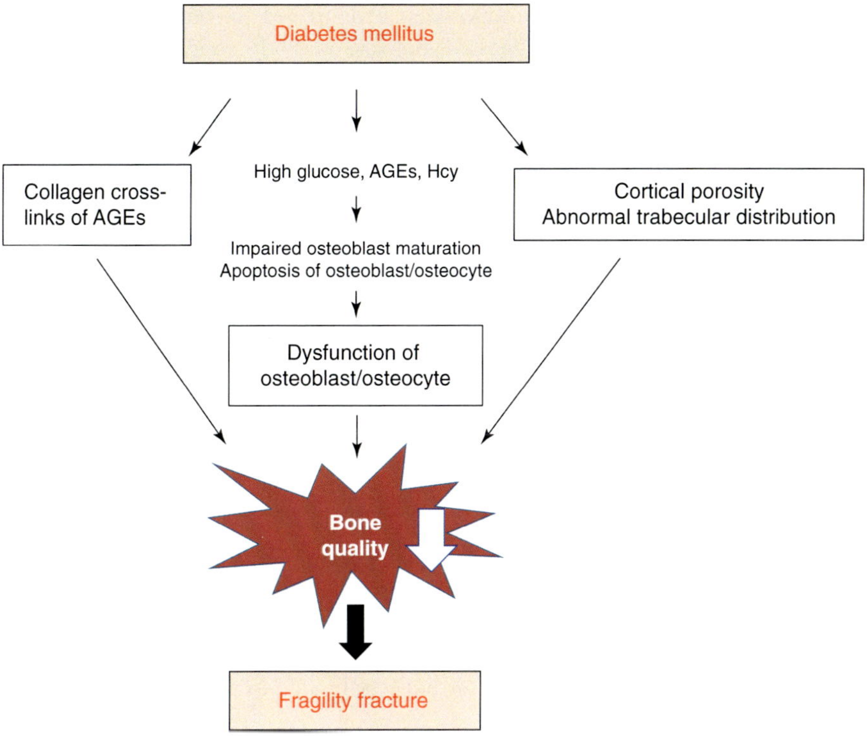

Fig. 10.3 Pathophysiology of diabetes-related bone fragility. Chronic hyperglycemia and increased oxidative stress by diabetes promote collagen cross-links of advanced glycation end products (AGEs). Hyperglycemia, AGEs, and Hcy inhibit osteoblastic differentiation and maturation and induce apoptosis of osteoblasts and osteocytes, resulting in dysfunction of osteoblast and osteocyte. Diabetes increases cortical porosity and abnormal trabecular distribution. These pathways contribute to the deterioration of bone quality and fragility fracture

of trabecular may be involved in the increased risk of fracture in diabetes. HbA1c levels and insulin resistance were reported to be associated with TBS; however, the mechanism of low TBS with high BMD is still unknown. A few clinical studies recently showed the usefulness of TBS to access the risk of fracture in patients with diabetes. Further longitudinal studies are needed to use TBS in clinical settings.

Taken all together, collagen cross-links of AGEs, dysfunction of osteoblasts with low bone turnover, and abnormal microstructure of trabecular and cortical bone are involved in bone fragility in diabetes mellitus (Fig. 10.3).

10.2 The Risk of Fall

Fragility fracture occurs after low-energy trauma such as falls and bumps, which wouldn't hurt a person with healthy bones, in patients with osteoporosis. It has been shown that diabetic patients have increased risk of falls. Thus, the increased risk of fracture is caused by not only weakened stiffness of bone itself but also high incidence of falls. It is suggested that loss of body weight, diabetic neuropathy, autonomic neuropathy, diabetic retinopathy with visual disturbance, renal dysfunction, insulin use, and hypoglycemia, etc. are associated with the increased risk of fall. Sarcopenia is one of diabetic complications (please see Chap. 11), and the presence of sarcopenia is also an important risk factor for the risk of fall. Like the dysfunction of osteoblasts, insulin and IGF-I action and pentosidine accumulation are associated with loss of muscle mass. Insulin and IGF-I are well known to have anabolic effects on muscle mass. Indeed, we previously showed that parameters of residual insulin secretion and serum IGF-I levels, but not HbA1c, are significantly and positively associated with skeletal muscle mass index in T2DM even after adjustment for age, duration of diabetes, renal function, and HbA1c [26, 27]. In addition, our *in vitro* studies have shown that AGEs directly inhibit myogenesis of myoblastic cells [28]. Previous lots of studies have revealed that vitamin D insufficiency and deficiency are associated with the increased risk of fall and muscle mass reduction, and supplementation of vitamin D decreases the incidence of fall. We previously reported that active vitamin D and eldecalcitol, which is an analogue of active vitamin D and is an available drug for the treatment of osteoporosis, enhanced myogenesis of myoblastic cells and protected against AGE-induced inhibition of myogenesis [28]. Since diabetic patients frequently have vitamin D insufficiency and deficiency, vitamin D status is very important for diabetes-related bone fragility regarding strength of bone and muscle.

Osteoporosis and sarcopenia are aging-related diseases associated with the deterioration of muscle and bone strength, resulting in frailty in elderly people. Sarcopenia and osteoporosis are traditionally viewed as separate entities that increase in prevalence with aging. However, accumulating evidence indicates that some pathological conditions such as accumulated AGEs and decreased IGF-I are involved in both diseases as described above. Recent studies have shown an interaction between muscle and bone tissues that has been recognized as the muscle-bone axis. Previous studies have shown that muscle tissue secretes various hormones called myokines and that bone also secretes various hormones such as osteocalcin. We have previously shown that osteoglycin (OGN) is an important factor linking muscle to bone. OGN is a small leucine-rich proteoglycan and initially isolated from bovine bone as an inducer of matrix mineralization. Our *in vitro* studies demonstrated that OGN suppressed the early stage of osteoblastogenesis, but enhanced the differentiation and mineralization of late-stage osteoblasts [29]. Also, we found that AGE treatment inhibited the expression of OGN in myoblasts and that active vitamin D recovered the AGE-induced suppression of OGN and sequentially inhibited osteoblastic differentiation [28].

Therefore, there are several common factors affecting bone and muscle as well as their interaction (Fig. 10.4). Especially, AGEs are important aggravating factors for the increased risk of fracture due to diabetes-related bone fragility and muscle weakness (Fig. 10.5).

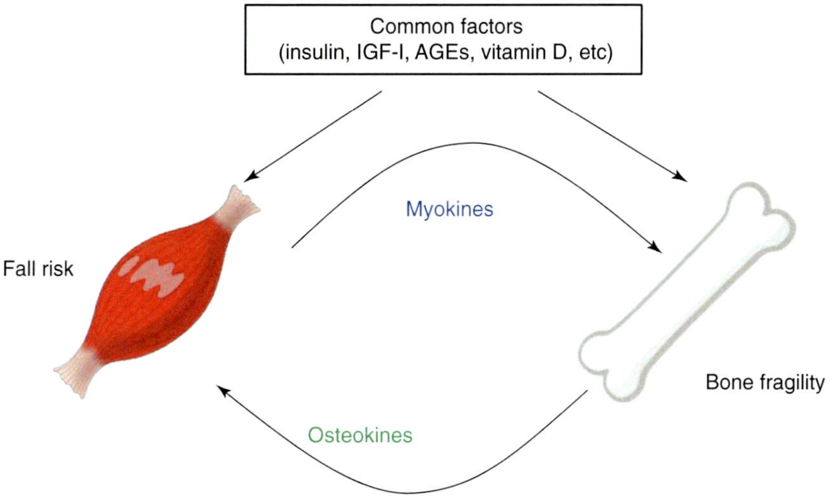

Fig. 10.4 Muscle function is involved in diabetes-related bone disease. Several common factors such as insulin, insulin-like growth factor (IGF)-I, AGEs, and vitamin D affect bone and muscle tissue. Muscle and bone are associated with each other through myokines and osteokines

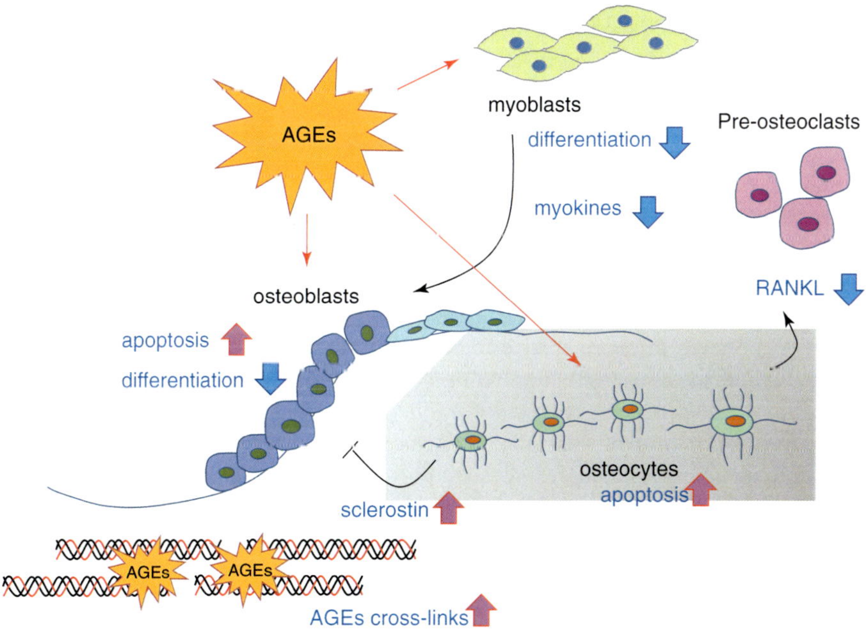

Fig. 10.5 Multifacet effects of advanced glycation end products (AGEs) on bone metabolism. AGEs induce apoptosis of osteoblasts and inhibit osteoblastic differentiation. AGEs induce apoptosis of osteocytes, enhance the expression of sclerostin, and decrease the expression of receptor activator of nuclear factor κB ligand (RANKL) in osteocytes, leading to inhibiting differentiation of osteoblasts and osteoclasts as well as decreasing bone turnover and remodeling. AGEs inhibit the differentiation of myoblasts and suppress the expression of myokines, resulting in suppression of osteoblastic differentiation. Production of AGE cross-links in bone matrix is promoted by diabetic condition

10.3 Treatments for Diabetes-Related Bone Fragility

A prospective population-based cohort study, the Rotterdam study, previously showed that HbA1c levels are associated with the incidence of fracture in T2DM patients [30]. Cox proportional hazard regression models adjusted for age, sex, height, and weight indicated that patients with inadequately controlled diabetes (HbA1c $\geq$ 7.5%) had 47–62% higher fracture risk than control subjects without diabetes (hazard ratio 1.47) and adequately controlled diabetes (HbA1c <7.5%, hazard ratio 1.62). Other groups also reported that poor controlled diabetes is associated with the increased risk of fracture although cutoff point is different from the Rotterdam study. Therefore, controlling blood glucose below 7.5% seems to be required for diabetes-related bone disease.

We and others previously reported that intensive glycemic control for 1–2 months significantly increased serum osteocalcin levels, while BAP was decreased [10], suggesting that lowering blood glucose can improve impaired osteoblastic maturation and reduce the risk of fracture in diabetes. However, of surprise, the action to control cardiovascular risk in diabetes (ACCORD) randomized trial revealed that intensive therapy targeting HbA1c < 6.0% did not affect 2-year percent change in BMD or the incidence of fracture (nonspine, hip, ankle, foot, proximal humerus, and distal forearm) or fall compared to standard therapy targeting HbA1c < 7.5% [31]. Several studies have shown that some antidiabetic drugs affect bone metabolism and fracture risk. Among them, insulin treatment and thiazolidines are known to be associated with the risk of fracture. Several studies including ours demonstrated that patients treated with insulin had higher risk of fracture [32]. In the ACCORD trial, many participants of intensive therapy received insulin treatment and had body weight gain and increased risk of hypoglycemia, which may affect bone metabolism and fracture risk. Therefore, approach of glycemic control should be considered, and further intervention trials are necessary to find out how we should treat diabetic patients with long-term diabetic duration in terms of reduction of fracture risk. On the other hand, peroxisome proliferator-activated receptor γ (PPARγ) is known to be a negative regulator of osteoblastogenesis. Activation of PPARγ inhibits the commitment of multipotential mesenchymal stem cells to osteoblastic lineage and induces adipogenesis. Indeed, several studies and meta-analyses have shown that treatment with thiazolidines decreases BMD and increases the risk of fracture in elderly women, but not men [32–34]. Treatment with sodium glucose cotransporter 2 (SGLT2) inhibitors is concerned to increase the risk of fracture because SGLT2 inhibitors increase calcium excretion along with glucose excretion in urine and induce loss of body weight, both of which may have negative impacts on bone. Although further studies are mandatory, we should take care of bone health when SGLT2 inhibitors are used. In contrast, several studies showed that incretin, especially glucose-dependent insulinotropic polypeptide (GIP), and dipeptidyl peptidase-4 (DPP-4) inhibitors as well as metformin may have favorable effects on bone. We previously demonstrated that serum DPP-4 levels were associated with the risk of multiple vertebral fractures in T2DM [35], and a meta-analysis showed that patients treated with DPP-4 inhibitors had lower incidence of fracture compared to other treatments [36]. Metformin is reported to enhance the differentiation of osteoblasts *in vitro* [37] and increase bone mass *in vivo* [38]. Several epidemiological studies showed that metformin treatment is associated with low risk of fracture. However, we don't have strong evidence about the effects of DPP-4 inhibitors and metformin on the risk of fracture in diabetic patients thus far.

10.4 Summary

In summary, it has been shown that the risk of fracture is significantly increased in both T1DM and T2DM. Thus, diabetes-related bone disease is one of important diabetic complications. Recent studies elucidate the mechanism of diabetes-related bone fragility, collagen cross-links of AGEs, dysfunction of osteoblasts with low bone turnover, and abnormal microstructure of trabecular and cortical bone. Also, sarcopenia associated with the risk of fall is important for protecting diabetic patients from osteoporotic fractures. In both T1DM and T2DM, BMD is not necessarily a good marker for the bone fragility and that BMD measurement seems to be less useful in diabetic patients. It is therefore an urgent task to seek suitable surrogate markers for diabetes-related bone disease, for example, HR-pQCT, TBS, and pentosidine levels in serum and urine. Because of no evidence that treatments for diabetes can improve diabetes-related bone fragility and reduce the risk of fracture, the use of anti osteoporotic drugs should be positively considered for diabetic patients with the increased risk of fracture such as presence of fracture, low BMD including osteopenia, poor glycemic control, long duration of diabetes, treatments with insulin and thiazolidines, and sarcopenia.

Disclosure Summary The authors have nothing to disclose.

References

1. Vestergaard P. Discrepancies in bone mineral density and fracture risk in patients with type 1 and type 2 diabetes—a meta-analysis. Osteoporos Int. 2007;18:427–44.
2. Janghorbani M, Van Dam RM, Willett WC, Hu FB. Systematic review of type 1 and type 2 diabetes mellitus and risk of fracture. Am J Epidemiol. 2007;166:495–505.
3. Yamamoto M, Yamaguchi T, Yamauchi M, Kaji H, Sugimoto T. Diabetic patients have an increased risk of vertebral fractures independent of bone mineral density or diabetic complications. J Bone Miner Res. 2009;24:702–9.
4. Yamaguchi T, Yamamoto M, Kanazawa I, Yamauchi M, Yano S, Tanaka N, Nitta E, Fukuma A, Uno S, Sho-no T, Sugimoto T. Quantitative ultrasound and vertebral fractures in patients with type 2 diabetes. J Bone Miner Metab. 2001;29:626–32.
5. Saito M, Fujii K, Mori Y, Marumo K. Role of collagen enzymatic and glycation induced cross-links as a determinant of bone quality in spontaneously diabetic WBN/Kob rats. Osteoporos Int. 2006;17:1514–23.

6. Yamamoto M, Yamaguchi T, Yamauchi M, Yano S, Sugimoto T. Serum pentosidine levels are positively associated with the presence of vertebral fractures in postmenopausal women with type 2 diabetes. J Clin Endocrinol Metab. 2008;93:1013–9.
7. Schwartz AV, Garnero P, Hillier TA, Sellmeyer DE, Strotmeyer ES, Feingold KR, Resnick HE, Tylavsky FA, Black DM, Cummings SR, Harris TB, Bauer DC. Health, aging, and body composition study. J Clin Endocrinol Metab. 2009;94:2380–6.
8. Farlay D, Armas LA, Gineyts E, Akhter MP, Recker RR, Boivin G. Nonenzymatic glycation and degree of mineralization are higher in bone from fractured patients with type 1 diabetes mellitus. J Bone Miner Res. 2016;31:190–5.
9. Liu C, Wo J, Zhao Q, Wang Y, Wang B, Zhao W. Association between serum total osteocalcin level and type 2 diabetes mellitus: a systematic review and meta-analysis. Horm Metab Res. 2015;47:813–9.
10. Kanazawa I, Yamaguchi T, Yamauchi M, et al. Adiponectin is associated with changes in bone markers during glycemic control in type 2 diabetes mellitus. J Clin Endocrinol Metab. 2009;94:3031–7.
11. Kanazawa I, Yamaguchi T, Yamamoto M, et al. Serum osteocalcin/bone-specific alkaline phosphatase ratio is a predictor for the presence of vertebral fractures in men with type 2 diabetes. Calcif Tissue Int. 2009;85:228–34.
12. Yamamoto M, Yamauchi M, Sugimoto T. Elevated sclerostin levels are associated with vertebral fractures in patients with type 2 diabetes mellitus. J Clin Endocrinol Metab. 2013;98:4030–7.
13. Ogawa N, Yamaguchi T, Yano S, Yamauchi M, Yamamoto M, Sugimoto T. The combination of high glucose and advanced glycation end-products (AGEs) inhibits the mineralization of osteoblastic MC3T3-E1 cells through glucose-induced increase in the receptor for AGEs. Horm Metab Res. 2007;39:871–5.
14. Notsu M, Yamaguchi T, Okazaki K, Tanaka K, Ogawa N, Kanazawa I, Sugimoto T. Advanced glycation end product 3 (AGE3) suppresses the mineralization of mouse stromal ST2 cells and human mesenchymal stem cells by increasing TGF-β expression and secretion. Endocrinology. 2014;155:2402–10.
15. Tanaka K, Yamaguchi T, Kaji H, Kanazawa I, Sugimoto T. Advanced glycation end products suppress osteoblastic differentiation of stromal cells by activation endoplasmic reticulum stress. Biochem Biophys Res Commun. 2013;438:463–7.
16. Tanaka K, Yamaguchi T, Kanazawa I, Sugimoto T. Effects of high glucose and advanced glycation end products on the expressions of sclerostin and RANKL as well as apoptosis in osteocyte-like MLO-Y4-A2 cells. Biochem Biophys Res Commun. 2015;461:193–9.
17. Li J, Zhang H, Yan L, Xie M, Chen J. Fracture is additionally attributed to hyperhomocysteinemia in men and premenopausal women with type 2 diabetes. J Diabetes Investig. 2014;5:236–41.
18. Herrmann M, Tami A, Wildemann B, Wolny M, Wagner A, Schorr H, Taban-Shomal O, Umanskaya N, Ross S, Garcia P, Hubner U, Hermann W. Hyperhomocysteinemia induces a tissue specific accumulation of homocysteine in bone by collagen binding and adversely affects bone. Bone. 2009;44:467–75.
19. Kanazawa I, Tomita T, Miyazaki S, Ozawa E, Yamamoto LA, Sugimoto T. Bazedoxifene ameliorates homocysteine-induced apoptosis and accumulation of advanced glycation end products by reducing oxidative stress in MC3T3-E1 cells. Calcif Tissue Int. 2017;100(3):286–97.
20. Takeno A, Kanazawa I, Tanaka K, Notsu M, Yokomoto M, Yamaguchi T, Sugimoto T. Activation of AMP-activated protein kinase protects against homocysteine-induced apoptosis of osteocytic MLO-Y4 cells by regulating the expressions of NADPH oxidase 1 (Nox1) and Nox2. Bone. 2015;77:135–41.
21. Fulzele K, Riddle RC, DiGirolamo DJ, Cao X, Wan C, Chen D, Faugere MC, Aja S, Hussain MA, Bruning JC, Clemens TL. Insulin receptor signaling in osteoblasts regulates postnatal bone acquisition and body composition. Cell. 2010;142:309–19.
22. Yakar S, Rosen CJ, Beamer WG, Ackert-Bicknell CL, Wu Y, Liu JL, Ooi GT, Setser J, Frystyk J, Boisclair YR, LeRoith D. Circulating levels of IGF-I directly regulate bone growth and density. J Clin Invest. 2002;110:771–81.

23. Kanazawa I, Yamaguchi T, Sugimoto T. Serum insulin-like growth factor-I is a marker for assessing the severity of vertebral fractures in postmenopausal women with type 2 diabetes mellitus. Osteoporos Int. 2011;22:1191–8.
24. Burghardt AJ, Issever AS, Schwartz AV, Davis KA, Masharani U, Majumdar Link TM. High-resolution peripheral quantitative computed tomographic imaging of cortical and trabecular bone microarchitecture in patients with type 2 diabetes mellitus. J Clin Endocrinol Metab. 2010;95:5045–55.
25. Dhaliwal R, Cibula D, Ghosh C, Weinstock RS, Moses AM. Bone quality assessment in type 2 diabetes mellitus. Osteoporos Int. 2014;25:1969–73.
26. Tanaka K, Kanazawa I, Sugimoto T. Elevated serum pentosidine and decreased serum IGF-I levels are associated with loss of muscle mass in postmenopausal women with type 2 diabetes mellitus. Exp Clin Endocrinol Diabetes. 2016;124:163–6.
27. Tanaka K, Kanazawa I, Sugimoto T. Reduction in endogenous insulin secretion is a risk factor of sarcopenia in men with type 2 diabetes mellitus. Calcif Tissue Int. 2015;97:385–90.
28. Tanaka K, Kanazawa I, Yamaguchi T, Yano S, Kaji H, Sugimoto T. Active vitamin D possesses beneficial effects on the interaction between muscle and bone. Biochem Biophys Res Commun. 2014;450:482–7.
29. Tanaka K, Matsumoto E, Higashimaki Y, Katagiri T, Sugimoto T, Seino S, Kaji H. Role of osteoglycin in the linkage between muscle and bone. J Biol Chem. 2012;287:11616–28.
30. Qei L, Zillikens MC, Dehghan A, Buitendijk GH, Castano-Betancourt MC, Estrada K, Stolk L, Oei EH, van Meurs JB, Janssen JA, Hofman A, van Leeuwen JP, Witteman JC, Pols HA, Uitterlinden AG, Klaver CC, Franco OH, Rivadeneira F. High bone mineral density and fracture risk in type 2 diabetes as skeletal complications of inadequate glucose control: the Rotterdam Study. Diabetes Care. 2013;36:1619–28.
31. Schwartz AV, Margolis KL, Sellmeyer DE, Vittinghoff E, Ambrosius WT, Bonds DE, Josse RG, Schnall AM, Simmons DL, Hue TF, Palermo L, Hamilton BP, Green JB, Atkinson HH, O'Connor PJ, Force RW, Bauer DC. Intensive glycemic control is not associated with fractures or falls in the ACCORD randomized trial. Diabetes Care. 2012;35:1525–31.
32. Kanazawa I, Yamaguchi T, Yamamoto M, Sugimoto T. Relationships between treatments with insulin and oral hypoglycemic agents versus the presence of vertebral fractures in type 2 diabetes mellitus. J Bone Miner Metab. 2010;28:554–60.
33. Kanazawa I, Yamaguchi T, Yano S, Yamamoto M, Yamauchi M, Kurioka S, Sugimoto T. Baseline atherosclerosis parameter could assess the risk of bone loss during pioglitazone treatment in type 2 diabetes mellitus. Osteoporos Int. 2010;21:2013–8.
34. Loke YK, Singh S, Furberg CD. Long-term use of thiazolidinediones and fractures in type 2 diabetes: a meta-analysis. CMAJ. 2009;180:32–9.
35. Notsu M, Kanazawa I, Tanaka S, Yamaguchi T, Sugimoto T. Serum dipeptidyl peptidase-4 is associated with multiple vertebral fractures in type 2 diabetes mellitus. Clin Endocrinol. 2016;84:332–7.
36. Monami M, Dicembrini I, Antenore A, Mannucci E. Dipeptidyl peptidase-4 inhibitors and bone fractures: a meta-analysis of randomized clinical trials. Diabetes Care. 2011;34:2474–6.
37. Kanazawa I, Yamaguchi T, Yano S, Yamauchi M, Sugimoto T. Metformin enhances the differentiation and mineralization of osteoblastic MC3T3-E1 cells via AMP kinase activation as well as eNOS and BMP-2 expression. Biochem Biophys Res Commun. 2008;375:414–9.
38. Gao Y, Li Y, Xue J, Jia Y, Hu J. Effect of the anti-diabetic drug metformin on bone mass in ovariectomized rats. Eur J Pharmacol. 2010;635:231–6.

Chapter 11
Diabetes and Sarcopenia

Masaki Mogi and Masatsugu Horiuchi

Abstract Diabetes induces muscle atrophy partly caused by an imbalance in contractile protein synthesis and degradation, hyperglycemia, bone marrow microenvironmental defects, and other changes. Muscle atrophy induces functional disability and promotes reduced physical activity. Muscle atrophy also enhances insulin resistance and impairs glucose metabolism. Moreover, sarcopenic obesity has been introduced as a syndrome in older subjects with reduced muscle mass and a change in fat distribution. Fat infiltration into muscle is associated with lower muscle strength and leg performance capacity. Furthermore, impairment of mitochondrial function may underlie the development and progression of both sarcopenia and diabetes. Such a vicious cycle of muscle atrophy and diabetes would worsen the quality of life of diabetic patients. Therefore, an interventional approach such as appropriate medication and exercise to break the bad relationship is needed.

Keywords Diabetes • Sarcopenia • Sarcopenic obesity • Insulin resistance • Mitochondria

11.1 Introduction

The number of elderly with diabetes is increasing unexpectedly. Aging is associated with increased fat mass and reduced muscle mass or strength, even in those with stable body weight. Such poor muscle quality is called "sarcopenia," and the copresence of sarcopenia and obesity is called "sarcopenic obesity," which was first described by Baumgartner et al. [1]. Aging is associated with an inactive lifestyle, which induces muscle atrophy from less exercise. Skeletal muscle atrophy has been linked to the development of insulin resistance and impaired glucose metabolism. On the other hand, type 2 diabetes mellitus (T2DM) induces muscle atrophy caused by an imbalance in contractile protein synthesis and degradation. T2DM and insulin

M. Mogi (✉) • M. Horiuchi
Department of Molecular Cardiovascular Biology and Pharmacology, Ehime University Graduate School of Medicine, Tohon, Ehime 791-0295, Japan
e-mail: mmogi@m.ehime-u.ac.jp

S.-i. Yamagishi (ed.), *Diabetes and Aging-related Complications*,
https://doi.org/10.1007/978-981-10-4376-5_11

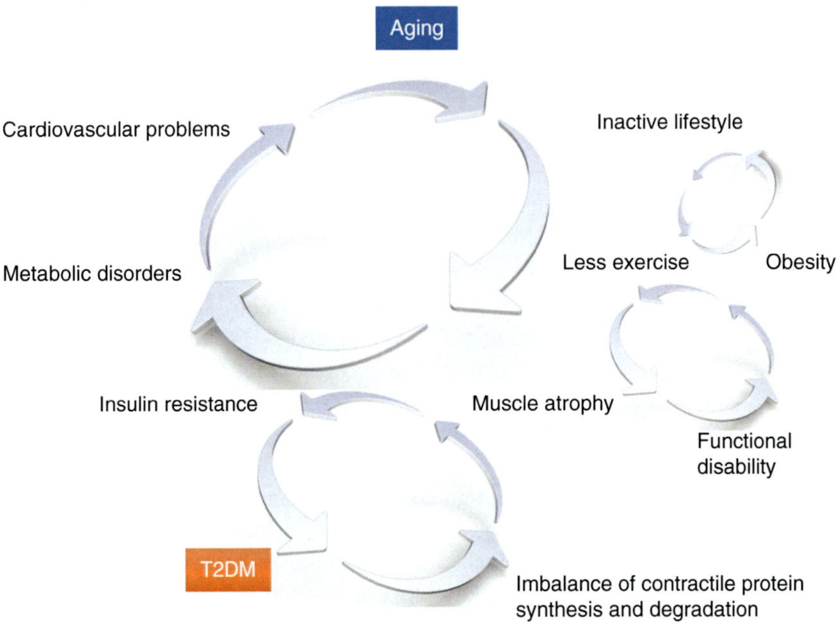

Fig. 11.1 Vicious cycles in elderly with T2DM. *T2DM* type 2 diabetes mellitus

resistance increase cardiovascular problems via vascular dysfunction and result in acceleration of aging. Muscle atrophy also leads to functional disability, which impairs physical activity and increases body weight, resulting in enhancement of muscle atrophy. For these reasons, the elderly with diabetes falls into the vicious cycles shown in Fig. 11.1. Sinclair et al. reviewed the relationship between diabetes and frailty [2]. T2DM accelerates the aging process and could provide an early pathophysiologic environment for frailty. Sarcopenia can be caused by several factors, such as genetic heritability, nutritional status, physical activity, insulin resistance, and proinflammatory cytokines [3, 4]. Thus, the close relationship between T2DM and sarcopenia may be induced by a common factor such as inflammation, malnutrition, physical inactivity, or insulin resistance (Fig. 11.2). Therefore, a preventive approach to muscle atrophy in older diabetic patients is very important to maintain their healthy lifestyle.

11.2 Sarcopenia with Diabetes

Buford et al. demonstrated accelerating factors for behaviors and diseases in sarcopenia (Fig. 11.3) [5]. Progression of sarcopenia is 30% faster in T2DM compared with age-matched nondiabetic subjects [6]. T2DM is one of the

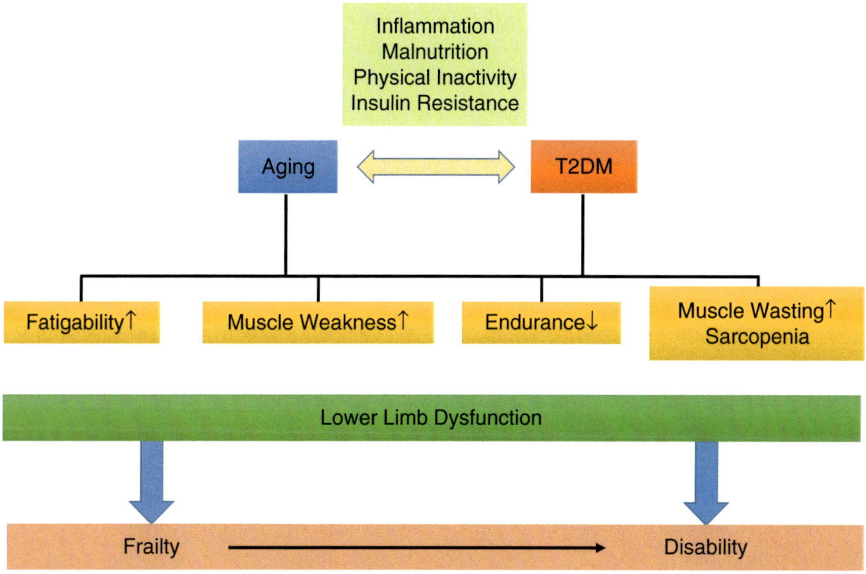

Fig. 11.2 Combined effects of aging and T2DM on frailty (modified from ref. [2]). *T2DM* type 2 diabetes mellitus

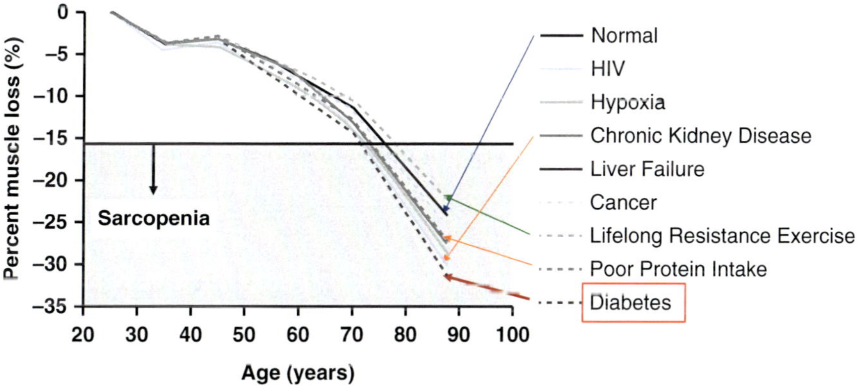

Fig. 11.3 Accelerating risk factors for sarcopenia (modified from ref. [5], with permission). *HIV* human immunodeficiency virus, *CKD* chronic kidney disease

strongest factors accelerating sarcopenia. Moreover, the prevalence of sarcopenia is higher in patients with T2DM than in nondiabetic subjects [7]. Interestingly, middle-aged and elderly women with diabetes exhibit a higher prevalence of sarcopenia than those without diabetes, while this difference was not significant in middle-aged men. Therefore, T2DM is an important predictor of sarcopenia, particularly in women [7]. On the other hand, Batsis et al. reported that the prevalence of sarcopenic obesity was 18.1% in women and 42.9% in men [8]. However, older women with sarcopenia have a higher all-cause mortality risk independent of obesity than older men, while sarcopenic obesity in women is not associated with mortality after adjusting for mobility limitations. For men, the risk of death with sarcopenia and sarcopenic obesity is not significant [8]. Although gender differences in sarcopenia in T2DM patients are not well known, there may be a sex-specific effect on sarcopenia. On the other hand, sarcopenia and central adiposity are associated with higher cardiovascular mortality and all-cause mortality [9]. Moreover, sarcopenia is associated with premature mortality in community-dwelling older adults [10]. Older adults with sarcopenic obesity have more adverse mid-life cardiometabolic risks, particularly diabetes 10 years earlier [11]. Therefore, prevention of sarcopenia is a valuable approach not only to improve quality of life in T2DM patients but also to reduce risks for all-cause mortality. However, the most important problem in clinical practice and research in sarcopenic obesity is the lack of a definition of sarcopenic obesity. Most studies are cross-sectional and present many different diagnostic criteria for sarcopenic obesity. Moreover, sarcopenic obesity is not the same as "sarcopenia with T2DM." Thus, more clinical research about the effect of sarcopenia in T2DM patients on cardiovascular disease and all-cause mortality is necessary.

11.3 Muscle Quality and Insulin Resistance

Hyperglycemia induces muscle protein loss through caspase 3- or 8-induced activation of double-stranded RNA-dependent protein kinase (PKR), leading to phosphorylation of eukaryotic initiation factor 2α (eIF2α) and depression of protein synthesis, together with PKR-mediated reactive oxygen species production, through p38 mitogen-activated protein kinase (MAPK) and increased protein degradation, as shown in Fig. 11.4 [12]. On the other hand, diabetes leads to multiple bone marrow microenvironmental defects, such as small vessel disease, nerve terminal pauperization, and impaired stem cell mobilization [13]. Fujimaki et al. reviewed the effect of diabetes on satellite cell activation and differentiation into myotubes [14]. T2DM promotes various impairment of satellite cell function such as proliferation and differentiation, possibly by an increase in oxidative stress; however, the molecular mechanisms of impairment of satellite cell function in diabetes are not well known.

Muscle quality deteriorates with aging, with loss of muscle mass and an increase in muscle atrophy, ectopic fat deposition, and intramuscular fibrosis (Fig. 11.5). Muscle atrophy and the development of insulin resistance have also been attributed to a decline in mitochondrial content and/or impairment of skeletal muscle mito-

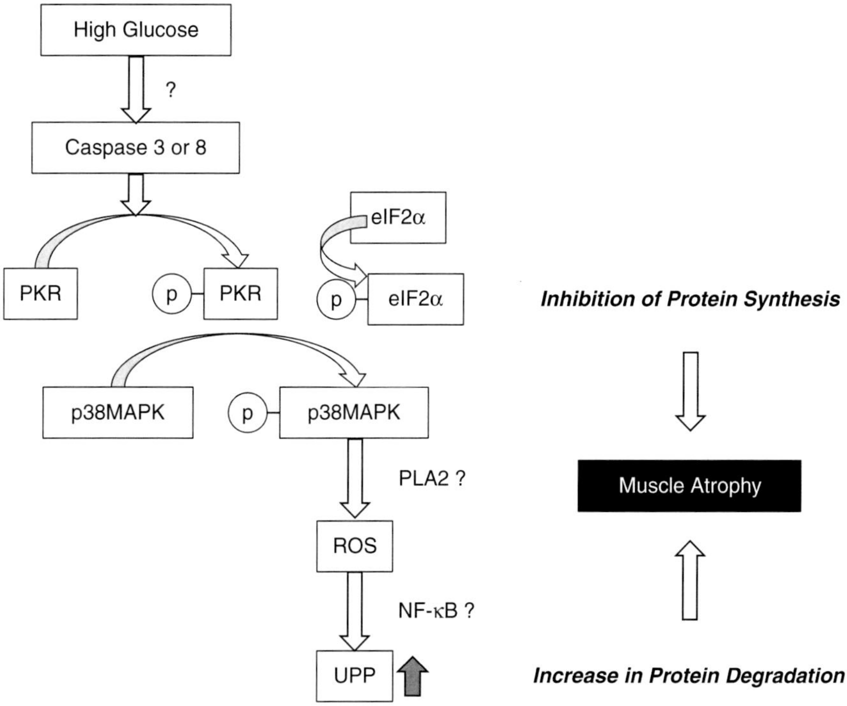

Fig. 11.4 Possible mechanism of muscle atrophy induced by hyperglycemia (modified from ref. [12]). *PKR* double-stranded RNA-dependent protein kinase, *eIF2α* eukaryotic initiation factor 2α, *p38MAPK* p38 mitogen-activated protein kinase, *PLA$_2$* phospholipase A_2, *ROS* reactive oxygen species, *NF-κB* nuclear factor-κB, *UPP* ubiquitin proteasome pathway. *Circled p* means phosphorylated proteins

chondrial function [15, 16]. Therefore, impairment of mitochondrial functioning may underlie the development and progression of both sarcopenia and T2DM. Mitochondrial dysfunction and the release of mitochondrial reactive oxygen species are considered a key factor in the development of muscle disuse atrophy [17]. One week of bed rest substantially reduces skeletal muscle mass and lowers whole-body insulin sensitivity [16]. Such an increase in insulin resistance is accompanied by a decline in muscle oxidative capacity, without alteration in skeletal muscle lipid content or saturation level, markers of oxidative stress, or capillary density. Exercise improves mitochondrial function by activating mitochondrial biogenesis and mitophagy [18]. On the other hand, muscle disuse atrophy is not accompanied by satellite cell content [19] and is not attenuated by dietary protein supplementation [20]. Therefore, exercise and prevention of short-term muscle disuse may be a better preventive approach in T2DM patients via maintenance of mitochondrial health.

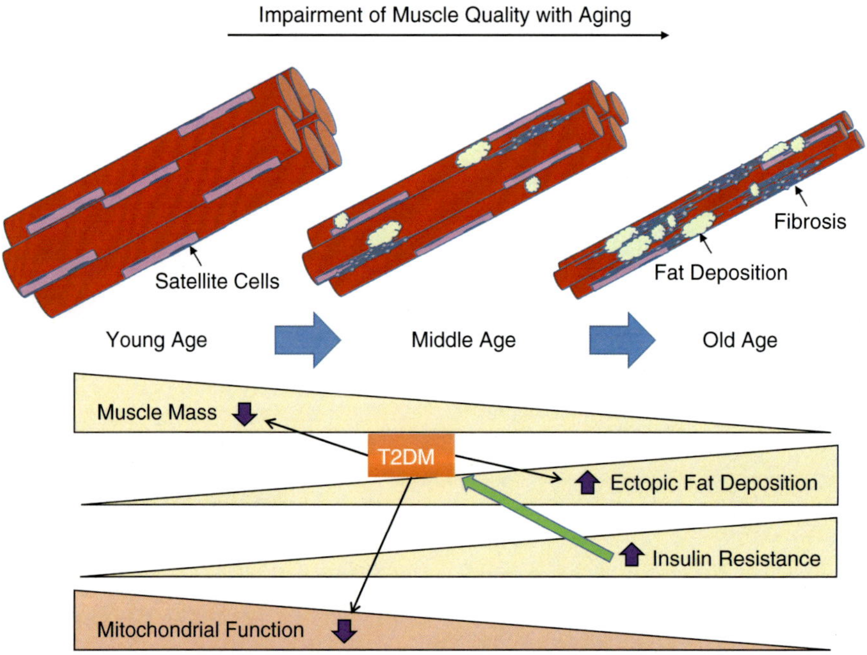

Fig. 11.5 Muscle quality and T2DM. Muscle quality deteriorates with aging, with loss of muscle mass and increase in muscle atrophy, ectopic fat deposition, and intramuscular fibrosis

11.4 Ectopic Fat Deposition

Aging is associated with progressive loss of subcutaneous fat and accumulation of visceral fat and ectopic fat deposition in the muscle (myosteatosis), liver, bone marrow, and elsewhere [21]. Goodpaster et al. reported that intermuscular fat was greater in subjects with T2DM than in subjects with normal glucose tolerance, despite similar amounts of subcutaneous thigh fat [22]. Fat infiltration into muscle is associated with lower muscle strength and leg performance capacity [23]. Moreover, Reinders et al. recently reported that an increase in muscle lean area, muscle quality, and strength was associated with lower mortality risk for men and women; on the other hand, an increase in intermuscular adipose tissue and intramuscular adipose tissue was associated with higher mortality risk for men [24]. Chest computed tomography demonstrated that skeletal muscle density in the brachialis muscle of KKAy is close to the density of fat (Fig. 11.6), indicating that the skeletal muscle is infiltrated with fat. Myosteatosis factors are not yet well defined; however, disuse, altered leptin signaling, sex steroid deficiency, and glucocorticoid treatment are reported to increase intramuscular fat [25]. We assessed muscle regeneration using a muscle injury model in obese diabetic mice [26]. Male wild-type mice (C57BL6) and obese-T2DM mice (KKAy) underwent intramuscular injection of cardiotoxin (CTX) into the tibia. Histological analysis of injured

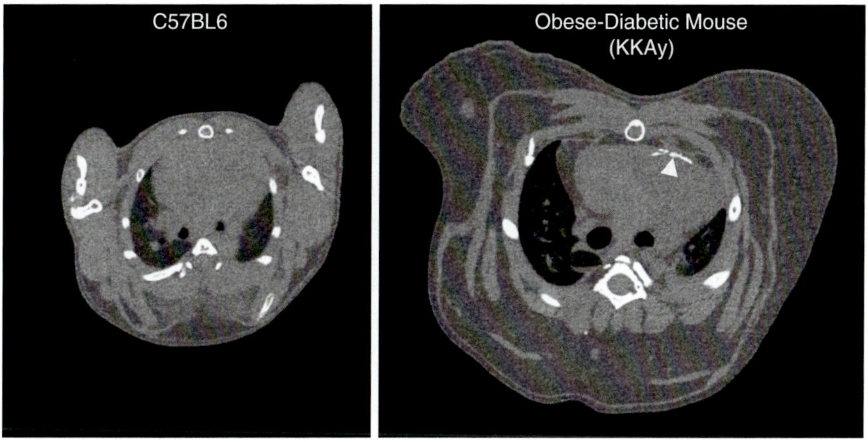

Fig. 11.6 Chest computed tomographic images of C57BL6 and KKAy (obese diabetic mouse)

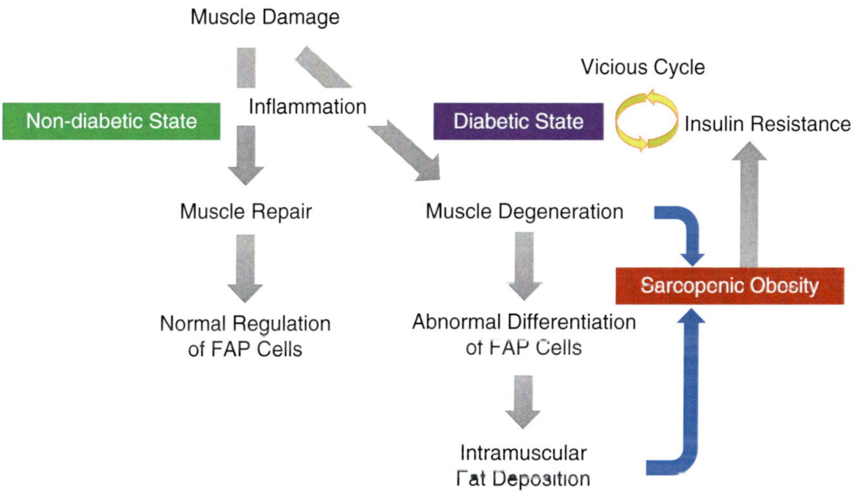

Fig. 11.7 Schematic comparison of muscle repair after muscle damage with and without diabetes (with reference to ref. [26]). *FAP* fibro-adipocyte progenitor

muscle 2 weeks after CTX injection showed significantly impaired muscle regeneration with replacement by fat deposition in KKAy. Ectopic fat was considered to be derived from fibro-adipocyte progenitors (FAP) evaluated by immunohistochemical staining, suggesting that diabetes enhanced sarcopenic obesity possibly due to abnormal FAP differentiation (Fig. 11.7). Therefore, one possible factor in myosteatosis is anomalous FAP differentiation under a diabetic condition. Prevention of intramuscular fat deposition with consideration of muscle degeneration is one of the critical targets to prevent sarcopenic obesity, focusing on abnormal FAP differentiation.

11.5 Epi-memory in the Skeletal Muscle

Early exposure to hyperglycemia predisposes individuals to the development of diabetic complications. Such a phenomenon is called "metabolic memory" or the "legacy effect." It is reported that skeletal muscle is also programmable and can remember early-life metabolic stimuli, affecting its function in adult life. Jacobsen et al. reported that only 5 days of high-fat feeding introduced widespread DNA methylation changes affecting 6508 of 14,475 genes [27]. Sharples et al. reviewed the role of epi-memory in the skeletal muscle [28] and reported that skeletal muscle cells have increased susceptibility to impaired differentiation after encountering TNF-α inflammatory stress in later proliferative life if the cells have experienced earlier, acute TNF-α stress [29]. Although the relation between diabetes and skeletal muscle is not well known, skeletal muscle memory with epigenetic modification is anticipated to be the next generation of targeted therapy to improve metabolic disorder-induced muscle dysfunction.

11.6 Therapeutic Approaches

To prevent muscle atrophy, different therapeutic approaches have been tried such as dietary supplementation; compounds with anabolic activity; anti-inflammatory drugs, modulating the energetic crisis of the skeletal muscle; muscle-wasting inhibitors; and exercise training [30]. Cetrone reviewed the effect of antidiabetic drugs on sarcopenia associated with T2DM [31]. Insulin therapy stimulated protein anabolism in younger but not older patients, who are in an insulin-resistant state characterizing the aging process, and failed to prevent atrophy [30]. In overweight/obese older men undergoing weight loss, pioglitazone increased visceral fat loss but did not improve skeletal muscle loss [32]. More marked muscle atrophy was found in glibenclamide-treated subjects [33]. However, no reports of atrophy were found in subjects receiving other sulfonylureas and glinides. There are no reports on the in vivo effects of metformin on skeletal muscle atrophy in humans and animals [31]. Very recently, a dipeptidyl peptidase-4 inhibitor was reported to improve exercise capacity and mitochondrial biogenesis in mice with heart failure by improvement of skeletal muscle abnormalities via activation of glucagon-like peptide-1 receptor signaling [34]. No evidence of direct muscle effects of sodium glucose co-transporter inhibitors has been found, to date.

On the other hand, exercise has been especially expected to break the vicious cycle of muscle atrophy in T2DM patients. Endurance exercise training stimulates modifying factors such as p38MAPK, AMP-activated protein kinase, and sirtuin 3 to activate specific transcriptional regulators such as peroxisome proliferator-activated receptor-gamma coactivator-1α (PGC-1α), resulting in an increase in mitochondrial volume and biogenesis [15]. Interestingly, Sharples et al. indicated that acute and chronic exercise stimuli can cause epigenetic modifications in skeletal muscle. Moreover, an exercise stimulus in the parents can be remembered by the offspring [28]. Although many beneficial effects of exercise have been reported, further clinical investigation is required to determine how to improve sarcopenia in T2DM patients by therapeutic exercise.

In conclusion, diabetes-induced sarcopenia impairs quality of life in T2DM patients with a vicious cycle of muscle atrophy with less activity and insulin resistance, resulting in poorer control of glucose metabolism.

References

1. Baumgartner RN. Body composition in healthy aging. Ann N Y Acad Sci. 2000;904:437–48.
2. Sinclair AJ, Rodriguez-Manas L. Diabetes and frailty: two converging conditions? Can J Diabetes. 2016;40(1):77–83. doi:10.1016/j.jcjd.2015.09.004.
3. Bauer JM, Sieber CC. Sarcopenia and frailty: a clinician's controversial point of view. Exp Gerontol. 2008;43(7):674–8. doi:10.1016/j.exger.2008.03.007.
4. Mithal A, Bonjour JP, Boonen S, Burckhardt P, Degens H, El Hajj Fuleihan G, et al. Impact of nutrition on muscle mass, strength, and performance in older adults. Osteoporos Int. 2013;24(5):1555–66. doi:10.1007/s00198-012-2236-y.
5. Buford TW, Anton SD, Judge AR, Marzetti E, Wohlgemuth SE, Carter CS, et al. Models of accelerated sarcopenia: critical pieces for solving the puzzle of age-related muscle atrophy. Ageing Res Rev. 2010;9(4):369–83. doi:10.1016/j.arr.2010.04.004.
6. Park SW, Goodpaster BH, Lee JS, Kuller LH, Boudreau R, de Rekeneire N, et al. Excessive loss of skeletal muscle mass in older adults with type 2 diabetes. Diabetes Care. 2009;32(11):1993–7. doi:10.2337/dc09 0264.
7. Kim TN, Park MS, Yang SJ, Yoo HJ, Kang HJ, Song W, et al. Prevalence and determinant factors of sarcopenia in patients with type 2 diabetes: the Korean Sarcopenic Obesity Study (KSOS). Diabetes Care. 2010;33(7):1497–9. doi:10.2337/dc09-2310.
8. Batsis JA, Mackenzie TA, Barre LK, Lopez-Jimenez F, Bartels SJ. Sarcopenia, sarcopenic obesity and mortality in older adults: results from the National Health and Nutrition Examination Survey III. Eur J Clin Nutr. 2014;68(9):1001–7. doi:10.1038/ejcn.2014.117.
9. Atkins JL, Whincup PH, Morris RW, Lennon LT, Papacosta O, Wannamethee SG. Sarcopenic obesity and risk of cardiovascular disease and mortality: a population-based cohort study of older men. J Am Geriatr Soc. 2014;62(2):253–60. doi:10.1111/jgs.12652.
10. Brown JC, Harhay MO, Harhay MN. Sarcopenia and mortality among a population-based sample of community-dwelling older adults. J Cachexia Sarcopenia Muscle. 2016;7(3):290–8. doi:10.1002/jcsm.12073.
11. Ma J, Hwang SJ, McMahon GM, Curhan GC, McLean RR, Murabito JM, et al. Mid-adulthood cardiometabolic risk factor profiles of sarcopenic obesity. Obesity (Silver Spring). 2016;24(2):526–34. doi:10.1002/oby.21356.
12. Russell ST, Rajani S, Dhadda RS, Tisdale MJ. Mechanism of induction of muscle protein loss by hyperglycaemia. Exp Cell Res. 2009;315(1):16–25. doi:10.1016/j.yexcr.2008.10.002.
13. Fadini GP, Ferraro F, Quaini F, Asahara T, Madeddu P. Concise review: diabetes, the bone marrow niche, and impaired vascular regeneration. Stem Cells Transl Med. 2014;3(8):949–57. doi:10.5966/sctm.2014-0052.
14. Fujimaki S, Wakabayashi T, Takemasa T, Asashima M, Kuwabara T. Diabetes and stem cell function. Biomed Res Int. 2015;2015:592915. doi:10.1155/2015/592915.
15. Russell AP, Foletta VC, Snow RJ, Wadley GD. Skeletal muscle mitochondria: a major player in exercise, health and disease. Biochim Biophys Acta. 2014;1840(4):1276–84. doi:10.1016/j.bbagen.2013.11.016.

16. Dirks ML, Wall BT, van de Valk B, Holloway TM, Holloway GP, Chabowski A, et al. One week of bed rest leads to substantial muscle atrophy and induces whole-body insulin resistance in the absence of skeletal muscle lipid accumulation. Diabetes. 2016;65(10):2862–75. doi:10.2337/db15-1661.
17. Petersen KF, Befroy D, Dufour S, Dziura J, Ariyan C, Rothman DL, et al. Mitochondrial dysfunction in the elderly: possible role in insulin resistance. Science. 2003;300(5622):1140–2. doi:10.1126/science.1082889.
18. Romanello V, Sandri M. Mitochondrial quality control and muscle mass maintenance. Front Physiol. 2015;6:422. doi:10.3389/fphys.2015.00422.
19. Snijders T, Wall BT, Dirks ML, Senden JM, Hartgens F, Dolmans J, et al. Muscle disuse atrophy is not accompanied by changes in skeletal muscle satellite cell content. Clin Sci (Lond). 2014;126(8):557–66. doi:10.1042/CS20130295.
20. Dirks ML, Wall BT, Nilwik R, Weerts DH, Verdijk LB, van Loon LJ. Skeletal muscle disuse atrophy is not attenuated by dietary protein supplementation in healthy older men. J Nutr. 2014;144(8):1196–203. doi:10.3945/jn.114.194217.
21. Buch A, Carmeli E, Boker LK, Marcus Y, Shefer G, Kis O, et al. Muscle function and fat content in relation to sarcopenia, obesity and frailty of old age--An overview. Exp Gerontol. 2016;76:25–32. doi:10.1016/j.exger.2016.01.008.
22. Goodpaster BH, Krishnaswami S, Resnick H, Kelley DE, Haggerty C, Harris TB, et al. Association between regional adipose tissue distribution and both type 2 diabetes and impaired glucose tolerance in elderly men and women. Diabetes Care. 2003;26(2):372–9.
23. Visser M, Kritchevsky SB, Goodpaster BH, Newman AB, Nevitt M, Stamm E, et al. Leg muscle mass and composition in relation to lower extremity performance in men and women aged 70 to 79: the health, aging and body composition study. J Am Geriatr Soc. 2002;50(5):897–904. doi:jgs50217 [pii].
24. Reinders I, Murphy RA, Brouwer IA, Visser M, Launer L, Siggeirsdottir K, et al. Muscle quality and myosteatosis: novel associations with mortality risk: The Age, Gene/Environment Susceptibility (AGES)-Reykjavik Study. Am J Epidemiol. 2016;183(1):53–60. doi:10.1093/aje/kwv153.
25. Hamrick MW, McGee-Lawrence ME, Frechette DM. Fatty infiltration of skeletal muscle: mechanisms and comparisons with bone marrow adiposity. Front Endocrinol (Lausanne). 2016;7:69. doi:10.3389/fendo.2016.00069.
26. Mogi M, Kohara K, Nakaoka H, Kan-No H, Tsukuda K, Wang XL, et al. Diabetic mice exhibited a peculiar alteration in body composition with exaggerated ectopic fat deposition after muscle injury due to anomalous cell differentiation. J Cachexia Sarcopenia Muscle. 2016;7(2):213–24. doi:10.1002/jcsm.12044.
27. Jacobsen SC, Brons C, Bork-Jensen J, Ribel-Madsen R, Yang B, Lara E, et al. Effects of short-term high-fat overfeeding on genome-wide DNA methylation in the skeletal muscle of healthy young men. Diabetologia. 2012;55(12):3341–9. doi:10.1007/s00125-012-2717-8.
28. Sharples AP, Stewart CE, Seaborne RA. Does skeletal muscle have an 'epi'-memory? The role of epigenetics in nutritional programming, metabolic disease, aging and exercise. Aging Cell. 2016;15(4):603–16. doi:10.1111/acel.12486.
29. Sharples AP, Polydorou I, Hughes DC, Owens DJ, Hughes TM, Stewart CE. Skeletal muscle cells possess a 'memory' of acute early life TNF-alpha exposure: role of epigenetic adaptation. Biogerontology. 2016;17(3):603–17. doi:10.1007/s10522-015-9604-x.
30. Fanzani A, Conraads VM, Penna F, Martinet W. Molecular and cellular mechanisms of skeletal muscle atrophy: an update. J Cachexia Sarcopenia Muscle. 2012;3(3):163–79. doi:10.1007/s13539-012-0074-6.
31. Cetrone M, Mele A, Tricarico D. Effects of the antidiabetic drugs on the age-related atrophy and sarcopenia associated with diabetes type II. Curr Diabetes Rev. 2014;10(4):231–7. doi:CDR-EPUB-62415 [pii].

32. Shea MK, Nicklas BJ, Marsh AP, Houston DK, Miller GD, Isom S, et al. The effect of pioglitazone and resistance training on body composition in older men and women undergoing hypocaloric weight loss. Obesity (Silver Spring). 2011;19(8):1636–46. doi:10.1038/oby.2010.327.
33. Mele A, Calzolaro S, Cannone G, Cetrone M, Conte D, Tricarico D. Database search of spontaneous reports and pharmacological investigations on the sulfonylureas and glinides-induced atrophy in skeletal muscle. Pharmacol Res Perspect. 2014;2(1):e00028. doi:10.1002/prp2.28.
34. Takada S, Masaki Y, Kinugawa S, Matsumoto J, Furihata T, Mizushima W, et al. Dipeptidyl peptidase-4 inhibitor improved exercise capacity and mitochondrial biogenesis in mice with heart failure via activation of glucagon-like peptide-1 receptor signalling. Cardiovasc Res. 2016;111(4):338–47. doi:10.1093/cvr/cvw182.

Chapter 12
Diabetes and Frailty

Mitsutaka Yakabe and Sumito Ogawa

Abstract Frailty is an age-related condition characterized by a decline in the reserve capacity of multiple physiological systems, which leads to geriatric syndromes, disability, and mortality. Frailty is often observed among diabetic patients. In the clinical practice for frail diabetic elderly, glycemic control should be personalized in order to minimize the risk of severe hypoglycemia and hyperglycemia. Other interventions for frailty with diabetes include nutrition, exercise, and avoiding polypharmacy.

Keywords Frailty • Fatigue • Falls • Geriatric syndrome

12.1 Introduction

Worldwide population aging is accelerating, and the most problematic expression of population aging is the clinical condition of frailty. Frailty develops as a consequence of age-related decline in multiple physiological systems, which results in a vulnerability to sudden health status changes triggered by relatively minor stressor events [1].

In this chapter, we describe the relationship between frailty and diabetes and the management of frailty with diabetes.

12.2 Definition of Frailty

Frailty is a dynamic, age-related condition characterized by a decline in the reserve capacity of multiple physiological systems [1]. When exposed to an apparently small stress, such as a new drug, minor illness, or minor surgery, a healthy elderly can almost entirely recover in a relatively short time. In a frail elderly, however, resistance to stressors is decreased. Therefore, the stress results in a striking and

M. Yakabe • S. Ogawa (✉)
Department of Geriatric Medicine, Graduate School of Medicine, The University of Tokyo, 7-3-1, Bunkyo-ku, Tokyo, Japan
e-mail: suogawa-tky@umin.ac.jp

S.-i. Yamagishi (ed.), *Diabetes and Aging-related Complications*,
https://doi.org/10.1007/978-981-10-4376-5_12

disproportionate change in health state—i.e., from independent to dependent, mobile to immobile, postural stability to proneness to falling, or lucid to delirious—and the person's functional ability might not recover to the previous level even after the stress was removed.

Frailty is supposed to be one of geriatric syndromes. It leads to increased risk of adverse health outcomes, such as low mobility, falls, functional decline, hospitalization, and death. The world is aging rapidly, and the number of frail elderly will lead to increased cost of healthcare and social security [2].

12.3 Clinical Presentations of Frailty

12.3.1 Fatigue

In older adults, fatigue is common and associated with functional deficits and survival. A simple question whether the patient "feels tired most of the time" could identify older adults with a higher risk of mortality [3].

12.3.2 Falls

Balance and gait impairment are major features of frailty and are important risk factors for falls. Spontaneous falls occur in severe frailty and are typically repeated, associated with fear of further falls that makes the patient less mobile [1].

12.3.3 Delirium

Delirium is characterized by the rapid onset of fluctuating confusion and impaired awareness. Delirium is related to reduced integrity of brain function and is independently associated with adverse outcomes [1].

12.3.4 Others

Frail elderly are susceptible to unintended weight loss, frequent infections, and fluctuating disability [1].

12.4 Pathophysiology of Frailty

Many organ systems have redundant capacity. A gradual decrease in physiological reserve occurs with aging. However, this decrease is accelerated in frailty and homeostatic mechanisms start to fail. Aging promotes cumulative decline in several physiological systems, the subsequent depletion of homeostatic reserve, and vulnerability to disproportionate changes in health status after minor stressor events. These complex aging mechanisms are determined by underlying genetic, epigenetic, and environmental factors [1].

In a cross-sectional study of 1002 women, abnormality in three or more systems among six different physiological systems (hematological, inflammatory, hormonal, adiposity, neuromuscular, and micronutrient) was a strong predictor of frailty. The brain, endocrine system, immune system, and skeletal muscle are intrinsically interrelated and are the organ systems that are best studied in the development of frailty [1].

12.4.1 The Frail Brain

Aging is associated with structural and physiological changes in the brain. In particular, the hippocampus could be affected by changes in synaptic function, protein transport, and mitochondrial function, which is involved in the pathophysiology of cognitive decline and Alzheimer's dementia. The aging brain is also characterized by structural and functional changes to microglial cells, which are activated by brain injury and local and systemic inflammation and become primed to small stimuli with aging, potentially causing damage and neuronal death [1].

12.4.2 The Frail Endocrine System

The brain and endocrine system are linked intrinsically through the hypothalamo-pituitary axis, which controls metabolism and energy use through the signaling action of hormones. During aging, production of three major circulating hormones decreases—(1) insulin-like growth factor-1 (IGF-1) and growth hormone, (2) sex hormones (estrogen and estradiol), and (3) adrenocortical hormones [1]. These could also be involved in the development of frailty.

12.4.3 The Frail Immune System

The aging immune system is characterized by a reduction in stem cells, changes in T-lymphocyte production, blunting of the B-cell-controlled antibody response, and reduced phagocytic activity of neutrophils, macrophages, and natural killer cells. This senescent immune system might function adequately in the quiescent state but might fail to respond appropriately to the stress of acute inflammation. Evidence suggests that chronic low-grade inflammation has a major role in the pathophysiology of frailty. Several inflammatory cytokines have been associated with frailty: interleukin-6 (IL-6), C-reactive protein (CRP), tumor necrosis factor-α (TNFα), and C-X-C motif chemokine ligand-10 (CXCL10) [1].

12.4.4 The Frail Skeletal Muscle (Sarcopenia)

Sarcopenia is a debilitating condition characterized by progressive loss of muscle mass, strength, and function. It is common in elderly and results in frailty, disability, and high mortality [4]. Sarcopenia is supposed to be an aspect of physical frailty. Fried et al. proposed the cycle of frailty, in which sarcopenia was one of the main potential causes of frailty [5]. In this cycle, sarcopenia and five components of frailty—weight loss, exhaustion, weakness, slowness, and low physical activity—are closely related and create a vicious circle (Fig. 12.1) [6].

For details about sarcopenia, see Chap. 11 ("Diabetes and Sarcopenia").

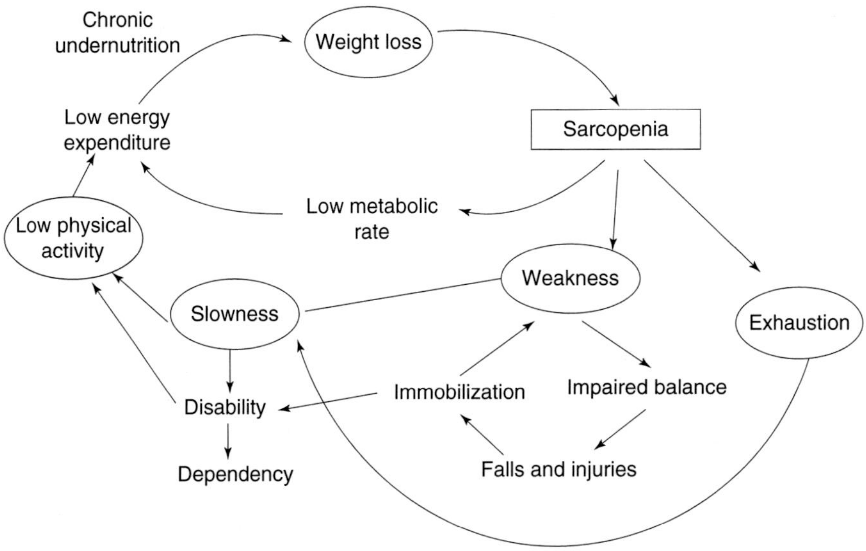

Fig. 12.1 The cycle of frailty (Adapted from Xue GL et al. [6])

12.5 Diagnostic Criteria of Frailty

Frailty is considered potentially reversible. Therefore, early detection of frailty and proper interventions are important. However, its assessment still lacks gold standard. Instruments for assessing frailty can be divided into two categories: the physical phenotype models and the multi-domain models.

An example of the physical phenotype models commonly used is Fried's criteria [5]. Fried et al. determined frailty by five physical components: (1) unintentional weight loss, (2) exhaustion, (3) weakness, (4) slowness, and (5) low physical activity. Persons are diagnosed as pre-frail when one or two of the five components are present, and they are diagnosed as frail when three or more are present. Based on Fried's criteria, the Women's Health and Aging Studies (WHAS) and Cardiovascular Health Study (CHS) also present frailty-defining criteria [7] (Table 12.1).

The multi-domain models are based on a broader concept of frailty and include the decline in the medical, psychological, cognitive, functional, and social domains.

Table 12.1 Proposed diagnostic criteria of frailty

Components	Fried's criteria	CHS	WHAS
Weight loss	Unintentional loss of ≥4.5 kg in the past year	Baseline: Lost >10 pounds unintentionally in last year Follow-up: (weight in previous year-current weight)/(weight in previous year) ≥0.05 and the loss was unintentional	Baseline: Either of: 1. (weight at age 60—weight at exam)/(weight at age 60) ≥0.1 2. BMI at exam <18.5 Follow-up: Either of : 1. BMI at exam <18.5 2. (weight in previous year-current weight)/(weight in previous year) ≥0.05 and the loss was unintentional
Exhaustion	Poor endurance and energy, self-reported from the Center for Epidemiologic Studies Depression Scale	Self-report of either of: 1. Felt that everything I did was an effort in the last week 2. Could not get going in the last week	Self-report of any of: 1. Low usual energy level1 (≤3, range 0–10) 2. Felt unusually tired in last 2 months 3. Felt unusually weak in the past 2 months
Low physical activity	Lowest quintile of kilocalories of physical activity during the past week, measured by the Minnesota Leisure Activity Scale	Women: Kcal < 270 on activity scale (18 items) Men: Kcal < 383 on activity scale (18 items)	Women: Kcal < 90 on activity scale (6 items) Men: Kcal <128 on activity scale (6 items)

(continued)

Table 12.1 (continued)

Components	Fried's criteria	CHS	WHAS
Slowness	Walking speed under the lowest quintile adjusted for sex and height	Walking 15 feet (4.57 m) at usual pace Women: Time ≥7 s for height ≤159 cm Time ≥6 s for height > 159 cm Men: Time ≥7 s for height ≤173 cm Time ≥6 s for height > 173 cm	Walking 4 m at usual pace Women: Speed ≤4.57/7 m/s for height ≤159 cm Speed ≤4.57/6 m/s for height > 159 cm Men: Speed ≤4.57/7 m/s for height ≤173 cm Speed ≤4.57/6 m/s for height > 173 cm
Weakness	Handgrip strength in the lowest 20% quintile adjusted for sex and body mass index	Grip strength Women: ≤17 kg for BMI ≤23 ≤17.3 kg for BMI 23.1–26 ≤ 18 kg for BMI 26.1–29 ≤21 kg for BMI >29 Men: ≤29 kg for BMI ≤24 ≤30 kg for BMI 24.1–26 ≤30 kg for BMI 26.1–	Grip strength: Same as in CHS

Adapted from Fried et al. [5] and Xue QL et al. [7]

One of the tools is the Kihon Checklist (KCL), which was established in Japan (Table 12.2) [8]. This score closely correlated with validated assessments of physical functions, nutritional state, cognitive function, depressive mood, and the number of frailty phenotypes defined by the CHS criteria. At a cutoff KCL score of 7/8, the sensitivity and specificity for estimating frailty were 89.5% and 80.7%, respectively. At a cutoff of 3/4 for pre-frail status, those for estimating pre-frail status were 70.3% and 78.3%, respectively.

12.6 The Relationship Between Type 2 Diabetes and Frailty

Diabetes has been associated with an increased risk of developing physical disability in elderly. Several studies have shown that diabetic patients aged 65 or over were more likely to be frail than nondiabetic elderly. These studies also reported that frail patients with diabetes had a higher mortality than non-frail patients, and the presence of frailty was an independent risk factor for mortality [9]. Diabetes mellitus is an independent fall risk factor among elderly nursing home residents [10]. Chronic conditions such as visual disturbances, diabetic complications, comorbidities, and depression could affect patients with diabetes and contribute to frailty.

Table 12.2 The Kihon checklist [8]

Question	Score
1. Do you go out by bus or train by yourself?	□0. YES □1. NO
2. Do you go shopping to buy daily necessities by yourself?	□0. YES □1. NO
3. Do you manage your own deposits and savings at the bank?	□0. YES □1. NO
4. Do you sometimes visit your friends?	□0. YES □1. NO
5. Do you turn to your family or friends for advice?	□0. YES □1. NO
6. Do you normally climb stairs without using handrail or wall for support?	□0. YES □1. NO
7. Do you normally stand up from a chair without any aids?	□0. YES □1. NO
8. Do you normally walk continuously for 15 min?	□0. YES □1. NO
9. Have you experienced a fall in the past year?	□1. YES □0. NO
10. Do you have a fear of falling while walking?	□1. YES □0. NO
11. Have you lost 2 kg or more in the past 6 months?	□1. YES □0. NO
12. Height, cm; weight, kg. If BMI (body mass index) is less than 18.5, this item is scored	□1. YES □0. NO
13. Do you have any difficulties eating tough foods compared to 6 months ago?	□1. YES □0. NO
14. Have you choked on your tea or soup recently?	□1. YES □0. NO
15. Do you often experience having a dry mouth?	□1. YES □0. NO
16. Do you go out at least once a week?	□0. YES □1. NO
17. Do you go out less frequently compared to last year?	□1. YES □0. NO
18. Do your family or your friends point out your memory loss? e.g., "You ask the same question over and over again"	□1. YES □0. NO
19. Do you make a call by looking up phone numbers?	□0. YES □1. NO
20. Do you find yourself not knowing today's date?	□1. YES □0. NO
21. In the last 2 weeks, have you felt a lack of fulfillment in your daily life?	□1. YES □0. NO
22. In the last 2 weeks, have you felt a lack of joy when doing the things you used to enjoy?	□1. YES □0. NO
23. In the last 2 weeks, have you felt difficulty in doing what you could do easily before?	□1. YES □0. NO
24. In the last 2 weeks, have you felt helpless?	□1. YES □0. NO
25. In the last 2 weeks, have you felt tired without a reason?	□1. YES □0. NO
	Total score /25

One study shows that frailty was associated with increased risk of incident type 2 diabetes in community-dwelling nondiabetic elderly [11]. Frail elderly are supposed to have higher oxidative stress, higher levels of proinflammatory cytokines, increased deoxyribonucleic acid damage, and shorter telomere length. These might play a role in the pathogenesis of type 2 diabetes.

As addressed in 13.5, psychological states such as depression are important aspects of frailty. One study reports that diabetic old men have a higher risk of depression than nondiabetic men and, interestingly, that the association of diabetes duration and the risk of depression is "J shaped" [12].

One mechanism that diabetes causes frailty might be that diabetes exacerbates inflammation. In a systematic review and meta-analysis of the relationship between inflammation and frailty, both frail and pre-frail elderly had significantly higher serum level of interleukin-6 and C-reactive protein (CRP) compared with non-frail elderly. Frailty and pre-frailty were also associated with elevated white blood cell and fibrinogen levels [13]. Another mechanism might be that sarcopenia and frailty may share the similar pathway for multiple pathologic processes in elderly. Sarcopenia may be an intermediate step in the development of frailty in patients with diabetes. For details about the relationship between frailty and sarcopenia, see Chap. 11 ("Diabetes and Sarcopenia").

12.7 Management of Frailty with Type 2 Diabetes

12.7.1 The Goal of Glycemic Control

There is no definite guideline for type 2 diabetes in frail elderly. Very tight glucose control may often be not desirable. An HbA1c less than 7% can increase the likelihood of hypoglycemia [14]. Fall risk markedly increased when HbA1c was 7% or below, regardless of frailty status [15].

In 2012, the American Diabetes Association (ADA) and the American Geriatrics Society (AGS) recommended a team approach to treat older patients with diabetes, including individualized treatment plans and education to patients and their caregivers. The goal of treatment is to establish acceptable glycemic control and minimize the risk of acute complications such as hypoglycemia and serious hyperglycemia [16]. Blood pressure and lipid control are also described. They are shown in Table 12.3.

According to the International Diabetes Federation, an HbA1c target of 7.0–8.0% is suitable for functionally independent older people with a reasonable life expectancy, and a target of $\leq$8.5% is appropriate for frail older people and those with dementia and a life expectancy of less than 10 years [17].

The DCPNS/PATH guidelines recommend that HbA1c should be maintained at or above 8% rather than below a specific level because lower HbA1c levels are associated with increased hypoglycemic events without accruing meaningful benefit for frail elderly [18]. The Italian Association of Medical Diabetologists has developed a guideline, in which six algorithms are proposed, and HbA1c <9.0% is recommended for elderly frail patients with mild/moderate hyperglycemia [19].

In 2016, the Japan Diabetes Society and the Japan Geriatrics Society announced a guideline for glycemic control in diabetes of the elderly (Table 12.4). Characteristics of the guideline are that it sets goals depending on the patients' physical and cognitive status. They say that the goals could be set flexibly.

These guidelines might be useful, but setting personalized goals independent of these guidelines could be acceptable.

Table 12.3 A framework for considering treatment goals for glycemia, blood pressure, and dyslipidemia in older adults with diabetes [16]

Patient characteristics/health status	Rationale	Reasonable A1C goal (a lower goal may be set for an individual if achievable without recurrent or severe hypoglycemia or undue treatment burden)	Fasting or preprandial glucose (mg/dL)	Bedtime glucose (mg/dL)	Blood pressure (mmHg)	Lipids
Healthy (few coexisting chronic illnesses, intact cognitive, and functional status)	Longer remaining life expectancy	<7.5%	90–130	90–150	<140/80	Statin unless contraindicated or not tolerated
Complex/intermediate (multiple coexisting chronic illnesses or 2+ instrumental ADL impairments or mild to moderate cognitive impairment)	Intermediate remaining life expectancy, high treatment burden, hypoglycemia vulnerability, fall risk	<8.0%	90–150	100–180	<140/80	Statin unless contraindicated or not tolerated
Very complex/poor health (Long-term care or end-stage chronic illnesses or moderate to severe cognitive impairment or 2+ ADL dependencies)	Limited remaining life expectancy makes benefit uncertain	<8.5%	100–180	110–200	<150/90	Consider likelihood of benefit with statin (secondary prevention more so than primary)

Table 12.4 The guideline by the Japan Diabetes Society and the Japan Geriatrics Society for glycemic control in diabetes of the elderly

Physical and cognitive status of patients		<Category 1> Normal cognitive function and normal ADL	<Category 2> "Mild cognitive impairment to mild dementia" or "lower IADL but normal BADL"	<Category 3> "Moderate to severe dementia" or "lower BADL" or "many comorbidities or multiple organ dysfunction"
Medication* with high risk of causing hypoglycemia used?	No	<7.0%	<7.0%	<8.0%
	Yes	6.5–7.4% (65–74 y.o.) 7.0–7.9% (over 75 y.o.)	7.0–7.9%	7.5–8.4%

*Insulin, sulfonylurea, or glinide

12.7.2 Medications

Elderly tend to have many morbidities and take many medicines. Polypharmacy is supposed to be a major cause of frailty in older persons. Prescriptions for frail elderly should be minimal. STOPP and START (Screening Tool of Older Persons' Potentially Inappropriate Prescriptions and Screening Tool to Alert Doctors to the Right Treatment) are screening tools that identify potentially inappropriate prescribing in older adults [20]. For example, anticholinergic medicines can cause cognitive decline and frailty. Overtreatment of blood pressure results in hypotension and falls. Clinicians who prescribe elderly patients should understand the effect of aging on physiology and pharmacokinetics, balance risks versus benefits, and listen to patient and caregiver concerns.

Treatment based on DPP-4 (dipeptidyl peptidase-4) inhibitors might be beneficial for frail elderly [21]. They ensure high rates of adequate glycemic control, are associated with a low risk of hypoglycemia, appear to have a neutral effect on body weight, and can potentially improve quality of life.

Sodium glucose co-transporter 2 (SGLT2) inhibitors have been developed and used in the treatment of type 2 diabetes. Effects of SGLT2 inhibitors on elderly people have not been well studied. According to a study about efficacy and safety of canagliflozin in individuals aged 75 or over, beneficial effects were observed, but overall incidence of adverse effects was higher in participants aged 75 or over than in those younger than 75 [22]. SGLT2 inhibitors could be a cause of weight loss. It should be recognized that frailty might not be a desirable indication for SGLT2 inhibitors.

One study shows that statin treatment was significantly associated with reduced 3-year mortality independently of age and multidimensional impairment in community-dwelling frail older patients with DM [23].

12.7.3 Nutrition and Weight Control

In general, diabetic patients should perform calorie restriction and control their weight in an appropriate range (e.g., BMI 18.5–25.0). However, this might not necessarily be applicable to frail elderly patients. Many older people do not consume sufficient amounts of dietary intake and protein. The current recommended dietary allowance (RDA) of dietary protein is 0.8 g/kg/day, but higher amount of protein might be needed for frail elderly. Caloric supplements between meals could increase weight and improve nutritional status. A review of guidelines recommends that elderly diabetic patients may have regular diets instead of diabetic diets, especially if they are in nursing homes [24].

Unintended weight loss and appetite loss are not rare in the elderly. Weight loss has been shown to be associated with accelerated mortality in older persons. It also leads to loss of muscle and bone, increasing frailty, falls, and hip fractures. When weight loss is observed in a frail elderly patient, there are various possible reasons, for example, internal diseases (such as cancers and infections), mental disorders (such as depression), medications, dysphagia, dental problems, eating problems, and social problems. Treatable causes of weight loss should not be overlooked.

12.7.4 Exercise

Resistance exercise involves muscles working hard against an applied force or weight such as in weight lifting. Aerobic exercise improves cardiovascular fitness and endurance capacity. Both exercises have been shown to prevent the decline in muscle mass and strength with age [9]. One resistance exercise training session per week could improve muscle strength.

12.7.5 Sarcopenia

Morley et al. suggested that the management of frailty in patients with diabetes initially should focus on the prevention of sarcopenia [25]. Until now, no pharmacologic agent has been proven to be as efficacious as nutrition plus exercise in order to prevent or treat sarcopenia, so this approach is the key strategy. For details, see Chap. 11 ("Diabetes and Sarcopenia").

12.7.6 Treatable Causes of Fatigue

Treatable causes of fatigue should be considered: they include vitamin B12 deficiency, hypoadrenalism, hypothyroidism, anemia, sleep apnea, hypotension, syncope, and depression. Treatment of sleep apnea in diabetic individuals results in lower blood pressure, better glycemic control, and an improvement in quality adjusted life years. Depression is more common in diabetic individuals, and psychological and pharmacological interventions positively affect depression and improve glycemic control. Diabetes is commonly associated with autonomic neuropathy, which leads to orthostatic hypotension, arrhythmias, and syncope.

12.8 Type 1 Diabetes and Frailty

Few studies have described the management of frailty with type 1 diabetes. Older adults with type 1 diabetes are a heterogeneous group. With long-duration diabetes, hypoglycemia is common, regardless of HbA1c level [26]. Individualized treatment plans using more complex insulin regimens and lower glycemic goals with frequent SMBG are recommended in healthy older adults. For frail elderly, however, it may be difficult to follow complex insulin regimens due to problems with cognition, mobility, vision, hearing, and depression. Guidelines for older individuals with type 1 diabetes are lacking, so the treatment could be based on the principles by the ADA and AGS [16]. The treatment regimens should be modified with the goal of minimizing hypoglycemia and severe hyperglycemia and maximizing quality of life [26].

12.9 Conclusions

Frailty is a serious problem in the era of world population aging. Especially in diabetic patients who are inclined to have comorbidities, early identification of frailty and proper interventions for frailty are important. Clinicians who examine diabetic elderly patients should be attentive to frailty and its complications, and personalized approach should be performed. Many clinical questions about frailty and diabetes remain unsolved. Further research is needed and more evidence should be established.

References

1. Clegg A, Young J, Iliffe S, Rikkert MO, Rockwood K. Frailty in elderly people. Lancet. 2013;381(9868):752–62. doi:10.1016/s0140-6736(12)62167-9.
2. Azzopardi RV, Vermeiren S, Gorus E, Habbig AK, Petrovic M, Van Den Noortgate N, et al. Linking frailty instruments to the international classification of functioning, disability, and health: a systematic review. J Am Med Dir Assoc. 2016;17(11):1066.e1–1066.e11. doi:10.1016/j.jamda.2016.07.023.
3. Hardy SE, Studenski SA. Fatigue predicts mortality in older adults. J Am Geriatr Soc. 2008;56(10):1910–4. doi:10.1111/j.1532-5415.2008.01957.x.

4. Yakabe M, Ogawa S, Akishita M. Clinical Manifestations and Pathophysiology of Sarcopenia. Biomedical Sciences. 2015;1(2):10–7. doi:10.11648/j.rnat.20150102.11.
5. Fried LP, Tangen CM, Walston J, Newman AB, Hirsch C, Gottdiener J, et al. Frailty in older adults: evidence for a phenotype. J Gerontol A Biol Sci Med Sci. 2001;56(3):M146–56.
6. Xue QL, Bandeen-Roche K, Varadhan R, Zhou J, Fried LP. Initial manifestations of frailty criteria and the development of frailty phenotype in the Women's Health and Aging Study II. J Gerontol A Biol Sci Med Sci. 2008;63(9):984–90.
7. Xue QL. The frailty syndrome: definition and natural history. Clin Geriatr Med. 2011;27(1):1–15. doi:10.1016/j.cger.2010.08.009.
8. Satake S, Senda K, Hong YJ, Miura H, Endo H, Sakurai T, et al. Validity of the Kihon Checklist for assessing frailty status. Geriatr Gerontol Int. 2016;16(6):709–15. doi:10.1111/ggi.12543.
9. Jang HC. Sarcopenia, frailty, and diabetes in older adults. Diabetes Metab J. 2016;40(3):182–9. doi:10.4093/dmj.2016.40.3.182.
10. Maurer MS, Burcham J, Cheng H. Diabetes mellitus is associated with an increased risk of falls in elderly residents of a long-term care facility. J Gerontol A Biol Sci Med Sci. 2005;60(9):1157–62.
11. Veronese N, Stubbs B, Fontana L, Trevisan C, Bolzetta F, De Rui M, et al. Frailty is associated with an increased risk of incident type 2 diabetes in the elderly. J Am Med Dir Assoc. 2016;17(10):902–7. doi:10.1016/j.jamda.2016.04.021.
12. Almeida OP, McCaul K, Hankey GJ, Yeap BB, Golledge J, Norman PE, et al. Duration of diabetes and its association with depression in later life: The Health In Men Study (HIMS). Maturitas. 2016;86:3–9. doi:10.1016/j.maturitas.2016.01.003.
13. Soysal P, Stubbs B, Lucato P, Luchini C, Solmi M, Peluso R, et al. Inflammation and frailty in the elderly: a systematic review and meta-analysis. Ageing Res Rev. 2016;31:1–8. doi:10.1016/j.arr.2016.08.006.
14. Sinclair A, Morley JE. How to manage diabetes mellitus in older persons in the 21st century: applying these principles to long term diabetes care. J Am Med Dir Assoc. 2013;14(11):777–80. doi:10.1016/j.jamda.2013.09.001.
15. Nelson JM, Dufraux K, Cook PF. The relationship between glycemic control and falls in older adults. J Am Geriatr Soc. 2007;55(12):2041–4. doi:10.1111/j.1532-5415.2007.01430.x.
16. Kirkman MS, Briscoe VJ, Clark N, Florez H, Haas LB, Halter JB, et al. Diabetes in older adults: a consensus report. J Am Geriatr Soc. 2012;60(12):2342–56. doi:10.1111/jgs.12035.
17. Sinclair A, Dunning T, Rodriguez-Manas L. Diabetes in older people: new insights and remaining challenges. Lancet Diabetes Endocrinol. 2015;3(4):275–85. doi:10.1016/s2213-8587(14)70176-7.
18. Mallery LH, Ransom T, Steeves B, Cook B, Dunbar P, Moorhouse P. Evidence-informed guidelines for treating frail older adults with type 2 diabetes: from the Diabetes Care Program of Nova Scotia (DCPNS) and the Palliative and Therapeutic Harmonization (PATH) program. J Am Med Dir Assoc. 2013;14(11):801–8. doi:10.1016/j.jamda.2013.08.002.
19. Ceriello A, Gallo M, Candido R, De Micheli A, Esposito K, Gentile S, et al. Personalized therapy algorithms for type 2 diabetes: a phenotype-based approach. Pharmacogenomics Pers Med. 2014;7:129–36. doi:10.2147/pgpm.s50288.
20. Hill-Taylor B, Walsh KA, Stewart S, Hayden J, Byrne S, Sketris IS. Effectiveness of the STOPP/START (Screening Tool of Older Persons' potentially inappropriate Prescriptions/Screening Tool to Alert doctors to the Right Treatment) criteria: systematic review and meta-analysis of randomized controlled studies. J Clin Pharm Ther. 2016;41(2):158–69. doi:10.1111/jcpt.12372.
21. Avogaro A, Dardano A, de Kreutzenberg SV, Del Prato S. Dipeptidyl peptidase-4 inhibitors can minimize the hypoglycaemic burden and enhance safety in elderly people with diabetes. Diabetes Obes Metab. 2015;17(2):107–15. doi:10.1111/dom.12319.
22. Sinclair AJ, Bode B, Harris S, Vijapurkar U, Shaw W, Desai M, et al. Efficacy and safety of canagliflozin in individuals aged 75 and older with type 2 diabetes mellitus: a pooled analysis. J Am Geriatr Soc. 2016;64(3):543–52. doi:10.1111/jgs.14028.

23. Pilotto A, Panza F, Copetti M, Simonato M, Sancarlo D, Gallina P, et al. Statin treatment and mortality in community-dwelling frail older patients with diabetes mellitus: a retrospective observational study. PLoS One. 2015;10(6):e0130946. doi:10.1371/journal.pone.0130946.
24. CADTH Rapid Response Reports. Diabetic diets for frail elderly long-term care residents with type II diabetes mellitus: a review of guidelines. Ottawa: Canadian Agency for Drugs and Technologies in Health Copyright (c) 2015 Canadian Agency for Drugs and Technologies in Health; 2015.
25. Morley JE, Malmstrom TK, Rodriguez-Manas L, Sinclair AJ. Frailty, sarcopenia and diabetes. J Am Med Dir Assoc. 2014;15(12):853–9. doi:10.1016/j.jamda.2014.10.001.
26. Dhaliwal R, Weinstock RS. Management of type 1 diabetes in older adults. Diabetes Spectr. 2014;27(1):9–20. doi:10.2337/diaspect.27.1.9.

Chapter 13
Diabetes and LOH Syndrome

Hisamitsu Ide, Mayuko Kanayama, and Shigeo Horie

Abstract Age-related declines in androgen levels lead to impaired organ function known as late-onset hypogonadism (LOH). Various diseases are considered to be involved in the emergence of LOH, among which are diabetes, metabolic syndrome, arteriosclerosis, hypertension, and hyperlipidemia. Testosterone increases insulin sensitivity in muscle through functional mitochondria in muscle tissue, while lowered testosterone conversely leads to reduced glucose uptake in muscle. Diabetes mellitus (DM) and LOH are deeply interrelated diseases requiring further clinical research results in areas including diagnosis and treatment.

13.1 Testosterone Production and Function

Male hormones (androgens) are comprised of testicular testosterone, dihydrotestosterone (DHT), dehydroepiandrosterone (DHEA, originating in the adrenal glands), and DHEA-sulfate (DHEA-S), among other components. When the hypothalamus synthesizes gonadotropin releasing hormones (GnRH), the anterior pituitary gland is stimulated and secretes gonadotrophic hormones luteinizing hormone (LH) and follicle-stimulating hormone (FSH). LH stimulates the testicular Leydig cells, promoting testosterone production (Fig. 13.1). FSH works together with testosterone to facilitate spermatogenesis by acting on Sertoli cells in the seminiferous tubules. In adults, testosterone is required to maintain muscle mass and strength while decreasing visceral fat, supporting hemopoiesis, and stimulating libido [1]. Testosterone is involved in higher brain functions such as concentration and risk determination [2]. Decreased testosterone leads to deteriorated insulin sensitivity and an increased risk of metabolic syndrome and diabetes (Fig. 13.2) [3]. Additional negative impacts

H. Ide
Department of Urology, Dokkyo Medical University Koshigaya Hospital,
2-1-50, Minamikoshigaya, Koshigaya, Saitama 343-8555, Japan
e-mail: ihisamit@dokkyomed.ac.jp

M. Kanayama • S. Horie (✉)
Department of Urology, Juntendo University, Graduate School of Medicine,
2-1-1, Hongo, Bunkyo-ku, Tokyo 113-8421, Japan
e-mail: shorie@juntendo.ac.jp

S.-i. Yamagishi (ed.), *Diabetes and Aging-related Complications*,
https://doi.org/10.1007/978-981-10-4376-5_13

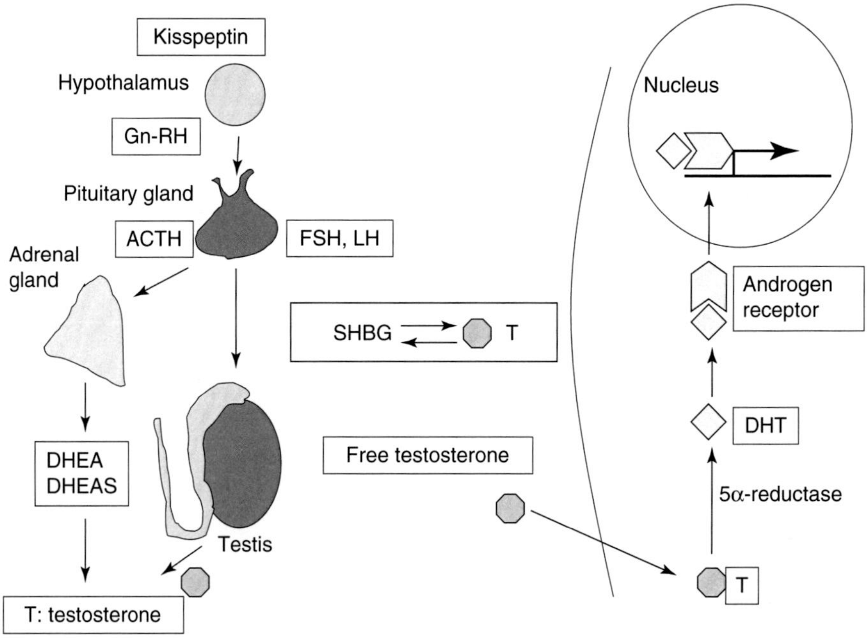

Fig. 13.1 The hypothalamic–pituitary–gonadal axis and testosterone production

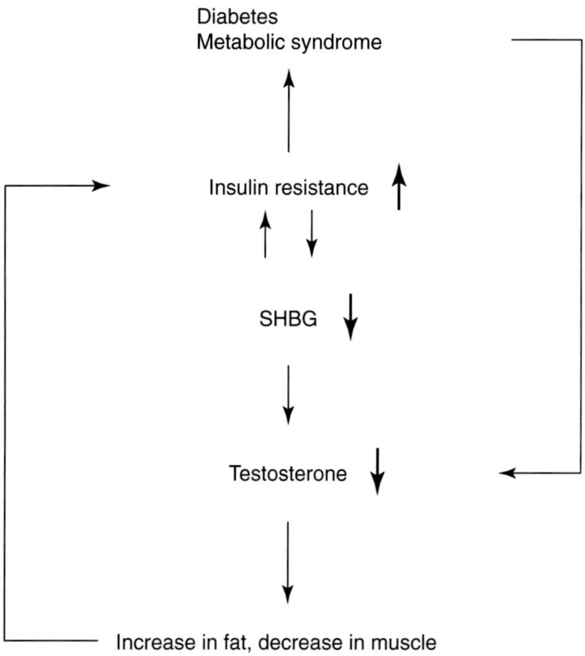

Fig. 13.2 Interaction of testosterone and insulin resistance

include worsening sexual and cognitive functions, mood disorder, increased visceral fat, decreased muscle mass, anemia, and reduced bone density, producing a considerable decline in QOL for men [4].

13.2 Action Mechanism of Testosterone Target Cells

Testosterone binds with SHBG (sex hormone-binding globulin), albumin, and other factors in the blood, with free testosterone (considered as the biologically active component) comprising approximately 2% of the aggregate (Fig. 13.1). 5α-Reductase functions to convert testosterone into active DHT in target tissues. Similarly, DHEA is believed to convert into testosterone and DHT. An androgen receptor (AR) for testosterone and DHT is a nuclear receptor which functions as a transcription factor when it binds with testosterone and DHT and participates in a variety of biological activities [5] (Fig. 13.1).

13.3 Testosterone Conversion Over Time

GnRH is secreted from the hypothalamus at the onset of puberty, stimulating testosterone production as LH and FSH are increasingly secreted from the anterior pituitary (Fig. 13.1). The peptide kisspeptin and the GPR54 receptor play major roles in GnRH secretion during puberty, as clarified by studies using knockout mice [6]. Many questions remain, however, such as how kisspeptin secretion increases during puberty. Testosterone levels continue to increase until the age of 20 or thereabouts, after which it begins to show a slow decline. Factors such as the age-related decrease in Leydig cells (responsible for testosterone production) and lessened GnRH secretion are responsible for a drop in testosterone levels, which fall 2–5% by age 40 and 30–70% by age 70 [7].

13.4 Testosterone and LOH

Age-related decreases in testosterone levels result in a disease known as late-onset hypogonadism syndrome (LOH). Diagnosis of hypogonadism is made when testosterone levels hit an approximate 300–350 ng/dL cutoff point. When 325 ng/dL is specified as the cutoff point, the percentage of men diagnosed as hypogonadism in their 50s, 60s, 70s, and 80s is reported to be 12%, 20%, 30%, and 50%, respectively [8]. Another report suggests that 38.7% of men aged 45 and above are diagnosed as hypogonadism when the cutoff point is specified as 300 ng/dL [9]. Analysis shows that when total serum testosterone levels drop to a threshold of 230–320 ng/dL as a result of LOH, likely symptoms include a decline in morning erections and libido as well as erectile dysfunction (ED) [10]. Therefore, concurrent emergence of these three symptoms strongly indicates the presence of LOH. Decreasing testosterone in aging males results in depression, sexual dysfunction, decreased cognitive function, osteoporosis, an increase in visceral fat, a decline in both insulin sensitivity and high-density lipoprotein (HDL) cholesterol, and an increase in both total cholesterol and low-density lipoprotein (LDL) cholesterol, all of which are risk factors for metabolic syndrome, eventually causing cardiovascular disease, diabetes, and respiratory illness [11–14].

13.5 Diagnosing LOH

While exact diagnostic criteria for LOH are yet to be defined, a reduced libido, an ED, and a decreased erection frequency are essential components in identifying the syndrome [10]. Differential diagnoses include mental disorders such as depression and psychosomatic illness. Since many LOH outpatients receive antidepressant medication, questionnaires aimed at diagnosing depression are used in outpatient screening. The psychiatric consultant is made immediately when a mental disorder such as depression deteriorates in patients harboring suicidal thoughts. Diseases such as metabolic syndrome, arteriosclerosis, diabetes, hypertension, and hyperlipidemia are also considered to be detrimental to LOH. Metabolic syndromes, which are identified by the concurrent appearance of obesity and two or more additional symptoms from among hyperglycemia, hypertension, and hyperlipidemia, further increase the risk of diabetes and cardiovascular disease. Moreover, as much as 65% of diabetic patients who died from cardiovascular disorder caused by hyperinsulinemia or obesity accompanied a decline in testosterone [15].Therefore, low testosterone in turn can be used as a predictive index of heart disease and diabetes in men of middle age and above [16].

We should measure both testosterone and free testosterone by blood tests. As testosterone level fluctuates during the day, blood should be collected during the morning hours between 7 and 11 am. Since antidepressants such as sulpiride may lower testosterone levels, it is essential to ascertain whether or not the patient is taking such medication. Measurements of LH and FSH are useful in helping differentiate primary and secondary hypogonadism. If LH and FSH show low values, prolactin measurement and MRI testing may be considered to help evaluate the pituitary gland. When deemed necessary, measurements of the following hormones should be taken: adrenal cortisol that fluctuates with stress and androgens DHEA and DHEA-S that are produced in the adrenal glands and may influence on LOH.

13.6 Treating LOH

The history of testosterone replacement therapy dates back to the nineteenth century. During the past decade, testosterone prescriptions in the United States have increased fourfold, growing 25–30% annually and its costs reaching 1.6 billion dollars by 2011 [17]. Pharmaceutical preparations of testosterone come in both injectable and ointment form. Chorionic gonadotrophin (hCG) is another type of testosterone replacement therapy [18]. Recently, 859 hypogonadism patients were reported to have participated in replacement therapy using testosterone gel in a multi-institutional study (Testim Registry in the United States, TriUS). The topical gel was prescribed over a 12-month period, elevating testosterone and free testosterone levels, improving sexual function, and alleviating depression [19, 20].

Side effects of frequent or protracted dosages of testosterone replacement therapy include, among others, polycythemia and acne. Participants of the Testosterone in Older Men (TOM) trial, particularly those of advanced age, are reported to experience an increase in cardiovascular disease as a result of testosterone replacement therapy [21]. Retrospective analysis of patients undergoing cardioangiography reportedly showed that those receiving testosterone replacement therapy had a statistically significant higher rate of cardiovascular disorder [22]. It was presumed that the larger volume of topical gel used in the TOM trial (compared to other studies) was one cause of increased cardiovascular disorders noted in this trial [17]. Meanwhile, recent meta-analyses show no added cardiovascular risk for patients taking forms of testosterone other than oral administrations [23]. Surely, dosage amounts and intervals should be optimized according to each patient's age and symptoms. Detailed medical diagnoses and management tools in the future may enable further adjustment of testosterone dosages based on individual patient's symptoms.

13.7 LOH and DM

A number of studies demonstrate relationships between testosterone levels and DM. Lower testosterone levels are associated with DM in men [24]. In addition, studies showed a consistent relationship between decreased level of SHBG, specific polymorphisms in SHBG gene, and risk of DM [25]. In androgen receptor disrupted mouse with impaired testosterone activity, male-specific obesity is observed as evidenced by an increase in subcutaneous and visceral adipose tissue and abnormal insulin resistance and glucose tolerance [26, 27]. Human epidemiological studies show that testosterone functions as an anti-obesity agent and inversely correlates with body weight and BMI. Accordingly, when body weight and BMI decrease, testosterone levels increase. It has been reported that total fat decreases in most clinical studies using testosterone replacement therapy [28].

In terms of blood sugar levels, a statistical analysis of age, BMI, abdominal girth, HDL cholesterol, and triglycerides in a lateral study of 2470 older men showed that a decrease in blood testosterone levels was an independent factor associated with insulin resistance [22]. Metabolic syndrome is identified by the concurrent presence of visceral fat accumulation and at least two additional symptoms from among hyperglycemia, hypertension, and dyslipidemia. In recent years, growing attention has focused on the increased risk of atherosclerotic disease—namely, cardiovascular disease—diagnosed by the concurrent presence of the four metabolic factors of obesity, hyperglycemia, hypertension, and dyslipidemia. Approximately 9.4 million Japanese men aged 40–74 suffer from cardiovascular disease, with another 10.2 million having latent symptoms, totaling 19.6 million individuals presumed to be affected. One in every two men is strongly suspected of experiencing or possessing latent symptoms of metabolic syndrome. Lateral [3], longitudinal [29], and meta-analysis [30] studies of testosterone and metabolic syndrome reported decreased levels of blood testosterone in patients with metabolic syndrome. In Japanese men of middle age and above, total testosterone levels decrease with an increase in metabolic factors (Fig. 13.3). Moreover, there is a close relationship between a decrease in total testosterone levels and metabolic factors in this population. As testosterone levels decrease, BMI, abdominal girth (Fig. 13.4a), blood pressure (Fig. 13.4b),

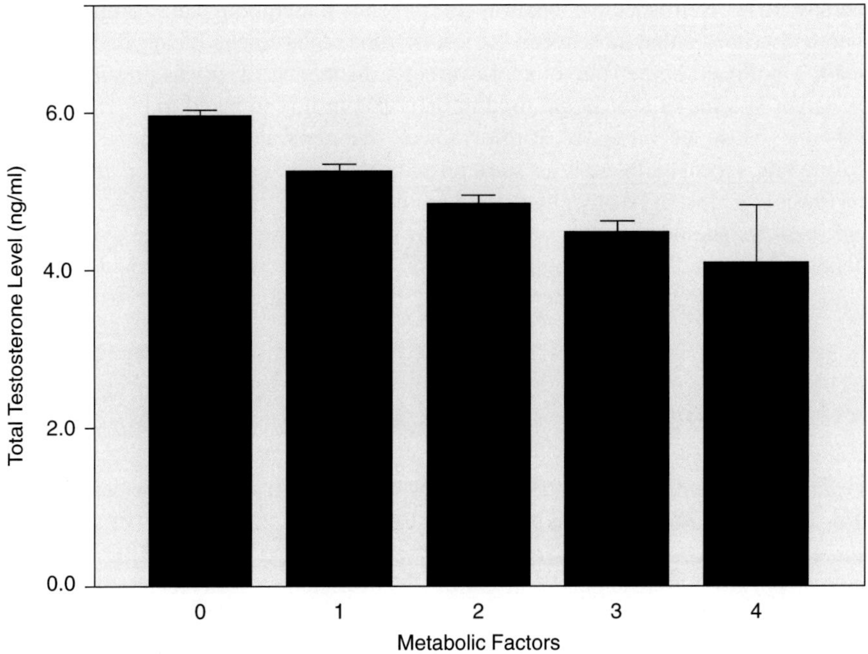

Fig. 13.3 The relationship of number of factors (obesity, hyperglycemia, hypertension, dyslipidemia) and testosterone level

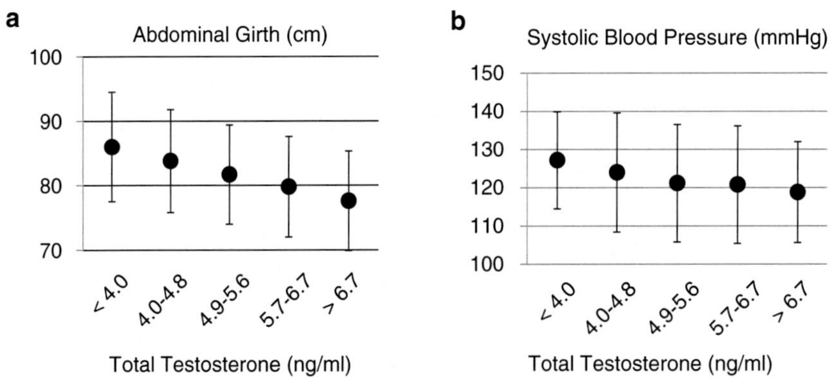

Fig. 13.4 The relationship of each metabolic factor and testosterone level

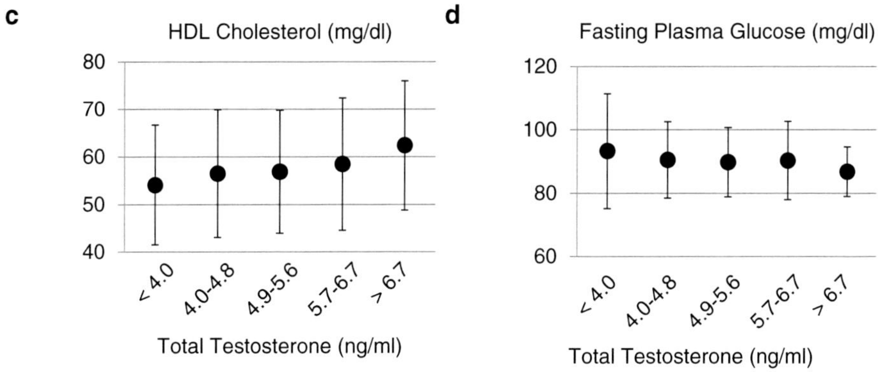

Fig. 13.4 (continued)

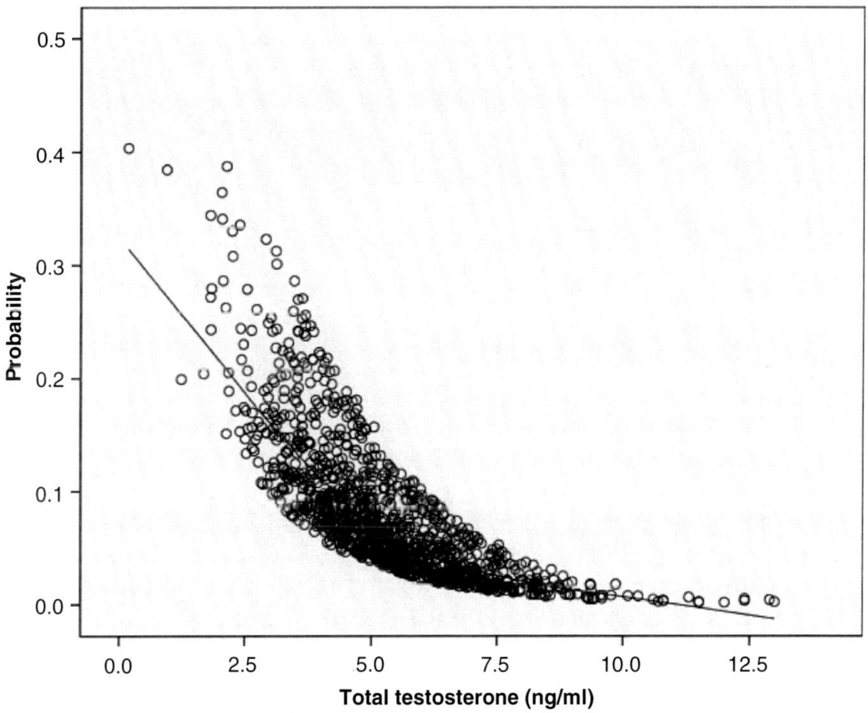

Fig. 13.5 Risk of metabolic syndrome and testosterone level

and triglycerides increase, HDL cholesterol decreases (Fig. 13.4c), and fasting plasma glucose (Fig. 13.4d) along with HbA1c increases. Testosterone and metabolic syndrome are inextricably linked, since a decrease in blood testosterone level appeared to elevate the risk of metabolic syndrome (Fig. 13.5) [31]. Accordingly, LOH patients are considered to have a high risk of metabolic syndrome.

13.8 Other Diseases Associated with LOH

Cardiovascular disease has a gender specificity attributed to estrogen, but in recent years, the male hormone has been suggested to play a role in the disease progression. Epidemiological studies in humans show that low testosterone levels are associated with the increased incidence rate of coronary artery disease [32]. Testosterone levels are associated with coronary artery disease in Japanese men of middle age and above and are shown to correlate with the recovery process as well [33].

ED is an impediment to sexual function arising from patients' physical condition, reaction to stress, and partner interrelationships. It is often correlated with diabetes, low testosterone, metabolic syndrome, and cardiovascular disease and greatly impairs patients' QOL [34].

Tumor-bearing patients with low testosterone are often characterized by a high frequency of weight loss, hypoalbuminemia, muscle loss, inflammation, pain, and opioid use, as well as by anxiety and depression [35]. Furthermore, low testosterone levels are reported to be associated with malignancy in patients with prostate cancer, which proliferates dependently with testosterone level. A data analysis of 235 prostate cancer patients who underwent prostate biopsies showed that, compared to those with Gleason scores under 7, patients with Gleason scores of 7 or higher (high-grade prostate cancer) had lower serum testosterone levels [36].

13.9 The Efficacy of Testosterone Replacement Therapy on DM

Numerous reports point to the beneficial effects of testosterone replacement therapy on metabolic factors. Many focus on the anti-obesity effects such as reduction of fat volume. Moreover, in terms of glucose metabolism, a 1-year administration of testosterone replacement therapy is shown to improve fasting plasma glucose and insulin sensitivity [37]. Recently, there are many reports that a 5-year administration of testosterone replacement therapy in males with low testosterone hyperlipidemia can gradually improve factors including body weight, fasting glucose, HbA1c, systolic/diastolic blood pressure, total cholesterol, and LDL cholesterol [38]. In fact, 20 hypogonadal men with metabolic syndrome were treated with testosterone replacement for 5 years and compared with 20 matched controls without the treatment [39]. From year one, body weight and abdominal girth decreased, and HbA1c and systolic/diastolic blood pressure improved significantly in the intervention group. Thus, researchers hope for the possibility of improvements in metabolic syndrome in LOH patients by administrating testosterone replacement therapy.

References

1. Bagatell CJ, Bremner WJ. Androgens in men: uses and abuses. N Engl J Med. 1996;334:707–14.
2. Coates JM, Herbert J. Endogenous steroids and financial risk taking on a London trading floor. Proc Natl Acad Sci U S A. 2008;105:6167–72.
3. Muller M, Grobbee DE, den Tonkelaar I, Lamberts SW, van der Schouw YT. Endogenous sex hormones and metabolic syndrome in aging men. J Clin Endocrinol Metab. 2005;90:2618–23.
4. Bhasin S, Cunningham GR, Hayes FJ, Matsumoto AM, Snyder PJ, Swerdloff RS, Montori VM. Testosterone therapy in adult men with androgen deficiency syndromes: an endocrine society clinical practice guideline. J Clin Endocrinol Metab. 2006;91:1995–2010.
5. Scher HI, Buchanan G, Gerald W, Butler LM, Tilley WD. Targeting the androgen receptor: improving outcomes for castration-resistant prostate cancer. Endocr Relat Cancer. 2004;11:459–76.
6. Kuohung W, Kaiser UB. GPR54 and KiSS-1: role in the regulation of puberty and reproduction. Rev Endocr Metab Disord. 2006;7:257–63.
7. Morley JE, Perry HM III. Andropause: an old concept in new clothing. Clin Geriatr Med. 2003;19:507–28.
8. Harman SM, Metter EJ, Tobin JD, Pearson J, Blackman MR. Longitudinal effects of aging on serum total and free testosterone levels in healthy men. Baltimore Longitudinal Study of Aging. J Clin Endocrinol Metab. 2001;86:724–31.
9. Mulligan T, Frick MF, Zuraw QC, Stemhagen A, McWhirter C. Prevalence of hypogonadism in males aged at least 45 years: the HIM study. Int J Clin Pract. 2006;60:762–9.
10. Wu FC, Tajar A, Beynon JM, Pye SR, Silman AJ, Finn JD, et al. Identification of late-onset hypogonadism in middle-aged and elderly men. N Engl J Med. 2010;363:123–35.
11. Nieschlag E, Swerdloff R, Behre HM, Gooren LJ, Kaufman JM, Legros JJ, et al. Investigation, treatment and monitoring of late-onset hypogonadism in males. ISA, ISSAM, and EAU recommendations. Eur Urol. 2005;48:1–4.
12. Shores MM, Sloan KL, Matsumoto AM, Moceri VM, Felker B, Kivlahan DR. Increased incidence of diagnosed depressive illness in hypogonadal older men. Arch Gen Psychiatry. 2004;61:162–7.
13. Bhasin S, Cunningham GR, Hayes FJ, Matsumoto AM, Snyder PJ, Swerdloff RS, et al. Testosterone therapy in adult men with androgen deficiency syndromes: an endocrine society clinical practice guideline. Clin Endocrinol Metab. 2006;91:1995–2010.
14. Shabsigh R, Katz M, Yan G, Makhsida N. Cardiovascular issues in hypogonadism and testosterone therapy. Am J Cardiol. 2005;96:67 M–72 M.
15. Zitzmann M. Testosterone deficiency, insulin resistance and the metabolic syndrome. Nat Rev Endocrinol. 2009;5:673–81.
16. Makinen JI, Huhtaniemi I. Androgen replacement therapy in late-onset hypogonadism: current concepts and controversies. Gerontology. 2011;57:193–202.
17. Spitzer M, Huang G, Basaria S, Travison TG, Bhasin S. Risks and benefits of testosterone therapy in older men. Nat Rev Endocrinol. 2013;9:414–24.
18. Nieschlag E. Testosterone treatment comes of age: new options for hypogonadal men. Clin Endocrinol (Oxf). 2006;65:275–81.
19. Khera M, Bhattacharya RK, Blick G, Kushner H, Nguyen D, Miner MM. Improved sexual function with testosterone replacement therapy in hypogonadal men: real-world data from the Testim Registry in the United States (TRiUS). J Sex Med. 2011;11:3204–13.
20. Khera M, Bhattacharya RK, Blick G, et al. The effect of testosterone supplementation on depression symptom in hypogonadal men form the Testim Registry in the US (TRiUS). Aging Male. 2012;15:14–21.

21. Basaria S, Coviello AD, Travison TG, et al. Adverse events associated with testosterone administration. N Engl J Med. 2010;363:109–22.
22. Vigen R, O'Donnell CI, Barón AE, et al. Association of testosterone therapy with mortality, myocardial infarction, and stroke in men with low testosterone levels. JAMA. 2013;310:1829–36.
23. Fernández-Balsells MM, Murad MH, Lane M, et al. Clinical review 1: Adverse effects of testosterone therapy in adult men: a systematicreview and meta-analysis. J Clin Endocrinol Metab. 2010;95:2560–75.
24. Ding EL, Song Y, Malik VS, et al. Sex differences of endogenous sex hormones and risk of type 2 diabetes: a systematic review and meta-analysis. JAMA. 2006;295:1288–99.
25. Le TN, Nestler JE, Strauss JF III, et al. Sex hormone-binding globulin and type 2 diabetes mellitus. Trends Endocrinol Metab. 2012;23:32–40.
26. Fan W, Yanase T, Nomura M, et al. Androgen receptor null male mice develop late-onset obesity caused by decreased energy expenditure and lipolytic activity but show normal insulin sensitivity with high adiponectin secretion. Diabetes. 2005;54:1000–8.
27. Lin HY, Xu Q, Yeh S, et al. Insulin and leptin resistance with hyperleptinemia in mice lacking androgen receptor. Diabetes. 2005;54:1717–25.
28. Allan CA, et al. Androgens and obesity. Curr Opin Endocrinol Diabetes Obes. 2010;17:224–32.
29. Laaksonen DE, Niskanen L, Punnonen K, et al. Testosterone and sex hormone-binding globulin predict the metabolic syndrome and diabetes in middle-aged men. Diabetes Care. 2004;27:1036–41.
30. Brand JS, van der Tweel I, Grobbee DE, et al. Testosterone, sex hormone-binding globulin and the metabolic syndrome: a systematic review and meta-analysis of observational studies. Int J Epidemiol. 2011;40:189–207.
31. Tsujimura A, Miyagawa Y, Takezawa K, et al. Is low testosterone concentration a risk factor for metabolic syndrome in healthy middle-aged men? Urology. 2013;82:814–9.
32. Kaushik M, et al. Cardiovascular disease and androgens: a review. Int J Cardiol. 2010;142:8–14.
33. Akishita M, et al. Low testosterone level as a predictor of cardiovascular events in Japanese men with coronary risk factors. Atherosclerosis. 2010;210:232–6.
34. Corona G, et al. The role of testosterone in erectile dysfunction. Nat Rev. Urol. 2010;7:46–56.
35. Vigano A, et al. Male hypogonadism associated with advanced cancer: a systematic review. Lancet Oncol. 2010;11:679–84.
36. Ide H, Yasuda M, Nishio K, et al. Development of a nomogram for predicting high-grade prostate cancer on biopsy: the significance of serum testosterone levels. Anticancer Res. 2008;28:2487–92.
37. Heufelder AE, Saad F, Bunck MC, et al. Fifty-two-week treatment with diet and exercise plus transdermal testosterone reverses the metabolic syndrome and improves glycemic control in men with newly diagnosed type 2 diabetes and subnormal plasma testosterone. J Androl. 2009;30:726–33.
38. Traish AM, Haider A, Doros G, et al. Long-term testosterone therapy in hypogonadal men ameliorates elements of the metabolic syndrome: an observational, long-term registry study. Int J Clin Pract. 2014;68:314–29.
39. Francomano D, Lenzi A, Aversa A. Effects of five-year treatment with testosterone undecanoate on metabolic and hormonal parameters in ageing men with metabolic syndrome. Int J Endocrinol. 2014;2014:527470.

Chapter 14
Diabetes and Female Sterility/Infertility

Kuniaki Ota, Hiroaki Ohta, and Sho-ichi Yamagishi

Abstract AGEs (advanced glycation end products) are pro-inflammatory molecules that trigger a state of intracellular oxidative stress and inflammation after binding to their cell membrane receptors, such as RAGE. The activation of the AGE-RAGE axis has been well known to play a role in type 2 diabetes mellitus (T2DM), obesity, metabolic syndrome (MetS), cardiovascular disease (CVD), aging, inflammation, and neurodegenerative disorders. AGEs might contribute to the etiology of polycystic ovary syndrome and infertility. This article explains for the relationship between the AGE-RAGE system and infertility as well as ovarian reserve in women of reproductive age.

Keywords Advanced glycation end products • Receptor for AGE • Polycystic ovarian syndrome • In vitro fertilization • Anti-Müllerian hormone

14.1 AGE-RAGE and Insulin Resistance

Polycystic ovarian syndrome (PCOS), while clinically heterogeneous, commonly exhibits hyperandrogenism and ovulatory dysfunction and is associated with obesity, insulin resistance, and subfertility [1, 2]. Overall, insulin resistance and the compensatory hyperinsulinemia affects some 65–70% of women with PCOS [3, 4], with 70–80% of obese (BMI >30) and 20–25% of lean (BMI <25) women exhibiting these characteristics. Part of the insulin resistance appears to be independent of obesity and related specifically to PCOS, with abnormalities of cellular mechanisms of insulin action and insulin receptor function having been documented [5, 6].

K. Ota, M.D., Ph.D. (✉) • H. Ohta
Department of Obstetrics and Gynecology, Nasu Red Cross Hospital,
1081-4 Nakadawara, Otawara, Tochigi 324-8686, Japan
e-mail: kuniakiota@gmail.com

S.-i. Yamagishi
Department of Pathophysiology and Therapeutics of Diabetic Vascular Complications,
Kurume University School of Medicine, Kurume 830-0011, Japan

S.-i. Yamagishi (ed.), *Diabetes and Aging-related Complications*,
https://doi.org/10.1007/978-981-10-4376-5_14

Other criteria that can be used include those from the National Institutes of Health (NIH) and the Androgen Excess Society (AES) [7]. PCOS has estimated prevalence of over 10% in women of childbearing age. Besides being associated with infertility, PCOS is also associated with a higher incidence of type 2 diabetes mellitus (T2DM) such as the status of insulin resistance.

On the other hand, AGEs have been proposed to be among the main intermediaries of several diseases such as type 2 diabetes mellitus (T2DM), obesity, metabolic syndrome (MetS), cardiovascular disease (CVD), aging, inflammation, and neurodegenerative disorders [8–10]. Along with the appreciation of these problems, there has been recognition that AGEs have a wider range of actions, including in reproduction.

Insulin resistant women with PCOS without hyperglycemia have elevated serum AGE levels and increased RAGE expression in their circulating monocytes [11]. Additionally, serum AGE levels are positively correlated with testosterone level, free androgen index, insulin, HOMA, and waist-to-hip ratio in women with PCOS without hyperglycemia [12]. Another study has shown that increased serum AGE level is a distinct finding in non-insulin resistant lean women with PCOS suggesting that serum AGEs are elevated in PCOS independently of the presence of insulin resistance [11].

Recent studies have demonstrated that RAGE- and AGE-modified proteins are expressed in human ovarian tissue [10, 13]. In ovarian tissue samples, women with PCOS have increased AGEs and RAGE expression in theca and granulosa cell layers compared with normal women [9]. Additionally, a differential qualitative distribution of AGE and RAGE subunit was observed in women with PCOS compared with healthy controls, where a more pronounced staining density of both AGE and RAGE was observed in the granulosa cell layer of PCOS ovaries [9].

The ovaries of women with PCOS have alterations in enzymes responsible for collagen synthesis [14]. Lysyl oxidase enzyme is one of the key enzymes in the ovary responsible for collagen and elastin cross-linking in the organization of ECM during follicular development [15]. A study has shown that the deposition of excess collagen in PCO tissue may, in part, be due to AGE-mediated stimulation of lysyl oxidase activity [16]. These results indicate that AGE signaling could regulate ovarian follicular ECM organization in PCOS. Other data demonstrated that AGEs could reduce the activity of some "good" detoxifying enzymes (such as glyoxalase-I) in the ovary of PCOS rats [17].

The AGE system has been shown to play a role in ovarian aging and reproduction [10, 13]. The accumulation of AGEs in the human ovary may account for a number of age-related features of ovarian dysfunction reflected by oxidative stress, such as impaired vascularization with its subsequent hypoxia and reduced intake of nutrients by granulosa cells [10, 18]. Prolonged exposure to AGEs, which are characterized by a long half-life, during reproductive life may cause subtle oxidative damage to follicles inside the ovary [19]. These alterations in the ovarian microenvironment may adversely impact granulosa cell metabolism, the assembly of antioxidant defense, and the development of adequate perifollicular vascularization, thus endangering follicular health and maturation. Markers of ovarian reserve, such as AMH, reflect ovarian aging. Studies pertaining to the effect of AGEs on ovarian aging have been reported [13, 16]; however, no studies to date have examined the relationship between the follicular AGE system and ovarian reserve measures, specifically granulosa cell AMH synthesis and release.

Because AGEs are elevated in the serum of women with PCOS, Christakou et al. [20] investigated whether oral contraceptives (OCPs) or metformin affect serum AGEs levels in women with PCOS. They randomized women with PCOS ($n = 109$) to receive either OCP or metformin (850 mg twice daily) for 6 months and determined serum AGE levels at baseline and after 3 and 6 months of treatment. Their results indicated that serum AGE levels were significantly reduced in all groups at 6 months of treatment compared with baseline, but the percentage reduction was significantly greater in the metformin group compared with the OCP group. Although they showed that metformin may be superior to OCP in reducing serum AGE levels, this does not necessarily mean that metformin is better than OCP in alleviating the cardiovascular risk associated with PCOS. Whether metformin lowers cardiovascular risks in PCOS women via the AGE-RAGE system remains to be determined.

14.2 AGE-RAGE and In Vitro Fertilization

Some researchers have already reported a relationship between the AGE-RAGE system and infertility included in in vitro fertilization (IVF) [13, 21, 22]. One of researchers measured the levels of toxic AGE (TAGE), pentosidine, and CML in blood and follicular fluid of 157 patients undergoing IVF [22]. They analyzed the association between these levels and assisted reproduction technology (ART) outcomes and pre-ART clinical factors. Their results elucidated that the accumulation of TAGE, pentosidine, and CML in the follicular fluid and TAGE in serum negatively correlated ($P < 0.05$) with follicular growth, fertilization, and embryonic development. Lower concentrations of pentosidine in the follicular fluid and TAGE in the serum were the most significant predictors for achievement of ongoing pregnancy, acting independently of conventional determinants, such as age and Day 3 FSH level. Additionally, elevation of serum TAGE >7.24 U/ml appeared to indicate ovarian dysfunction causing diminished fertility, even at a young age (<40 years old) or with normal FSH during menses (below 10 IU/l). These data explain that there is a clinical evidence for an important role of AGE accumulation in ovarian dysfunction and poorer outcome in women with elevated AGEs and undergoing IVF [22].

Another study evaluated sRAGE, as decoy receptor, levels in serum, and follicular fluid of 33 women under IVF program [21]. The control group of serum samples was collected from 35 healthy females. Their results indicated that sRAGE levels of follicular fluid were several times higher than serum levels ($P < 0.001$). Additionally, it was found that serum levels of sRAGE in women after controlled ovarian hyperstimulation (COH) were significantly lower than in controls ($P = 0.045$). They also found a significant negative correlation between serum sRAGE levels and the number of stimulated follicles ($r = 20.71$, $P = 0.01$) and retrieved oocytes ($r = 20.54$, $P = 0.048$). Women in that study who conceived following IVF showed significantly higher sRAGE levels in the follicular fluid compared with women who did not conceive ($P = 0.031$). A similar study evaluated follicular fluid and plasma sRAGE levels in 28 participants who underwent IVF and found a positive correlation between follicular fluid and plasma sRAGE levels and a borderline positive correlation between follicular fluid sRAGE and the number of collected oocytes ($r = 0.25$; $P = 0.05$). These data speculate that the decoy sRAGE, via binding circulating and follicular fluid AGEs, might be able to serve as a useful biological marker of the follicular environment [13].

14.3 AGE-RAGE and Anti-Müllerian Hormone

Anti-Müllerian hormone (AMH) is a very sensitive indicator of the ovarian follicular content. AMH is produced by granulosa cells of preantral and small antral follicles, and its main physiological role seems to be the inhibition of the initial follicular recruitment from the primordial to the antral pool [23]. It has been extensively studied in assisted reproductive therapy processes. It is now well established that AMH is the more accurate marker of the ovarian reserve [24].

One researcher showed that there was a positive correlation between follicular fluid sRAGE and follicular fluid AMH protein levels ($r = 0.5$, $P = 0.008$) while, in contrast, RT-PCR results showed no correlation between follicular fluid sRAGE and AMH or AMHR-II mRNA levels, suggesting that sRAGE has an effect on AMH release rather than AMH synthesis in granulosa cells. The potential accumulation of AGEs in the ovary may account for compromised efficiency of vascularization and for activation of oxidative stress response through interaction with cellular RAGE [18]. Similar to sRAGE, follicular fluid AMH reflects ovarian health and constitutes a useful biological marker of the follicular environment [25]. Within follicles, AMH is expressed exclusively by granulosa cells with mitotic activity [25, 26] presumably because it interacts with mitogenic growth factors during follicle development. Therefore, a positive relationship between intrafollicular AMH and sRAGE concentrations suggests that AGEs play a role in the inhibition of cellular proliferation or a role in enhancing granulosa cell apoptosis. It is unclear whether the AMH system has a role in the mechanistic effect of sRAGE on the number of oocytes retrieved. It is well known that AMH release inhibits, in paracrine fashion, the depletion of the oocyte pool by slowing down growth followed by atresia of follicles containing the oocytes [27]. Thus, clearly a favorable interrelationship exists between sRAGE and AMH in the follicular environment. Altogether, the AGE-RAGE system could represent a potential therapeutic target in women with a diagnosis of diminished ovarian reserve undergoing ART.

14.4 AGE-RAGE and Recurrent Pregnancy Miscarriage

It is estimated that 20–30% of pregnant women may experience one or more spontaneous pregnancy losses [28]. Recurrent pregnancy losses (RPL) are often defined as three or more consecutive pregnancy losses prior to 20 weeks' gestation [28], and more than 500,000 women per year have experienced recurrent pregnancy losses in the United States [29].

The outcomes for approximately half the patients remain unexplained with current medical practice patterns, and they are classified as idiopathic or unexplained RPL [30]. Therefore, identifying new biomarkers for RPL is urgently needed for the proper diagnosis and management of RPL.

We investigated whether sRAGE is increased in women with PRL and which anthropometric, metabolic, and inflammatory variables are independently correlated with sRAGE in women with idiopathic RPL [31]. We measured the levels of AGE-RAGE, anthropometric, metabolic, and inflammatory immune markers as AGE-RAGE related factor in blood of 63 women with RPL. Levels of sRAGE were statistically significantly higher in RPL patients than in control patients (1528.9 ± 704.5 vs. 1149.9 ± 447.4 pg/mL). In the multivariate analysis, the levels of insulin, plasminogen activator inhibitor-1, the resistance index of the uterine radial artery, and the ratio of tumor necrosis factor-a/interleukin-10 producing T helper cells were statistically significantly associated with the serum sRAGE level. We concluded that elevated levels of serum sRAGE are associated with RPL. The soluble receptor for advanced glycation end products might contribute to RPL by reducing uterine blood flow and subsequently causing ischemia in the fetus via inflammatory and thrombotic reactions. Furthermore, our data suggest that sRAGE may be a novel biomarker of RPL and that RAGE might be a therapeutic target for this devastating disorder.

References

1. Dunaif A. Insulin resistance and the polycystic ovary syndrome: mechanism and implications for pathogenesis. Endocr Rev. 1997;18:774–800.
2. Moran L, Teede H. Metabolic features of the reproductive phenotypes of polycystic ovary syndrome. Hum Reprod Update. 2009;15:477–88.
3. Dunaif A, Segal KR, Futterweit W, Dobrjansky A. Profound peripheral insulin resistance, independent of obesity, in polycystic ovary syndrome. Diabetes. 1989;38:1165–74.
4. DeFronzo RA, Tobin JD, Andres R. Glucose clamp technique: a method for quantifying insulin secretion and resistance. Am J Physiol. 1979;237:E214–23.
5. Ovesen P, Moller J, Ingerslev HJ, et al. Normal basal and insulin-stimulated fuel metabolism in lean women with the polycystic ovary syndrome. J Clin Endocrinol Metab. 1993;77:1636–40.
6. Dunaif A, Graf M, Mandeli J, Laumas V, Dobrjansky A. Characterization of groups of hyperandrogenic women with acanthosis nigricans, impaired glucose tolerance, and/or hyperinsulinemia. J Clin Endocrinol Metab. 1987;65:499–507.

7. March WA, Moore VM, Willson KJ, Phillips DI, Norman RJ, Davies MJ. The prevalence of polycystic ovary syndrome in a community sample assessed under contrasting diagnostic criteria. Hum Reprod. 2010;25:544–51.
8. Yamagishi S, Nakamura K, Imaizumi T. Advanced glycation end products (AGEs) and diabetic vascular complications. Curr Diabetes Rev. 2005;1:93–106.
9. Diamanti-Kandarakis E, Piperi C, Patsouris E, et al. Immunohistochemical localization of advanced glycation end-products (AGEs) and their receptor (RAGE) in polycystic and normal ovaries. Histochem Cell Biol. 2007;127:581–9.
10. Tatone C, Amicarelli F. The aging ovary—the poor granulosa cells. Fertil Steril. 2013;99:12–7.
11. Diamanti-Kandarakis E, Katsikis I, Piperi C, et al. Increased serum advanced glycation end-products is a distinct finding in lean women with polycystic ovary syndrome (PCOS). Clin Endocrinol (Oxf). 2008;69:634–41.
12. Burghen GA, Givens JR, Kitabchi AE. Correlation of hyperandrogenism with hyperinsulinism in polycystic ovarian disease. J Clin Endocrinol Metab. 1980;50:113–6.
13. Fujii EY, Nakayama M. The measurements of RAGE, VEGF, and AGEs in the plasma and follicular fluid of reproductive women: the influence of aging. Fertil Steril. 2010;94:694–700.
14. Henmi H, Endo T, Nagasawa K, et al. Lysyl oxidase and MMP-2 expression in dehydroepiandrosterone-induced polycystic ovary in rats. Biol Reprod. 2001;64:157–62.
15. Harlow CR, Rae M, Davidson L, Trackman PC, Hillier SG. Lysyl oxidase gene expression and enzyme activity in the rat ovary: regulation by follicle-stimulating hormone, androgen, and transforming growth factor-beta superfamily members in vitro. Endocrinology. 2003;144:154–62.
16. Papachroni KK, Piperi C, Levidou G, et al. Lysyl oxidase interacts with AGE signalling to modulate collagen synthesis in polycystic ovarian tissue. J Cell Mol Med. 2010;14:2460–9.
17. Kandaraki E, Chatzigeorgiou A, Piperi C, et al. Reduced ovarian glyoxalase-I activity by dietary glycotoxins and androgen excess: a causative link to polycystic ovarian syndrome. Mol Med. 2012;18:1183–9.
18. Tatone C, Amicarelli F, Carbone MC, et al. Cellular and molecular aspects of ovarian follicle ageing. Hum Reprod Update. 2008;14:131–42.
19. de Bruin JP, Dorland M, Spek ER, et al. Age-related changes in the ultrastructure of the resting follicle pool in human ovaries. Biol Reprod. 2004;70:419–24.
20. Christakou C, Diamanti-Kandarakis E. Structural, biochemical and non-traditional cardiovascular risk markers in PCOS. Curr Pharm Des. 2013;19:5764–74.
21. Malickova K, Jarosova R, Rezabek K, et al. Concentrations of sRAGE in serum and follicular fluid in assisted reproductive cycles—a preliminary study. Clin Lab. 2010;56:377–84.
22. Jinno M, Takeuchi M, Watanabe A, et al. Advanced glycation end-products accumulation compromises embryonic development and achievement of pregnancy by assisted reproductive technology. Hum Reprod. 2011;26:604–10.
23. Weenen C, Laven JS, Von Bergh AR, et al. Anti-Mullerian hormone expression pattern in the human ovary: potential implications for initial and cyclic follicle recruitment. Mol Hum Reprod. 2004;10:77–83.
24. La Marca A, Broekmans FJ, Volpe A, Fauser BC, Macklon NS. ESHRE Special Interest Group for Reproductive Endocrinology—AMH Round Table. Anti-Mullerian hormone (AMH): what do we still need to know? Hum Reprod. 2009;24:2264–75.
25. Hirobe S, He WW, Lee MM, Donahoe PK. Mullerian inhibiting substance messenger ribonucleic acid expression in granulosa and Sertoli cells coincides with their mitotic activity. Endocrinology. 1992;131:854–62.
26. Hirobe S, He WW, Gustafson ML, MacLaughlin DT, Donahoe PK. Mullerian inhibiting substance gene expression in the cycling rat ovary correlates with recruited or graafian follicle selection. Biol Reprod. 1994;50:1238–43.
27. Durlinger AL, Gruijters MJ, Kramer P, et al. Anti-Mullerian Hormone Inhibits Initiation of Primordial Follicle Growth in the Mouse Ovary. Endocrinology. 2002;143:1076–84.

28. Li TC, Makris M, Tomsu M, Tuckerman E, Laird S. Recurrent miscarriage: aetiology, management and prognosis. Hum Reprod Update. 2002;8:463–81.
29. Bick RL. Recurrent miscarriage syndrome due to blood coagulation protein/platelet defects: prevalence, treatment and outcome results. DRW Metroplex Recurrent Miscarriage Syndrome Cooperative Group. Clin Appl Thromb Hemost. 2000;6:115–25.
30. Jaslow CR, Carney JL, Kutteh WH. Diagnostic factors identified in 1020 women with two versus three or more recurrent pregnancy losses. Fertil Steril. 2010;93:1234–43.
31. Ota K, Yamagishi S, Kim M, et al. Elevation of soluble form of receptor for advanced glycation end products (sRAGE) in recurrent pregnancy losses (RPL): possible participation of RAGE in RPL. Fertil Steril. 2014;102:782–9.

Chapter 15
Diabetes and Periodontitis

Takanori Shinjo and Fusanori Nishimura

Abstract Periodontal disease is known as the sixth complication of diabetes. Recently, many clinical and epidemiologic reports have shown that local periodontal inflammation induces systemic micro-inflammation, contributing to insulin resistance and increasing the risk of cardiovascular diseases. We have used in vitro and in vivo studies to address the amplification mechanism of periodontal inflammation from the viewpoint of adipocyte–macrophage interaction. Our studies suggest that inflammatory cytokines, such as tumor necrosis factor-alpha (TNFα), are secreted from monocytes and macrophages that are stimulated by periodontal pathogen-derived Toll-like receptor ligands, such as lipopolysaccharides (LPS). TNFα then activates both adipocytes and infiltrated macrophages, thereby amplifying micro-inflammation through the synergistic production of inflammatory cytokines, including interleukin-6 and monocyte chemoattractant protein-1. Additionally, the expression of chemokine (C-C motif) ligand 19 (CCL19), involved in homing of dendritic cells, was found to be markedly upregulated in adipocytes co-cultured with LPS-stimulated macrophages. In vivo studies suggest that CCR7-CCL19 signaling possibly plays a critical role in adipose tissue metabolism through infiltration of immune cells, such as dendritic cells. Furthermore, the Hiroshima study, a clinical intervention study on diabetic patients receiving periodontal treatment, clearly showed that periodontal treatment combined with local oral antibiotic administration could improve glycated hemoglobin levels in subjects with a high-sensitivity C-reactive protein level > 500 ng/ml and a body mass index of approximately 25 kg/m^2. A series of our studies suggests that periodontal treatment could improve glycemic control in diabetic patients with mild obesity.

Keywords Periodontal disease • Micro-inflammation • Adipocyte–macrophage interaction • Glycated hemoglobin • Antibiotics

T. Shinjo • F. Nishimura (✉)
Section of Periodontology, Division of Oral Rehabilitation,
Faculty of Dental Science, Kyushu University, Fukuoka,
3-1-1 Maidashi, Higashi-ku, Fukuoka City, Fukuoka 812-8582, Japan
e-mail: fusanori@dent.kyushu-u.ac.jp

S.-i. Yamagishi (ed.), *Diabetes and Aging-related Complications*,
https://doi.org/10.1007/978-981-10-4376-5_15

15.1 Periodontal Disease: Local and Systemic Aspects

Periodontal disease is a localized oral infectious and inflammatory disease caused by gram-negative obligate anaerobes. It is divided into gingivitis and periodontitis. The pathology in the former is inflammation of the gingiva; in the latter, the inflammation has progressed from the gingiva to the periodontal tissues, such as alveolar bone, resulting in destruction. Based on the age of onset and the degree of progression, periodontitis is roughly categorized into two types: aggressive and chronic periodontitis. Aggressive periodontitis is characterized by young onset (teenage years to the thirties) and rapid destruction of the periodontal tissues. However, aggressive periodontitis is a rare disorder; its incidence rate is estimated to be only 0.05–0.1%. On the other hand, most patients suffer from chronic periodontitis, which used to be called "adult periodontitis." This is characterized by indolent progression in patients over 35 years of age. The morbidity rate of chronic periodontitis increases with age. In Japan, 86.7% of 45–49-year-olds suffer from chronic periodontitis [1], and chronic periodontitis is the most frequent cause of tooth loss in patients over 40 years old [2]. Immunoreaction to periodontal pathogens results in production of inflammatory cytokines such as interleukin (IL)-1, IL-6, and tumor necrosis factor-alpha (TNFα), thereby leading to progression of periodontal disease with tissue destruction. Furthermore, these bioactive substances (periodontal pathogens and their products) have been shown to induce micro-inflammation throughout the body in cases of advanced periodontitis [3]. This has brought periodontal disease into the spotlight.

15.2 Relationship Between Diabetes and Periodontal Disease

15.2.1 Periodontal Disease in Diabetic Patients

Periodontal disease has been reported as the sixth complication of diabetes mellitus, in addition to microvascular disease and macroangiopathy [4]. Many factors, such as increased rates of specific bacteria requiring glucose, neutrophilic dysfunction, inhibition of collagen synthesis, adipokines, and advanced glycation end products (AGEs), are reported to be associated with the higher susceptibility to periodontal disease in diabetic patients [5].

A meta-analysis showed that periodontal disease was significantly exacerbated in patients with both type 1 and 2 diabetes (T1DM and T2DM) [6]. Some cohort studies on T1DM showed that progression of periodontal disease was aggravated in patients with poor glycemic control [7–9]. In terms of T2DM, a large-scale epidemiologic study conducted among Pima Indians, a population with an extremely high rate of diabetes-related morbidity, indicated that the incidence of periodontal disease in the diabetic group was approximately 2.6-fold higher than that of the nondiabetic group aged older than 15 years [10]. Further, a study using data from the third National Health and Nutrition Examination Survey (NHANES III) database investigated the association between glycemic control and severity of periodontal disease. In this report, the odds ratios of severe periodontal disease in the T2DM groups with a glycated hemoglobin (HbA1c) level ≥ 9.0% (NGSP) and <9.0%, relative to the nondiabetic group, were 2.90 and 1.56, respectively [11]. These studies suggest that both T1DM and T2DM are exacerbating factors for periodontal disease.

15.2.2 Diabetes in Patients with Periodontal Disease

Many cohort studies have shown that periodontal disease affects the onset of diabetes and glycemic control. Studies analyzing data from NHANES indicated that the prevalence of diabetes in patients with periodontal disease was twofold higher than that in patients without periodontal disease [12, 13]. Additionally, a cohort study surveying health in Pomerania, Germany, over a 15-year period reported that, in the fifth year, HbA1c in nondiabetic patients with severe periodontitis at baseline tended to be elevated in comparison with patients without periodontitis [14]. Furthermore, a cohort study in Hisayama town showed that the prevalence of periodontal disease was significantly higher among patients who had developed glucose intolerance during the 10-year follow-up period than among patients who had not [15].

15.3 Effect of Periodontal Inflammation on the Whole Body

15.3.1 Periodontitis as Factor Promoting Atherosclerosis

The progression of atherosclerosis and onset of ischemic heart disease are largely associated with classical risk factors such as obesity, hyperglycemia, hyperinsulinemia, hypertriglyceridemia, hyper-LDL-cholesterolemia, and hypo-HDL-cholesterolemia [16]. However, these factors alone do not provide sufficient cause; hence, micro-inflammation is being evaluated as another factor. For example, minor elevations in C-reactive protein (CRP) within the normal limit, known as high-sensitivity CRP (hsCRP), have been shown to increase the risk of future onset of or mortality related to coronary heart disease (CHD) two- to threefold in people free from systemic problems [17, 18]. These reports suggest that micro-inflammation is a factor promoting atherosclerosis, as increases in hsCRP reflect the presence of micro-inflammation.

It is known that hsCRP increases in patients with severe periodontal disease and decreases with administration of periodontal treatment [19], supporting the view that severe periodontal disease induces systemic micro-inflammation. Periodontitis-induced increases in CRP are reported to match the CRP levels associated with a twofold increase in the risk of CHD onset or mortality in the Japanese population [17, 19] (Fig.15.1). Research conducted in Japan and abroad has reported the risk of

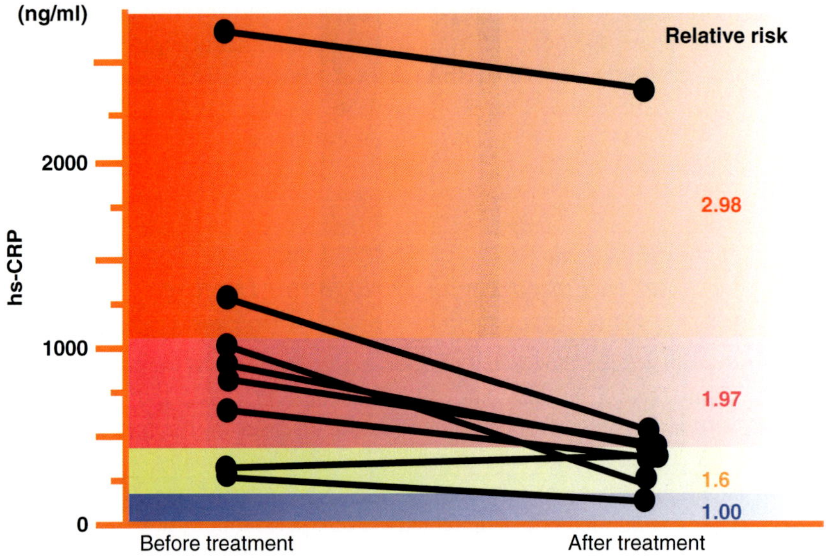

Fig. 15.1 Periodontal treatment-induced decrease in CRP and relative risk of ischemic heart disease (IHD). Our data, indicating that hsCRP was increased by periodontitis and decreased by periodontal treatment [19], is collated with data investigating the correlation between CRP levels at baseline and relative risk of IHD in the Hiroshima study [15]. The data is reproduced with permission from American Academy of Periodontology, and image is reprinted from Biology of Anti-Aging (Medical Review Co., Ltd)

CHD to be 1.5–2-fold higher in patients with periodontitis than in controls [17, 20]. Therefore, increases in hsCRP as a result of periodontal disease are reasonably consistent with the epidemiologic data. Even though the extent of inflammation in periodontitis is not as much as that in acute rheumatism or extreme obesity with a body mass index (BMI) >30 kg/m^2, periodontal disease-induced micro-inflammation is considered to affect persistent atherosclerosis.

15.3.2 Periodontitis as an Insulin Resistance-Inducing Factor

As micro-inflammation is demonstrated to induce insulin resistance in diabetic patients, periodontal disease, a systemic micro-inflammation-inducing disease, is considered to adversely affect insulin resistance. We have reported that short-term, intensive, antimicrobial periodontal disease treatment improved insulin resistance in T2DM patients with periodontitis [21]. We also found that this treatment decreased blood concentrations of TNFα, a representative inflammatory cytokine that contributes to insulin resistance, and lowered HbA1c in accordance with improvements in insulin sensitivity [19]. These reports support the view that severe periodontal disease contributes to inducing systemic micro-inflammation, exacerbating insulin resistance.

15.4 Amplification Mechanism of Periodontal Inflammation: Investigations Based on Adipocyte–Macrophage Interaction Theory

15.4.1 Effect of Periodontal Inflammation on Interaction Between Adipocytes and Macrophages

As mentioned above, chronic periodontal disease induces systemic micro-inflammation. On the other hand, obesity is one of the most common diseases inducing systemic micro-inflammation. In contrast to many obese Westerners who show severe adiposity phenotypes, most obese Asians, including the Japanese, show mild phenotypes. Moreover, many Asian patients with T2DM do not fall into the obesity category (BMI >25 kg/m^2). However, patients with a BMI of approximately 25 kg/m^2 are known to be most susceptible to increases in hsCRP induced by periodontal disease [22].

Why are these patients susceptible to increases in hsCRP? Visceral adipose tissue is considered as a key to understanding this subject. Many studies have clarified that mature adipose tissue produces large amounts of adipokines; these play an important role in the pathogenesis of the metabolic syndrome [23, 24]. A recent report indicated that adipokine production from mature adipose tissue was enhanced by interaction between infiltrated macrophages and adipocytes (adipocyte–macrophage interaction theory) (Fig. 15.2) [25]. In addition, both macrophages and adipocytes

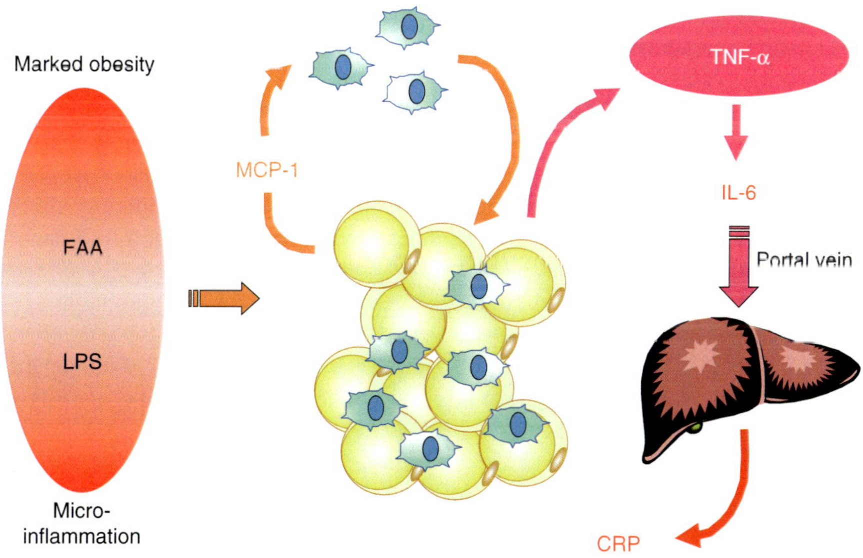

Fig. 15.2 Amplification of the inflammatory reaction mediated by the interaction between adipocytes and macrophages**.** Adipocytes activated through TLR-4 signal produce MCP-1 and IL-6: MCP-1 is considered to induce further infiltration of macrophages into adipose tissue. IL-6 is considered to enter the liver via portal vein, where it promotes CRP production. The image is reprinted from Biology of Anti-Aging

are reported to express Toll-like receptor (TLR)-2 and TLR-4 on their plasma membranes; free fatty acid released through lipolysis in mature adipocytes acts as ligands for these receptors [25].

Meanwhile, we evaluated the hypothesis that peripheral monocyte-derived macrophages activated by periodontal pathogens infiltrated into adipose tissue, thereby amplifying local periodontal inflammation through macrophage–adipocyte interaction, because periodontal disease is caused by gram-negative obligate anaerobe-induced infection. First, we confirmed adipokine production from adipocytes co-cultured with LPS-stimulated macrophages in vitro. We found that IL-6 and monocyte chemoattractant protein-1 (MCP-1) production from co-cultured adipocytes increased more than 100-fold in comparison with single-cultured adipocytes [25]. As IL-6 is known to be a representative cytokine inducing CRP production from hepatocytes, adipose tissue-derived IL-6 was suggested to be involved in CRP production through inflow into the liver via the portal vein. On the other hand, MCP-1 was considered to promote further monocyte/macrophage migration toward adipose tissue [25].

15.4.2 Global Analysis for Differentially Expressed Gene Clusters in Adipocytes Co-cultured with LPS-Stimulated Macrophages

Because under co-culture of adipocytes and macrophages, adipokine production was found to markedly increase when both cells were stimulated with TLR ligands such as LPS, we attempted to analyze gene clusters differentially expressed in the presence of LPS, using a DNA microarray. We confirmed remarkable changes in the genes involved in insulin resistance and increase in cardiovascular risk [24]. For example, glucose transporter 4 expression was markedly downregulated while a suppressor of cytokine signaling, known as inhibitory factor of insulin signaling, was upregulated, indicating promotion of insulin resistance. On the other hand, expression of plasminogen activator inhibitor-1 and serum amyloid A (SAA) was shown to increase, suggesting these adipokines are involved in the facilitation of atherosclerosis. Furthermore, expression of MCP-1 and regulated on activation, normal T cell expressed and secreted (RANTES) were also upregulated. With regard to LPS signaling-related genes, the expression of TLR-2, TLR-4, CD14, and LPS-binding protein (LBP) in adipocytes was found to increase markedly.

Then, we determined whether these results in vitro were reflected in in vivo using ob/ob and high-fat diet (HFD)-fed mice. In brief, these mice were injected with LPS via a tail vein, and the dynamics of SAA, LBP, and RANTES in the blood were observed. We found that blood concentrations of SAA, LBP, and RANTES in these mice increased significantly 1 day after LPS injection, compared with controls [26]. Together, these studies suggest that induction of inflammation in mature adipose tissue promotes the infiltration of monocytes and macrophages into adipose tissue and a possibility that inflammatory responses induced by gram-negative bacteria are excessively induced by increased levels of LBP in obesity. In addition, mature adipose tissue was clarified to be an important source of cytokines and adipokines.

15.4.3 Influence of Amplified Micro-inflammation Through Adipose Tissue on Migration of Dendritic Cells

Moreover, like RANTES, we found that the expression of chemokine (C-C motif) ligand 19 (CCL19), involved in homing of dendritic cells (DCs), was markedly upregulated in adipocytes co-cultured with LPS-stimulated macrophages. While adipocytes in single culture secreted little CCL19, secretion of CCL19 was increased in adipocytes co-cultured with macrophages. In addition, we confirmed that CCL19 production increased remarkably in an LPS-injected obese model mouse [27]. We investigated the role of CCL19 in obesity and insulin resistance using mice lacking C-C chemokine receptor type 7 (CCR7), a receptor for CCL19. In this study, CCR7-deficient (CCR7KO) and wild type (WT) mice were fed with a normal diet (ND) and HFD for 16 weeks. The HFD-fed CCR7KO mice gained body weight at the same rate as the ND-fed mice, despite same food intake as other groups. Subsequently, by means of the intraperitoneal glucose tolerance test and insulin tolerance test, we confirmed that CCR7KO mice maintained normal glucose tolerance. In addition, HFD-fed WT mice were observed to gain weight in adipose tissue and the liver, and induction of adipocyte enlargement and advanced liver steatosis were observed. This was not observed in HFD-fed CCR7KO mice, in whom adipose tissue was not infiltrated by inflammatory cells and levels of gene expression of inflammatory cytokines were the same as those in ND-fed mice. We also found that CD11c-positive cells were observed in HFD-fed WT mice but not in HFD-fed CCR7KO mice, suggesting the possibility that DCs infiltration triggered obesity and subsequent inflammation in adipose tissue, as CD11c is a marker for mature DCs.

CCL19 is known to be involved not only in homing mature DCs to the lymph nodes but also in migration of neutrophils and lymphocytes [28]. However, we confirmed that gene expression of neutrophil and lymphocyte markers was slightly raised while CD11b and CD11c expression was highly upregulated in inflamed adipose tissue, indicating that CCL19-mediated infiltrated cells consisted mainly of DCs. These results suggest that CCL19-CCR7 signaling plays an important role in induction of inflammation and insulin resistance in adipose tissue. The physiologic significance of high CCL19 expression in obese adipose tissue remains unclear, but high CCL19 expression in adipose tissue conceivably contributes to the pseudo-homing of mature DCs into adipose tissue.

Next, we investigated avoidant mechanisms of obesity in HFD-fed CCR7KO mice; two possibilities were suggested. One was involvement of adiponectin, known to promote energy expenditure through increase of AMP kinase activity. The blood adiponectin level was found to increase significantly in HFD-fed CCR7KO mice, suggesting that adiponectin increased energy expenditure. The other possibility was that thermogenesis resulted in transduction from intake energy to thermal energy. We attempted a cold exposure test to evaluate thermogenesis in each group following a cold challenge by measuring rectal temperature. CCR7KO mice were shown to maintain rectal temperature, indicating promotion of thermogenesis. Future studies are needed to quantitatively and qualitatively assess the involvement of adipose tissue in thermogenesis.

In conclusion, our studies suggest that people with inflammation in adipose tissue are prone to developing obesity due to the influence of energy expenditure. Conversely, obesity-promoting mechanisms might be activated in obese patients. We believe that it is important to elucidate the mechanism of weight control in terms of inflammation for future study.

15.5 Suggestions from Clinical Intervention Studies

15.5.1 The Hiroshima Study

As mentioned above, severe periodontal disease induces systemic micro-inflammation although it is a local oral infection. Recently, the findings of many worldwide reports that periodontal treatment improves inflammation and decreases HbA1c in patients with T2DM were supported and summarized by meta-analysis and systematic review. Thereafter, both practice guidelines of the Japan Diabetes Society and the Japanese Society of Periodontology recommended that diabetic patients should receive periodontal treatment from the viewpoint that periodontal treatment may improve HbA1c levels [29, 30].

Then, a detailed investigation was needed to answer questions about what kind of periodontal treatment should be given to diabetic patients to improve glycemic control and at what degree of periodontal disease should such treatment be initiated. So we conducted an intervention study called the Hiroshima study [15]. In this study, T2DM patients with periodontal disease were divided into two groups: a high hsCRP (>500 ng/ml) and low hsCRP (<500 ng/ml) group. Each group was subdivided into two groups: one received conventional nonsurgical periodontal treatment combined with local antibiotic administration (corresponding to group A with high hsCRP and group C with low hsCRP); the other group received nonsurgical periodontal treatment only (corresponding to group B with high hsCRP and group D with low hsCRP). Patients who refused periodontal treatment were set as controls and divided into two groups: group E with high hsCRP and group F with low hsCRP (Fig. 15.3). Based on a report from the Hisayama study investigating correlations between CRP at baseline and risk of myocardial infarction (MI), hsCRP >500 ng/ml, the threshold for a twofold increased risk of MI, was used to define high hsCRP.

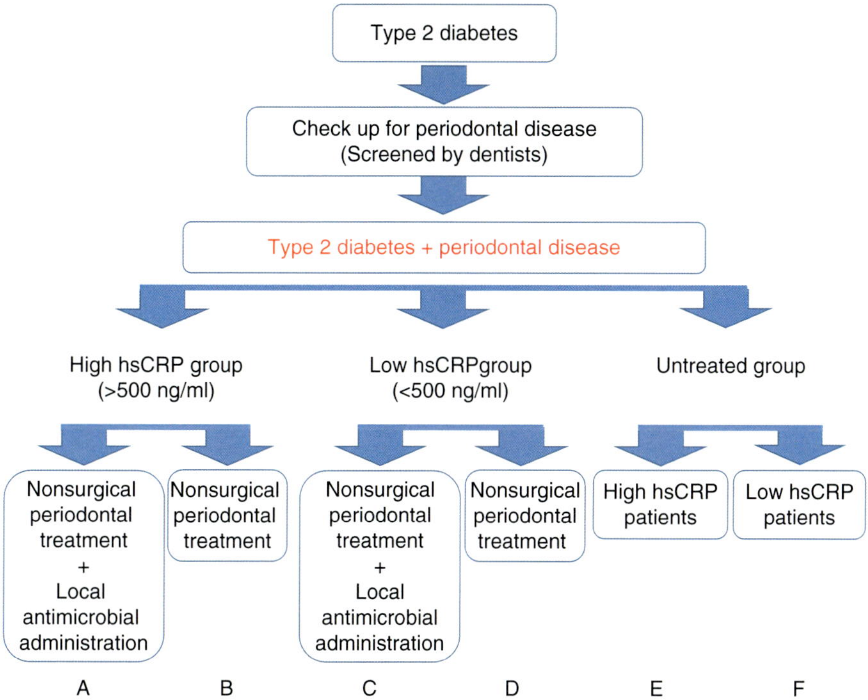

Fig. 15.3 Overview of the Hiroshima study investigating the effect of periodontal treatment on improvement of glycemic control in patients with T2DM**.** The image is reprinted from Trailblazing Studies of Intestinal and Oral Microflora in Systemic Diseases (CMC Publishing Co., Ltd)

While groups A and B (with high hsCRP at baseline) showed decreases in CRP and HbA1c levels after receiving periodontal treatment in a simple before-and-after comparison, the HbA1c levels in groups receiving periodontal treatment combined with local antibiotic administration were only confirmed to significantly improve in multiple group comparison. Interestingly, no change in HbA1c levels was observed in groups with low baseline hsCRP; regardless of the presence or absence of antibiotic administration, systemic inflammation was not induced even in those patients with severe periodontal disease. Neither CRP nor HbA1c levels were shown to change in groups that did not receive periodontal treatment (Table 15.1). Logistic regression analysis showed that periodontal treatment combined with local antibiotic administration as a starting point for intervention was found to influence HbA1c improvement most significantly. Namely, it was likely that the periodontal treatment in T2DM contributed to reducing systemic inflammation.

Then, despite their severity of periodontal disease is similar, what is the difference between subjects with high hsCRP and low hsCRP? Interestingly, the statistically significant difference between both was ascertained in only BMI; the high hsCRP group had a higher BMI than the low hsCRP group. Of note, there was a

Table 15.1 Summary of results in Hiroshima study

	Age	Sex (M:F)	BMI (kg/m^2)	hsCRP (ng/ml)		HbA1c (%)	
				Initial	Follow-up	Initial	Follow-up
A (*N* = 42)	66.79 (9.71)	(29:13)	25.11 (3.11)	1946.24 (2188.34)	552.0 (343.05)**	7.40 (1.17)	6.91 (0.86)**
B (*N* = 33)	67.18 (9.28)	(10:23)	23.61 (3.09)	1826.52 (1904.15)	907.82 (863.19)**	7.43 (1.17)	7.13 (0.96)*
C (*N* = 38)	65.82 (9.67)	(17:21)	23.78 (2.98)	237.24 (121.42)	271.71 (162.34)	6.92 (1.39)	6.89 (1.49)
D (*N* = 47)	66.21 (10.10)	(28:19)	23.15 (3.36)	226.09 (113.12)	384.43 (366.02)*	7.00 (0.97)	6.93 (0.88)
E (*N* = 62)	62.71 (13.62)	(37.25)	25.24 (4.00)	2231.02 (1909.77)	2140.31 (2164.37)	7.17 (0.99)	7.1 (1.01)
F (*N* = 56)	62.80 (10.50)	(27:29)	23.21 (2.79)	250.93 (125.04)	305.64 (196.69)	6.79 (0.93)	6.82 (0.95)

Statistical analyses for the differences between hsCRP and HbA1c values before and after periodontal treatment, and between 1 month and 3 months in the control group were performed by Wilcoxon's rank test. Data is expressed as mean standard deviation

*$P < 0.05$

**$P < 0.001$

slight but significant difference in BMI between both groups: the BMI in the high hsCRP subjects was approximately 25 kg/m^2 while that in low hsCRP subjects was approximately 23 kg/m^2. It was unlikely that subjects with a high hsCRP and increased BMI had more muscle mass than those with low hsCRP, as both groups suffered from T2DM. Therefore, subjects with high hsCRP were considered to have more mature adipose tissue.

Subjects with hsCRP >500 ng/ml were divided into two groups: patients received conventional nonsurgical periodontal treatment with (A) or without (B) local antibiotic administration. Subjects with hsCRP ≤500 ng/ml were divided into two groups: patients received conventional nonsurgical periodontal treatment with (C) or without (D) local antibiotic administration. Untreated subjects were also divided into two groups: patients with hsCRP >500 ng/ml (E) and ≤500 ng/ml (F) at baseline. The table is summarized from [22].

15.5.2 Reports from the Journal of the American Medical Association

A report entitled "The effect of nonsurgical periodontal therapy on hemoglobin A1c levels in persons with type 2 diabetes and chronic periodontitis: a randomized clinical trial" was published in the *Journal of the American Medical Association* (JAMA) at the end of 2013 [31]. This report stated that even though many clinical studies had reported that periodontal treatment may improve HbA1c levels in T2DM patients, evidence that chronic periodontitis was on the causal pathway of diabetes was observational, limited, and inconsistent.

Briefly, outpatient medical and dental clinics and communities of five academic medical centers in the United States participated in this randomized clinical trial. Participants were men and women with T2DM, aged ≥35 years, with no changes made to their diabetes medication(s) within the last 3 months and with an HbA1c level 7.0–8.9% at screening, who had ≥16 teeth and who had not received periodontal treatment in the preceding 6 months (total $n = 514$). Participants were divided into two groups: the treated group received nonsurgical periodontal therapy including scaling and root planning (SRP), oral hygiene instructions, chlorhexidine mouth washing, and supportive periodontal therapy (SPT) after 3 and 6 months, while the non-treated group did not. Changes in HbA1c in both groups were observed between baseline (just before periodontal treatment) and after 3 and 6 months. Surprisingly, this paper concluded that "Nonsurgical periodontal therapy did not improve glycemic control in patients with type 2 diabetes and moderate to advanced chronic periodontitis," exploding the conventional consensus. Specifically, HbA1c levels in the non-treated group were shown to increase by 0.11 ± 1.0%, and, instead of decreasing, the HbA1c levels in the treated group increased by 0.17 ± 1.0%. The authors concluded no significant difference between the groups [31].

15.5.3 Rebuttal Paper Against the Report of JAMA

A rebuttal paper was published against this JAMA paper in the Journal of Evidence-Based Dental Practice the next year. In this rebuttal paper, the authors described three major concerns with the JAMA paper [32]. The first concern was that no significant effect of periodontal treatment would be expected because baseline HbA1c levels were already close to the goal for good glycemic control. In general, the HbA1c goal is set at <7% in most patients; however, it is sometimes set at <8% in certain patients. In the JAMA paper, at baseline the average HbA1c in the treated group was 7.84% and that in untreated group was 7.77%. Besides, HbA1c in 60.3% of the treated group and 63.8% of the untreated group was <8%, indicating that the rest (~40%) of the subjects had an HbA1c >8%. Regardless of periodontal treatment, the effect size of improvement of glycemic control of any intervention depends on the HbA1c at baseline, that is, it is easy to imagine that the higher the HbA1c at baseline, the larger the potential improvement shown, and vice versa.

The second concern was that the effect of periodontal treatment was not accurately demonstrated because the treatment failed to reach the accepted standard of care. In principle, whether periodontal treatment was successful or not was objectively evaluated by measuring clinical parameters such as pocket probing depth (PPD), bleeding on probing, plaque score, and clinical attachment gain. In the JAMA paper, at the end of the study, each subject in the treated group still had on average 20.1% of sites with PPD ≥4 mm, and half of those (10.2% of sites) were ≥5 mm; 41.6% of all sites bled on probing, a relatively high rate. In terms of plaque score (a parameter of remaining dental plaque causing periodontitis), the average score was observed to change from 86.7% at baseline to only 72.1%, suggesting unsuccessful improvement. These parameters meant that most of the periodontal treatment provided in this study was inadequate. It is clear that inadequate periodontal treatment could not result in adequate improvement in HbA1c.

The third concern was that pronounced obesity would mask any decrease in inflammatory response caused by successful periodontal treatment. The mean BMI of the treated group was extremely high: 34.7 ± 7.5 kg/m^2. Previously, a study in the United States called the Atherosclerosis Risk Communities (ARIC) showed that while hsCRP in patients with a BMI of 20–29 kg/m^2 was associated with a twofold increase in severe periodontitis compared with control, the difference in hsCRP between both was gradually reduced in accordance with increases in BMI; finally, no difference was shown in patients whose BMI was ≥35 kg/m^2 [33]. In addition, the Periodontitis and Vascular Events (PAVE) multicenter clinical study reported that obese patients maintained a systemic inflammatory state after receiving periodontal treatment [34]. Furthermore, the aforementioned Hiroshima study clearly showed improvements in HbA1c following periodontal treatment in subjects with mild obesity. Taken together, the authors stated that in the JAMA paper, although no effect of periodontal therapy on the reduction of the systemic inflammatory burden was reported, it was possible that most of the subjects were resistant to the elimination of periodontal disease-related systemic inflammation due to the overwhelming influence of their obesity-related systemic inflammatory load.

15.6 Summary

Periodontal disease is thought to amplify inflammation through mature adipose tissue and to induce systemic micro-inflammation, thereby contributing to insulin resistance, resulting in exacerbation of diabetes (Fig. 15.4). Although many aspects of the mechanism remain unclear, there is no doubt that mechanism underlying the effects of periodontal disease on the whole body will be elucidated in more detail.

Moreover, from the results of many clinical studies including those aforementioned, it is likely that reducing obesity is important to allow sufficient improvement of glycemic control from the provision of periodontal treatment. In particular, patients with mild obesity are likely to gain glycemic control benefits from periodontal treatment. In the future, multicenter clinical studies targeting various obese and diabetic patients, supported with good-quality periodontal treatment in accordance with guidelines, are necessary to elucidate further the evidence for the effects of periodontal treatment on diabetic therapy.

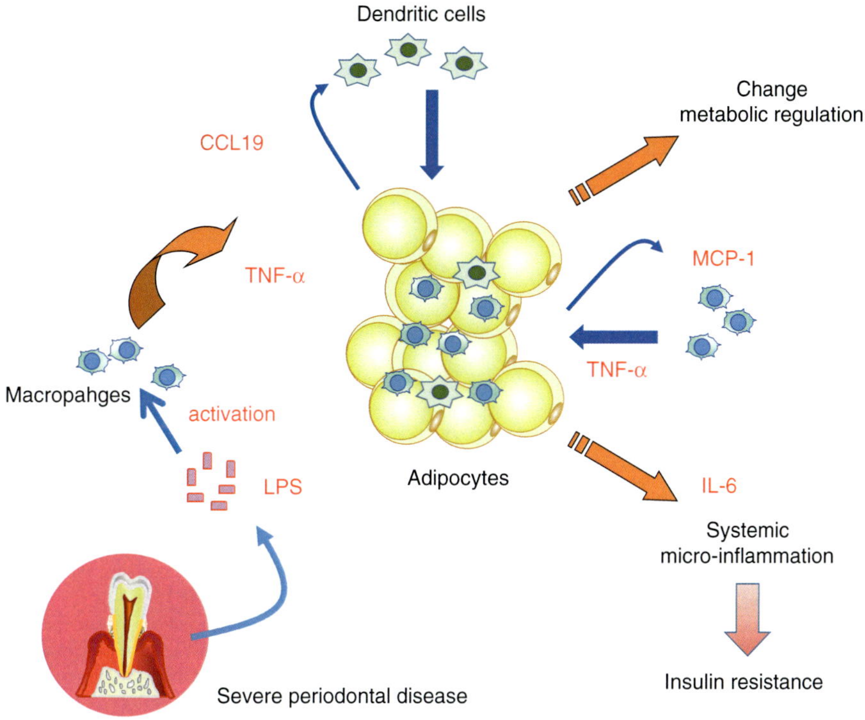

Fig. 15.4 Assumed mechanism of systemic amplification of periodontal inflammation. In severe periodontitis, TLR ligands are considered to flow into blood continuously, resulting in activation of the immune system. Immune cells are thought to infiltrate into adipose tissue, where they contribute to not only enhancing inflammation in adipose tissue but also, possibly, influence energy metabolism

References

1. Japan Society for Oral Health. Survey of dental diseases report in fiscal 2011; 2011.
2. Aida J, Ando Y, Akhter R, Aoyama H, Masui M, Morita M. Reasons for permanent tooth extractions in Japan. J Epidemiol. 2006;16:214–9.
3. Prabhu A, Michalowicz BS, Mathur A. Detection of local and systemic cytokines in adult periodontitis. J Periodontol. 1996;67:515–22.
4. Löe H. Periodontal disease. The sixth complication of diabetes mellitus. Diabetes Care. 1993;16:329–34.
5. Preshaw PM, Alba AL, Herrera D, Jepsen S, Konstantinidis A, Makrilakis K, et al. Periodontitis and diabetes: a two-way relationship. Diabetologia. 2012;55:21–31.
6. Khader YS, Dauod AS, El-Qaderi SS, Alkafajei A, Batayha WQ. Periodontal status of diabetics compared with nondiabetics: a meta-analysis. J Diabetes Complications. 2006;20:59–68.
7. Firatli E. The relationship between clinical periodontal status and insulin-dependent diabetes mellitus. Results after 5 years. J Periodontol. 1997;68:136–40.
8. Seppälä B, Seppälä M, Ainamo J. A longitudinal study on insulin-dependent diabetes mellitus and periodontal disease. J Clin Periodontol. 1993;20:161–5.

9. Tervonen T, Karjalainen K. Periodontal disease related to diabetic status. A pilot study of the response to periodontal therapy in type 1 diabetes. J Clin Periodontol. 1997;24:505–10.
10. Nelson RG, Shlossman M, Budding LM, Pettitt DJ, Saad MF, Genco RJ, et al. Periodontal disease and NIDDM in Pima Indians. Diabetes Care. 1990;13:836–40.
11. Tsai C, Hayes C, Taylor GW. Glycemic control of type 2 diabetes and severe periodontal disease in the US adult population. Community Dent Oral Epidemiol. 2002;30:182–92.
12. Soskolne WA, Klinger A. The relationship between periodontal disease and diabetes: an overview. Ann Periodontol. 2001;6:91–8.
13. Demmer RT, Jacobs DR Jr, Desvarieux M. Periodontal disease and incident type 2 diabetes: results from the First National Health and Nutrition Examination Survey and its epidemiologic follow-up study. Diabetes Care. 2008;31:1373–9.
14. Demmer RT, Desvarieux M, Holtfreter B, Jacobs DR Jr, Wallaschofski H, Nauck M, et al. Periodontal status and A1C change: longitudinal results from the study of health in Pomerania (SHIP). Diabetes Care. 2010;33:1037–43.
15. Saito T, Shimazaki Y, Kiyohara Y, Kato I, Kubo M, Iida M, et al. The severity of periodontal disease is associated with the development of glucose intolerance in non-diabetics: the Hisayama study. J Dent Res. 2004;83:485–90.
16. Ginsberg HN. Insulin resistance and cardiovascular disease. J Clin Invest. 2000;106:453–8.
17. Arima H, Kubo M, Yonemoto K, Doi Y, Ninomiya T, Tanizaki Y, et al. High-sensitivity C-reactive protein and coronary heart disease in a general population of Japanese: the Hisayama study. Arterioscler Thromb Vasc Biol. 2008;28:1385–91.
18. Ridker PM. High-sensitivity C-reactive protein: potential adjunct for global risk assessment in the primary prevention of cardiovascular disease. Circulation. 2001;103:1813–8.
19. Iwamoto Y, Nishimura F, Soga Y, Takeuchi K, Kurihara M, Takashiba S, et al. Antimicrobial periodontal treatment decreases serum C-reactive protein, tumor necrosis factor-alpha, but not adiponectin levels in patients with chronic periodontitis. J Periodontol. 2003;74:1231–6.
20. Madianos PN, Bobetsis GA, Kinane DF. Is periodontitis associated with an increased risk of coronary heart disease and preterm and/or low birth weight births? J Clin Periodontol. 2002;29:22–36.
21. Iwamoto Y, Nishimura F, Nakagawa M, Sugimoto H, Shikata K, Makino H, et al. The effect of antimicrobial periodontal treatment on circulating tumor necrosis factor-alpha and glycated hemoglobin level in patients with type 2 diabetes. J Periodontol. 2001;72:774–8.
22. Munenaga Y, Hiroshima Study Group, Yamashina T, Tanaka J, Nishimura F. Improvement of glycated hemoglobin in Japanese subjects with type 2 diabetes by resolution of periodontal inflammation using adjunct topic antibiotics: results from the Hiroshima Study. Diabetes Res Clin Pract. 2013;100:53–60.
23. Guilheme A, Virbasius JV, Puri V, Czech MP. Adipocyte dysfunctions linking obesity to insulin resistance and type 2 diabetes. Nat Rev Mol Cell Biol. 2008;9:367–77.
24. Yamashita A, Soga Y, Iwamoto Y, Asano T, Li Y, Abiko Y, et al. DNA microarray analyses of gene expressed differentially in 3 T3-L1 adipocytes co-cultured with murine macrophage cell line RAW264.7 in the presence of the toll-like receptor 4 ligand bacterial endotoxin. Int J Obes. 2008;32:1725–9.
25. Yamashita A, Soga Y, Iwamoto Y, Yoshizawa S, Iwata H, Kokeguchi S, et al. Macrophage-adipocyte interaction: marked interleukin-6 production by lipopolysaccharide. Obesity. 2007;15:2549–52.
26. Nakarai H, Yamashita A, Nagayasu S, Iwashita M, Kumamoto S, Ohyama H, et al. Adipocyte-macrophage interaction may mediate LPS-induced low-grade inflammation: potential link with metabolic complications. Innate Immun. 2012;18:164–70.
27. Sano T, Iwashita M, Nagayasu S, Yamashita A, Shinjo T, Hashikata A, et al. Protection from diet-induced obesity and insulin resistance in mice lacking CCL19-CCR7 signaling. Obesity. 2015;23:1460–71.
28. Von Andrian UH, Mempel TR. Homing and cellular traffic in lymph nodes. Nat Rev Immunol. 2003;3:867–78.

29. The Japan Diabetes Society. Diabetes and periodontitis. In: Evidence-based practice guideline for the treatment for diabetes in Japan 2013. Japan: Academic; 2013.
30. Japanese Society of Periodontology. Guideline for the periodontal treatment for diabetic patients. Revision of second edition. Japan: Academic; 2014, p. 29–34.
31. Engebretson SP, Hyman LG, Michalowicz BS, Schoenfeld ER, Gelato MC, Hou W, et al. The effect of non-surgical periodontal therapy on hemoglobin A1c levels in persons with type 2 diabetes and chronic periodontitis: a randomized clinical trial. JAMA. 2013;310:2523–32.
32. Borgnakke WS, Chapple IL, Genco RJ, Armitage G, Bartold PM, D'Aiuto F, et al. The multicenter randomized controlled trial (RCT) published by the journal of the American Medical Association (JAMA) on the effect of periodontal therapy on glycated hemoglobin (HbA1c) has fundamental problems. J Evid Based Dent Pract. 2014;14:127–32.
33. Slade GD, Ghezzi EM, Heiss G, Beck JD, Riche E, Offenbacher S. Relationship between periodontal disease and C-reactive protein among adults in the Atherosclerosis Risk in Communities study. Arch Intern Med. 2003;163:1172–9.
34. Offenbacher S, Beck JD, Moss K, Mendoza L, Paquette DW, Barrow DA, et al. Results from the Periodontitis and Vascular Events (PAVE) Study: a pilot multicentered, randomized, controlled trial to study effects of periodontal therapy in a secondary prevention model of cardiovascular disease. J Periodontol. 2009;80:190–201.

Chapter 16
Diabetes and Advanced Glycation End Products

Sho-ichi Yamagishi

Abstract The reaction of sugars, such as glucose and glyceraldehyde, with amino groups of proteins and lipids is enhanced under hyperglycemic conditions. As a result, the formation and accumulation of senescent macroprotein derivatives called advanced glycation end products (AGEs) have been known to progress in diabetes. Modification of proteins by AGEs alters their tertiary structure and physiological function, thereby causing multiple organ damage in diabetes. Further, engagement of the cell surface receptor RAGE with AGEs evokes oxidative stress and inflammatory reactions in a variety of tissues, being involved in the development and progression of numerous diabetes-associated disorders, including cardiovascular disease, osteoporosis, Alzheimer's disease, and cancer growth and metastasis. In this chapter, I briefly review the pathophysiological role of AGEs and their receptor RAGE system in diabetes- and aging-related complications, especially focusing on cardiovascular disease and osteoporosis.

Keywords AGEs • Aging • Diabetes • RAGE

16.1 Introduction

According to the recent report of Diabetes Atlas, about 415 million people worldwide had diabetes in 2015 [1]. The prevalence of diabetes is estimated to be 9%, and one person dies from diabetes every 6 s all over the world [1]. The global figure of people with diabetes is projected to increase to 642 million in 2040. Now, diabetes is a major health burden. Although cardiovascular disease (CVD) is the leading cause of death in diabetes, other aging-associated disorders, such as osteoporosis, Alzheimer's disease, and various kinds of cancers, are highly prevalent in patients with both type 1 and type 2 diabetes [2–7]. As a result, average life span is

S.-i. Yamagishi
Department of Pathophysiology and Therapeutics of Diabetic Vascular Complications, Kurume University School of Medicine, Kurume 830-0011, Japan
e-mail: shoichi@med.kurume-u.ac.jp

S.-i. Yamagishi (ed.), *Diabetes and Aging-related Complications*,
https://doi.org/10.1007/978-981-10-4376-5_16

significantly reduced in diabetic patients compared with non-diabetic individuals; Emerging Risk Factors Collaboration revealed that 40-year-old diabetic patients without known CVD at the time of enrollment died 6.3 years younger than non-diabetic subjects [8–11].

Large clinical trials have substantiated the concept of "metabolic memory" in the increased risk of vascular complications and death in type 1 and type 2 diabetic patients [12–14]. This means that cumulative diabetic exposure is mainly involved in the pathogenesis of diabetes-associated complications. There is a growing body of evidence that advanced glycation end products (AGEs) play a role in CVD, osteoporosis, Alzheimer's disease, and cancer growth and metastasis as well [2–7]. Moreover, the unique biochemical nature and mode of actions of AGEs may provide the mechanistic basis to understand why former diabetic exposure has contributed to current progression of vascular complications and increased mortality in patients with diabetes [12–14]. In this chapter, I briefly review the pathophysiological role of AGEs and their receptor RAGE system in diabetes- and aging-related complications, especially focusing on cardiovascular disease and osteoporosis.

16.2 AGEs

A nonenzymatic reaction between sugars, such as glucose, fructose, and glyceraldehyde, and the amino groups of proteins, lipids, and nucleic acids is enhanced under diabetic conditions to form reversible Schiff bases and then Amadori products [15–22]. These early glycation products undergo rearrangement, dehydration, condensation, and other complex reactions to become irreversibly cross-linked, heterogeneous macroprotein derivatives called AGEs [15–22]. The abovementioned process of nonenzymatic glycation is also known as Maillard reaction because L.C. Maillard, a French chemist, discovered a century ago that brown fluorescent products were generated when amino acids were heated with reducing sugars [15–22]. Since then, food chemists have long studied this process as a source of flavor, color, and texture changes in cooked or stored foods. But, in the late 1970s, it was realized that this process could also occur in human body [23, 24].

The formation and accumulation of AGEs in various tissues and organs have been known to progress at a physiological normal aging and at an extremely accelerated rate under hyperglycemic and/or oxidative stress conditions [15–24]. Modification of proteins by AGEs alters their tertiary structure and physiological function, thereby causing multiple organ damage in diabetes [2–7, 15–24]. Furthermore, engagement of the cell surface receptor RAGE with AGEs evokes oxidative stress and inflammatory reactions in a variety of tissues, being involved in the development and progression of numerous diabetes-associated disorders, including cardiovascular disease, osteoporosis, Alzheimer's disease, and cancer growth and metastasis [2–7, 25–32]. AGEs are slowly degraded and remain for a long time in diabetic vessels and tissues even after achieving good glycemic control [33, 34]. In addition, AGEs have been shown to upregulate RAGE expression and induce

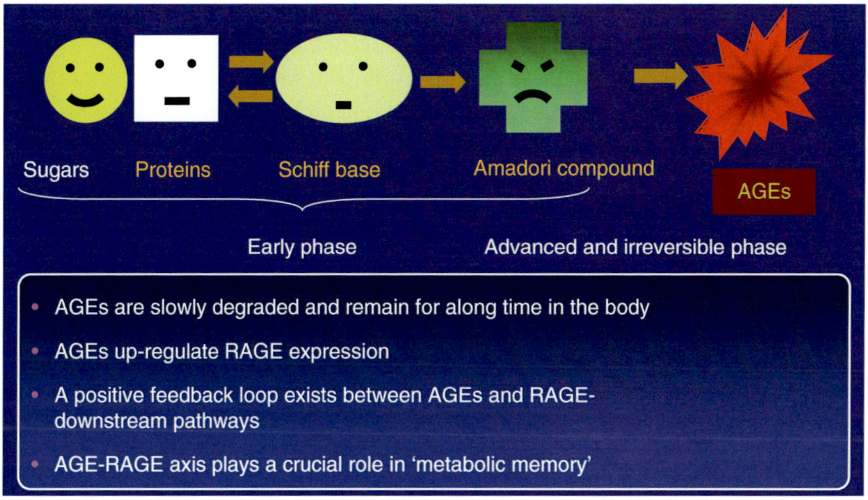

Fig. 16.1 Formation of AGEs and activation of RAGE

sustained activation of nuclear factor-κB [25–32]. Therefore, the AGE-RAGE-induced oxidative stress generation further potentiates the formation and accumulation of AGEs and subsequent RAGE overexpression, making a positive feedback loop between AGEs and RAGE-downstream pathways. These observations suggest that activation of the AGE-RAGE axis may play a crucial role in the phenomenon of "metabolic memory" (Fig. 16.1).

16.3 AGEs and CVD

AGEs evoke oxidative stress generation and subsequently elicit inflammatory and thrombotic reactions in endothelial cells (ECs) through the interaction of RAGE via activation of NADPH oxidase [35, 36]. AGE-induced, nuclear factor-κB-dependent transcriptional gene expression of chemokines and growth factors, such as monocyte chemoattractant protein-1 and platelet-derived growth factor-B, contributes to vascular inflammation and smooth muscle cell proliferation and migration, thereby promoting the progression of atherosclerosis [37, 38].

AGE-RAGE interaction not only reduces the production of nitric oxide (NO) by ECs but also inactivates NO to generate peroxynitrite, a highly toxic product of NO with superoxide anion [39, 40]. Moreover, AGEs increase asymmetric dimethylarginine (ADMA), an endogenous inhibitor of NO synthase by various types of cells, including ECs [41–44]. The generation of ADMA is stimulated, whereas its degradation is suppressed by the AGE-RAGE axis [41–44]. Since NO is recognized as an endogenous atheroprotective factor by exerting anti-inflammatory, antiproliferative, and antithrombotic effects on ECs, activation of the AGE-RAGE system may contribute to endothelial dysfunction, an initial step of atherosclerosis [41–44]. Indeed, we have recently found that plasma ADMA levels are positively associated with serum AGE levels and inversely correlated with endothelial function determined by flow-mediated vasodilatation in end-stage renal disease patients due to diabetic nephropathy [44]. The ratio of AGEs to soluble RAGE is correlated with impaired endothelial function in non-diabetic individuals as well [45]. Furthermore, we have demonstrated that circulating AGE levels are independently associated with vascular inflammation evaluated by [(18)F]fluorodeoxyglucose positron emission tomography, which are correlated with endothelial dysfunction in high-risk patients for CVD, thus suggesting that vascular inflammation evoked by AGEs may also be involved in impairment of endothelial function in these patients [46–48]. AGE-RAGE axis also inhibits adhesion, spreading, proliferation, and migration of endothelial progenitor cells [49, 50]. Since serum AGE levels are inversely associated with number and migratory activity of endothelial progenitor cells [51], AGEs could also impair EC repair.

Atherothrombosis, characterized by atherosclerotic lesion disruption with superimposed thrombus formation, is thought to be the major cause of acute coronary syndrome [52, 53]. AGE-RAGE interaction inhibits prostacyclin production in ECs, whereas it evokes platelet activation and aggregation, stimulates procoagulant activity, and stabilizes arterial thrombi by suppressing the fibrinolytic activity [54–61]. Plaque neovascularization promoted by AGE-RAGE axis may also cause plaque rupture and intraplaque hemorrhage, which could lead to acute coronary syndrome [62–65]. Circulating AGE levels are associated with thrombogenic markers such as plasminogen activator inhibitor-1 and fibrinogen in a general population as well [66, 67].

We have found that AGEs decrease gene expression levels of adenosine triphosphate-binding membrane cassette transporter A1 and G1 in THP-1 macrophages and subsequently suppress cholesterol efflux from THP-1 macrophages to apolipoprotein AI and HDL-cholesterol, respectively [68]. The findings suggest that the AGE-RAGE axis may impair reverse cholesterol transport and promote foam cell formation within the atherosclerotic lesions in diabetes [68, 69].

Administration of a recombinant soluble form of RAGE consisting of the extracellular ligand-binding domain has been shown not only to suppress the development of atherosclerosis but also to stabilize established atherosclerosis in diabetic apolipoprotein E-null mice [70, 71]. The treatment with soluble RAGE resulted in decreased atherosclerotic lesion area in apolipoprotein E-deficient db/db mice, a murine model of type 2 diabetes [72]. Diabetic RAGE(-/-)/apolipoprotein E (apoE) (-/-) mice also exhibited significantly reduced atherosclerotic plaque area, which was associated with attenuation of leukocyte recruitment, decreased expression of pro-inflammatory mediators, reduced oxidative stress, and AGE accumulation [73].

We have recently found that DNA aptamer that can bind with high affinity and specificity to AGEs (AGE-aptamer) inhibits neointima formation after balloon angioplasty in association with the reduced expression of AGEs, RAGE, and an oxidative stress marker, 8-hydroxy-2′-deoxyguanosine in balloon-injured arteries [74]. Compared with control aptamer, AGE-aptamer significantly suppresses smooth muscle cell proliferation, macrophage infiltration, and platelet-derived growth factor-BB expression in balloon-injured carotid arteries as well [74].

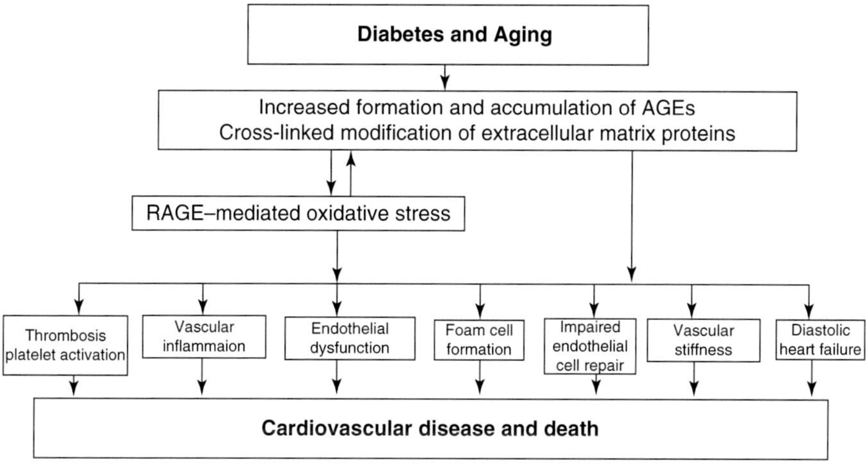

Fig. 16.2 Role of AGE-RAGE axis in CVD

It should be noted that cross-linked modification of extracellular matrix proteins by AGE increases vascular and myocardial stiffness and impairs structural integrity and physiological function of multiple organ systems, thus being involved in arterial stiffness, arterial fibrillation, isolated systolic hypertension, and diastolic heart failure [3, 4]. The role of AGE-RAGE axis in CVD is summarized in Fig. 16.2.

16.4 AGEs and Osteoporosis

The risk of osteoporosis-related bone fractures is elevated in both type 1 and type 2 diabetic patients [75–78]. Although bone mineral density (BMD) is decreased in patients with type 1 diabetes, it cannot entirely explain the increased risk of osteoporotic bone fractures in these patients. Furthermore, BMD is increased *rather than* reduced in type 2 diabetes [78–81]. These observations suggest that bone quality and microstructure are also impaired in diabetes, making the relative risk of bone fracture much higher than that calculated based on BMD. Moreover, the Rotterdam study showed that risk of bone fracture was higher only in already established and treated type 2 diabetic patients but not subjects in newly diagnosed diabetes compared with non-diabetic individuals [82]. Therefore, cumulative diabetic exposure may also be involved in osteoporosis-related bone fractures in diabetes.

AGE-RAGE axis induces apoptotic cell death of osteoblasts via oxidative stress generation [83, 84]. Furthermore, AGE-modified type 1 collagen decreases adhesion of osteoblasts and inhibits its proliferation and spreading through intracellular reactive oxygen species production [85]. Since AGE modification of collagen in the bone matrix is accelerated under diabetes, it may play a role in reduced BMD in diabetes [86, 87]. Although there is some controversy about the pathological role of AGEs in osteoclast function, AGEs or RAGE-downstream pathway have been reported to activate osteoclasts or promote osteoclastogenesis, enhancing bone resorptive activity, which may also lead to decreased BMD and reduced bone biomechanical strength in diabetes [88–90].

In vitro glycation of human tibial cancellous bone cores increases the microdamage and reduces the fracture resistance [91]. AGE-modified collagen impairs lysyl oxidase-dependent physiological collagen cross-links by osteoblast cells, which could stimulate bone collagen degradation [92, 93]. Moreover, decreased bone mechanical properties are associated with AGE accumulation levels in the bone collagen of diabetic rats [94]. Trabecular AGE levels in human vertebrae are also inversely correlated with whole bone strength [95]. These observations suggest that mechanical integrity of the collagen network in the bone might deteriorate with diabetes and/or age due to enhanced accumulation of bone AGEs, being involved in osteoporosis in these subjects [96].

Serum levels of pentosidine, one of the well-characterized AGEs, are significantly increased in postmenopausal type 2 diabetic women with vertebral fractures compared with those without fractures and associated with the presence of vertebral fractures, which is totally independent of BMD [97]. Schwartz et al. reported that elevation in urinary pentosidine levels was independently correlated with increased clinical fracture incidence as well as vertebral fracture prevalence in elderly patients with type 2 diabetes [98].

16.5 AGEs and Aging

A lifelong restriction of AGE-rich diet reduces oxidative stress generation and AGE accumulation as well as RAGE expression, resulting in extension of life span in mice [99]. Furthermore, oral intake of AGE-containing foods has been shown to determine the biological effects of calorie-restricted diet, such as oxidant stress generation, risk of age-related diseases, and mortality in mice [100]. These findings suggest that restriction of AGE-rich diet may be a novel therapeutic target for slowing the aging process and achieving a successful life.

The Baltimore Longitudinal Study of Aging showed that serum carboxymethyllysine (CML), one of the dominant AGEs contained in foods, was independently associated with progression of renal dysfunction in community-dwelling adults [101]. Furthermore, high circulating CML levels were reported to predict cardiovascular disease mortality among older community-dwelling women [102]. In nondiabetic adults aged 65 and older residing in Tuscany, Italy, those with plasma CML in the highest tertile had greater all cause and CVD as well [103]. Dietary AGEs may be a modifiable risk factor for diabetes- and aging-related complications.

16.6 Conclusions

Accumulation of AGEs via endogenous and exogenous pathway and resultant activation of RAGE downstream signaling may play a role in the pathogenesis of various diabetes- and aging-related disorders. Inhibition of the AGE formation, reduction of intake of AGE-rich diet, and blockade of the AGE-RAGE-induced oxidative stress system may be a novel target for antiaging medicine.

Acknowledgments This work was supported in part by Grants-in-Aid for Scientific Research (B) from the Ministry of Education, Culture, Sports, Science, and Technology of Japan. No potential conflicts of interest relevant to this article were reported.

References

1. International Diabetes Federation. IDF diabetes atlas. 7th ed. Brussels: International Diabetes Federation; 2016.
2. Yamagishi S, Imaizumi T. Diabetic vascular complications: pathophysiology, biochemical basis and potential therapeutic strategy. Curr Pharm Des. 2005;11:2279–99.
3. Yamagishi S. Potential clinical utility of advanced glycation end product cross-link breakers in age- and diabetes-associated disorders. Rejuvenation Res. 2012;15:564–72.
4. Yamagishi S, Fukami K, Matsui T. Evaluation of tissue accumulation levels of advanced glycation end products by skin autofluorescence: a novel marker of vascular complications in high-risk patients for cardiovascular disease. Int J Cardiol. 2015;185:263–8.
5. Yamagishi S, Matsui T, Fukami K. Role of receptor for advanced glycation end products (RAGE) and its ligands in cancer risk. Rejuvenation Res. 2015;18:48–56.
6. Takeuchi M, Yamagishi S. Possible involvement of advanced glycation end-products (AGEs) in the pathogenesis of Alzheimer's disease. Curr Pharm Des. 2008;14:973–8.
7. Yamagishi S. Role of advanced glycation end products (AGEs) in osteoporosis in diabetes. Curr Drug Targets. 2011;12:2096–102.
8. Emerging Risk Factors Collaboration, Seshasai SR, Kaptoge S, Thompson A, Di Angelantonio E, Gao P, Sarwar N, Whincup PH, Mukamal KJ, Gillum RF, Holme I, Njølstad I, Fletcher A, Nilsson P, Lewington S, Collins R, Gudnason V, Thompson SG, Sattar N, Selvin E, Hu FB, Danesh J. Diabetes mellitus, fasting glucose, and risk of cause-specific death. N Engl J Med. 2011;364:829–41.
9. Loukine L, Waters C, Choi BC, Ellison J. Impact of diabetes mellitus on life expectancy and health-adjusted life expectancy in Canada. Popul Health Metr. 2012;10:7.
10. Turin TC, Murakami Y, Miura K, Rumana N, Kadota A, Ohkubo T, Okamura T, Okayama A, Ueshima H. NIPPON DATA80 Research Group: diabetes and life expectancy among Japanese-NIPPON DATA80. Diabetes Res Clin Pract. 2012;96:e18–22.
11. Rhodes ET, Prosser LA, Hoerger TJ, Lieu T, Ludwig DS, Laffel LM. Estimated morbidity and mortality in adolescents and young adults diagnosed with Type 2 diabetes mellitus. Diabet Med. 2012;29:453–63.
12. Diabetes Control and Complications Trial (DCCT)/Epidemiology of Diabetes Interventions and Complications (EDIC) Research Group, Lachin JM, White NH, Hainsworth DP, Sun W, Cleary PA, Nathan DM. Effect of intensive diabetes therapy on the progression of diabetic retinopathy in patients with type 1 diabetes: 18 years of follow-up in the DCCT/EDIC. Diabetes. 2015;64:631–42.
13. Nathan DM, DCCT/EDIC Research Group. The diabetes control and complications trial/epidemiology of diabetes interventions and complications study at 30 years: overview. Diabetes Care. 2014;37:9–16.
14. Cefalu WT, Rosenstock J, LeRoith D, Blonde L, Riddle MC. Getting to the "heart" of the matter on diabetic cardiovascular disease: "thanks for the memory". Diabetes Care. 2016;39:664–7.
15. Vlassara H, Brownlee M, Cerami A. Accumulation of diabetic rat peripheral nerve myelin by macrophages increases with the presence of advanced glycosylation endproducts. J Exp Med. 1984;160:197–207.

16. Brownlee M, Cerami A, Vlassara H. Advanced glycosylation end products in tissue and the biochemical basis of diabetic complications. N Engl J Med. 1988;318:1315–21.
17. Dyer DG, Blackledge JA, Thorpe SR, Baynes JW. Formation of pentosidine during nonenzymatic browning of proteins by glucose. Identification of glucose and other carbohydrates as possible precursors of pentosidine in vivo. J Biol Chem. 1991;266:11654–60.
18. Grandhee SK, Monnier VM. Mechanism of formation of the Maillard protein cross-link pentosidine. Glucose, fructose, and ascorbate as pentosidine precursors. J Biol Chem. 1991;266:11649–53.
19. Bucala CA. Advanced glycosylation: chemistry, biology, and implications for diabetes and aging. Adv Pharmacol. 1992;23:1–34.
20. Glomb MA, Monnier VM. Mechanism of protein modification by glyoxal and glycoaldehyde, reactive intermediates of the Maillard reaction. J Biol Chem. 1995;70:10017–26.
21. Vlassara H, Palace MR. Diabetes and advanced glycation endproducts. J Intern Med. 2002;251:87–101.
22. Rahbar S, Figarola JL. Novel inhibitors of advanced glycation endproducts. Arch Biochem Biophys. 2003;419:63–79.
23. Rahbar S, Blumenfeld O, Ranney HM. Studies of an unusual hemoglobin in patients with diabetes mellitus. Biochem Biophys Res Commun. 1969;36:838–43.
24. Stevens VJ, Vlassara H, Abati A, Cerami A. Nonenzymatic glycosylation of hemoglobin. J Biol Chem. 1977;252:2998–3002.
25. Bierhaus A, Hofmann MA, Ziegler R, Nawroth PP. AGEs and their interaction with AGE-receptors in vascular disease and diabetes mellitus. I. The AGE concept. Cardiovasc Res. 1998;37:586–600.
26. Schmidt AM, Stern D. Atherosclerosis and diabetes: the RAGE connection. Curr Atheroscler Rep. 2000;2:430–6.
27. Ward MS, Fortheringham AK, Cooper ME, Forbes JM. Targeting advanced glycation endproducts and mitochondrial dysfunction in cardiovascular disease. Curr Opin Pharmacol. 2013;13:654–61.
28. Yamagishi S, Fukami K, Matsui T. Crosstalk between advanced glycation end products (AGEs)-receptor RAGE axis and dipeptidyl peptidase-4-incretin system in diabetic vascular complications. Cardiovasc Diabetol. 2015;14:2.
29. Fukami K, Taguchi K, Yamagishi S, Okuda S. Receptor for advanced glycation endproducts and progressive kidney disease. Curr Opin Nephrol Hypertens. 2015;24:54–60.
30. Yamagishi S, Nakamura N, Suematsu M, Kaseda K, Matsui T. Advanced glycation end products: a molecular target for vascular complications in diabetes. Mol Med. 2015;21(Suppl 1):S32–40.
31. Ramasamy R, Shekhtman A, Schmidt AM. The multiple faces of RAGE—opportunities for therapeutic intervention in aging and chronic disease. Expert Opin Ther Targets. 2016;20:431–46.
32. Yamagishi S, Matsui T. Pathologic role of dietary advanced glycation end products in cardiometabolic disorders, and therapeutic intervention. Nutrition. 2016;32:157–65.
33. Wolffenbuttel BH, Giordano D, Founds HW, Bucala R. Long-term assessment of glucose control by haemoglobin-AGE measurement. Lancet. 1996;347:513–5.
34. Hricik DE, Wu YC, Schulak A, Friedlander MA. Disparate changes in plasma and tissue pentosidine levels after kidney and kidney-pancreas transplantation. Clin Transplant. 1996;10:568–73.
35. Yamagishi S, Maeda S, Matsui T, Ueda S, Fukami K, Okuda S. Role of advanced glycation end products (AGEs) and oxidative stress in vascular complications in diabetes. Biochim Biophys Acta. 2012;1820:663–71.
36. Yamagishi S, Matsui T. Pigment epithelium-derived factor (PEDF) and cardiometabolic disorders. Curr Pharm Des. 2014;20:2377–86.
37. Inagaki Y, Yamagishi S, Okamoto T, Takeuchi M, Amano S. Pigment epithelium-derived factor prevents advanced glycation end products-induced monocyte chemoattractant protein-1

production in microvascular endothelial cells by suppressing intracellular reactive oxygen species generation. Diabetologia. 2003;46:284–7.
38. Yamagishi S, Matsui T. Smooth muscle cell pathophysiology and advanced glycation end products (AGEs). Curr Drug Targets. 2010;11:875–81.
39. Yamagishi S, Ueda S, Matsui T, Nakamura K, Imaizumi T, Takeuchi M, Okuda S. Pigment epithelium-derived factor (PEDF) prevents advanced glycation end products (AGEs)-elicited endothelial nitric oxide synthase (eNOS) reduction through its anti-oxidative properties. Protein Pept Lett. 2007;14:832–5.
40. Soro-Paavonen A, Zhang WZ, Venardos K, Coughlan MT, Harris E, Tong DC, Brasacchio D, Paavonen K, Chin-Dusting J, Cooper ME, Kaye D, Thomas MC, Forbes JM. Advanced glycation end-products induce vascular dysfunction via resistance to nitric oxide and suppression of endothelial nitric oxide synthase. J Hypertens. 2010;28:780–8.
41. Ueda S, Yamagishi S, Yokoro M, Okuda S. Role of asymmetric dimethylarginine in cardiorenal syndrome. Curr Pharm Des. 2014;20:2448–55.
42. Ojima A, Ishibashi Y, Matsui T, Maeda S, Nishino Y, Takeuchi M, Fukami K, Yamagishi S. Glucagon-like peptide-1 receptor agonist inhibits asymmetric dimethylarginine generation in the kidney of streptozotocin-induced diabetic rats by blocking advanced glycation end product-induced protein arginine methyltranferase-1 expression. Am J Pathol. 2013;182:132–41.
43. Ishibashi Y, Matsui T, Ueda S, Fukami K, Okuda S, Yamagishi S. Irbesartan inhibits advanced glycation end product-induced increase in asymmetric dimethylarginine level in mesangial cells through its anti-oxidative properties. Int J Cardiol. 2014;176:1120–2.
44. Ando R, Ueda S, Yamagishi S, Miyazaki H, Kaida Y, Kaifu K, Yokoro M, Nakayama Y, Obara N, Fukami K, Takeuchi M, Okuda S. Involvement of advanced glycation end product-induced asymmetric dimethylarginine generation in endothelial dysfunction. Diab Vasc Dis Res. 2013;10:436–41.
45. Kajikawa M, Nakashima A, Fujimura N, Maruhashi T, Iwamoto Y, Iwamoto A, Matsumoto T, Oda N, Hidaka T, Kihara Y, Chayama K, Goto C, Aibara Y, Noma K, Takeuchi M, Matsui T, Yamagishi S, Higashi Y. Ratio of serum levels of AGEs to soluble form of RAGE is a predictor of endothelial function. Diabetes Care. 2015;38:119–25.
46. Tahara N, Yamagishi S, Takeuchi M, Honda A, Tahara A, Nitta Y, Kodama N, Mizoguchi M, Kaida H, Ishibashi M, Hayabuchi N, Matsui T, Imaizumi T. Positive association between serum level of glyceraldehyde-derived advanced glycation end products and vascular inflammation evaluated by [(18)F]fluorodeoxyglucose positron emission tomography. Diabetes Care. 2012;35:2618–25.
47. Honda A, Tahara N, Nitta Y, Tahara A, Igata S, Bekki M, Nakamura T, Sugiyama Y, Kaida H, Kurata S, Fujimoto K, Abe T, Enomoto M, Adachi H, Narula J, Yamagishi SI, Fukumoto Y. Vascular Inflammation Evaluated by [18F]-Fluorodeoxyglucose-Positron Emission Tomography/Computed Tomography Is Associated With Endothelial Dysfunction. Arterioscler Thromb Vasc Biol. 2016;36(9):1980–8. doi:10.1161/ATVBAHA.116.307293.
48. Yamagishi SI. Structural abnormality or vascular dysfunction? A road to ruin. J Atheroscler Thromb. 2016;23(11):1255–6. doi:10.5551/jat.ED047.
49. Chen Q, Dong L, Wang L, Kang L, Xu B. Advanced glycation end products impair function of late endothelial progenitor cells through effects on protein kinase Akt and cyclooxygenase-2. Biochem Biophys Res Commun. 2009;381:192–7.
50. Scheubel RJ, Kahrstedt S, Weber H, Holtz J, Friedrich I, Borgermann J, Silber RE, Simm A. Depression of progenitor cell function by advanced glycation endproducts (AGEs): potential relevance for impaired angiogenesis in advanced age and diabetes. Exp Gerontol. 2006;41:540–8.
51. Ueda S, Yamagishi S, Matsui T, Noda Y, Ueda S, Jinnouchi Y, Sasaki K, Takeuchi M, Imaizumi T. Serum levels of advanced glycation end products (AGEs) are inversely associated with the number and migratory activity of circulating endothelial progenitor cells in apparently healthy subjects. Cardiovasc Ther. 2012;30:249–54.

52. Takenaka K, Yamagishi S, Matsui T, Nakamura K, Imaizumi T. Role of advanced glycation end products (AGEs) in thrombogenic abnormalities in diabetes. Curr Neurovasc Res. 2006;3:73–7.
53. Yamagishi SI, Matsui T. Anti-atherothrombogenic properties of PEDF. Curr Mol Med. 2010;10:284–91.
54. Yamagishi S, Fujimori H, Yonekura H, Yamamoto Y, Yamamoto H. Advanced glycation endproducts inhibit prostacyclin production and induce plasminogen activator inhibitor-1 in human microvascular endothelial cells. Diabetologia. 1998;41:1435–41.
55. Yamagishi S, Matsui T, Takenaka K, Nakamura K, Takeuchi M, Inoue H. Pigment epithelium-derived factor (PEDF) prevents platelet activation and aggregation in diabetic rats by blocking deleterious effects of advanced glycation end products (AGEs). Diabetes Metab Res Rev. 2009;25:266–71.
56. Yamagishi S, Matsui T, Nakamura K, Takenaka K. Pigment epithelium-derived factor (PEDF) inhibits collagen-induced platelet activation by reducing intraplatelet nitrotyrosine levels. Int J Cardiol. 2010;140:121–2.
57. Yamagishi S, Matsui T, Ueda S, Takeuchi M. Pigment epithelium-derived factor (PEDF) inhibits diabetes- or advanced glycation end product (AGE)-induced platelet CD40 ligand overexpression in rats. Int J Cardiol. 2010;144:283–5.
58. Bierhaus A, Illmer T, Kasper M, Luther T, Quehenberger P, Tritschler H, Wahl P, Ziegler R, Müller M, Nawroth PP. Advanced glycation end product (AGE)-mediated induction of tissue factor in cultured endothelial cells is dependent on RAGE. Circulation. 1997;96:2262–71.
59. Ishibashi Y, Matsui T, Ueda S, Fukami K, Yamagishi S. Advanced glycation end products potentiate citrated plasma-evoked oxidative and inflammatory reactions in endothelial cells by up-regulating protease-activated receptor-1 expression. Cardiovasc Diabetol. 2014;13:60.
60. Ishibashi Y, Matsui T, Yamagishi S. Apixaban exerts anti-inflammatory effects in mesangial cells by blocking thrombin/protease-activated receptor-1 system. Thromb Res. 2014;134:1365–7.
61. Ishibashi Y, Matsui T, Fukami K, Ueda S, Okuda S, Yamagishi SI. Rivaroxaban inhibits oxidative and inflammatory reactions in advanced glycation end product-exposed tubular cells by blocking thrombin/protease-activated receptor-2 system. Thromb Res. 2015;135:770–3.
62. Moulton KS. Plaque angiogenesis and atherosclerosis. Curr Atheroscler Rep. 2001;3:225–33.
63. Yamagishi S, Imaizumi T. Pericyte biology and diseases. Int J Tissue React. 2005;27:125–35.
64. Yamagishi S, Yonekura H, Yamamoto Y, Katsuno K, Sato F, Mita I, Ooka H, Satozawa N, Kawakami T, Nomura M, Yamamoto H. Advanced glycation end products-driven angiogenesis in vitro. Induction of the growth and tube formation of human microvascular endothelial cells through autocrine vascular endothelial growth factor. J Biol Chem. 1997;272:8723–30.
65. Yamagishi S, Nakamura K, Matsui T, Inagaki Y, Takenaka K, Jinnouchi Y, Yoshida Y, Matsuura T, Narama I, Motomiya Y, Takeuchi M, Inoue H, Yoshimura A, Bucala R, Imaizumi T. Pigment epithelium-derived factor inhibits advanced glycation end product-induced retinal vascular hyperpermeability by blocking reactive oxygen species-mediated vascular endothelial growth factor expression. J Biol Chem. 2006;281:20213–20.
66. Enomoto M, Adachi H, Yamagishi S, Takeuchi M, Furuki K, Hino A, Hiratsuka A, Takajo Y, Imaizumi T. Positive association of serum levels of advanced glycation end products with thrombogenic markers in humans. Metabolism. 2006;55:912–7.
67. Yamagishi S, Adachi H, Takeuchi M, Enomoto M, Furuki K, Matsui T, Nakamura K, Imaizumi T. Serum level of advanced glycation end-products (AGEs) is an independent determinant of plasminogen activator inhibitor-1 (PAI-1) in nondiabetic general population. Horm Metab Res. 2007;39:845–8.
68. Ishibashi Y, Matsui T, Takeuchi M, Yamagishi S. Rosuvastatin blocks advanced glycation end products-elicited reduction of macrophage cholesterol efflux by suppressing NADPH oxidase activity via inhibition of geranylgeranylation of Rac-1. Horm Metab Res. 2011;43:619–24.
69. Khera AV, Cuchel M, de la Llera-Moya M, Rodrigues A, Burke MF, Jafri K, French BC, Phillips JA, Mucksavage ML, Wilensky RL, Mohler ER, Rothblat GH, Rader DJ. Cholesterol

efflux capacity, high-density lipoprotein function, and atherosclerosis. N Engl J Med. 2011;364:127–35.
70. Park L, Raman KG, Lee KJ, Lu Y, Ferran LJ Jr, Chow WS, Stern D, Schmidt AM. Suppression of accelerated diabetic atherosclerosis by the soluble receptor for advanced glycation end products. Nat Med. 1998;4:1025–31.
71. Bucciarelli L, Wendt T, Qu W, Lu Y, Lalla E, Rong LL, Goova MT, Moser B, Kislinger T, Lee DC, Kashyap Y, Stern DM, Schmidt AM. RAGE blockade stabilizes established atherosclerosis in diabetic apolipoprotein E-null mice. Circulation. 2002;106:2827–35.
72. Wendt T, Harja E, Bucciarelli L, Qu W, Lu Y, Rong LL, Jenkins DG, Stein G, Schmidt AM, Yan SF. RAGE modulates vascular inflammation and atherosclerosis in a murine model of type 2 diabetes. Atherosclerosis. 2006;185:70–7.
73. Soro-Paavonen A, Watson AM, Li J, Paavonen K, Koitka A, Calkin AC, Barit D, Coughlan MT, Drew BG, Lancaster GI, Thomas M, Forbes JM, Nawroth PP, Bierhaus A, Cooper ME, Jandeleit-Dahm KA. Receptor for advanced glycation end products (RAGE) deficiency attenuates the development of atherosclerosis in diabetes. Diabetes. 2008;57:2461–9.
74. Ojima A, Oda E, Higashimoto Y, Matsui T, Yamagishi S. DNA aptamer raised against advanced glycation end products inhibits neointimal hyperplasia in balloon-injured rat carotid arteries. Int J Cardiol. 2014;171:443–6.
75. Drake MT, Murad MH, Mauck KF, Lane MA, Undavalli C, Elraiyah T, Stuart LM, Prasad C, Shahrour A, Mullan RJ, Hazem A, Erwin PJ, Montori VM. Clinical review. Risk factors for low bone mass-related fractures in men: a systematic review and meta-analysis. J Clin Endocrinol Metab. 2012;97:1861–70.
76. Merlotti D, Gennari L, Dotta F, Lauro D, Nuti R. Mechanisms of impaired bone strength in type 1 and 2 diabetes. Nutr Metab Cardiovasc Dis. 2010;20:683–90.
77. Kurra S, Siris E. Diabetes and bone health: the relationship between diabetes and osteoporosis-associated fractures. Diabetes Metab Res Rev. 2011;27:430–5.
78. Vestergaard P. Discrepancies in bone mineral density and fracture risk in patients with type 1 and type 2 diabetes—a meta-analysis. Osteoporos Int. 2007;18:427–44.
79. Hofbauer LC, Brueck CC, Singh SK, Dobnig H. Osteoporosis in patients with diabetes mellitus. J Bone Miner Res. 2007;22:1317–28.
80. Pietschmann P, Patsch JM, Schernthaner G. Diabetes and bone. Horm Metab Res. 2010;42:763–8.
81. Isidro ML, Ruano B. Bone disease in diabetes. Curr Diabetes Rev. 2010;6:144–55.
82. De Liefde II, van der Klift M, de Laet CE, van Daele PL, Hofman A, Pols HA. Bone mineral density and fracture risk in type-2 diabetes mellitus: the Rotterdam Study. Osteoporos Int. 2005;16:1713–20.
83. Mercer N, Ahmed H, Etcheverry SB, Vasta GR, Cortizo AM. Regulation of advanced glycation end product (AGE) receptors and apoptosis by AGEs in osteoblast-like cells. Mol Cell Biochem. 2007;306:87–94.
84. Schurman L, McCarthy AD, Sedlinsky C, Gangoiti MV, Arnol V, Bruzzone L, Cortizo AM. Metformin reverts deleterious effects of advanced glycation end products (AGEs) on osteoblastic cells. Exp Clin Endocrinol Diabetes. 2008;116:333–40.
85. McCarthy AD, Etcheverry SB, Bruzzone L, Lettieri G, Barrio DA, Cortizo AM. Non-enzymatic glycosylation of a type I collagen matrix: effects on osteoblastic development and oxidative stress. BMC Cell Biol. 2001;2:16.
86. Katayama Y, Akatsu T, Yamamoto M, Kugai N, Nagata N. Role of nonenzymatic glycosylation of type I collagen in diabetic osteopenia. J Bone Miner Res. 1996;11:931–7.
87. Katayama Y, Celic S, Nagata N, Martin TJ, Findlay DM. Nonenzymatic glycation of type I collagen modifies interaction with UMR 201-10B preosteoblastic cells. Bone. 1997;21:237–42.
88. Miyata T, Notoya K, Yoshida K, Horie K, Maeda K, Kurokawa K, Taketomi S. Advanced glycation end products enhance osteoclast-induced bone resorption in cultured mouse unfractionated bone cells and in rats implanted subcutaneously with devitalized bone particles. J Am Soc Nephrol. 1997;8:260–70.

89. Zhou Z, Immel D, Xi CX, Bierhaus A, Feng X, Mei L, Nawroth P, Stern DM, Xiong WC. Regulation of osteoclast function and bone mass by RAGE. J Exp Med. 2006;203:1067–80.
90. Ding KH, Wang ZZ, Hamrick MW, Deng ZB, Zhou L, Kang B, Yan SL, She JX, Stern DM, Isales CM, Mi QS. Disordered osteoclast formation in RAGE-deficient mouse establishes an essential role for RAGE in diabetes related bone loss. Biochem Biophys Res Commun. 2006;340:1091–7.
91. Tang SY, Vashishth D. Non-enzymatic glycation alters microdamage formation in human cancellous bone. Bone. 2010;46:148–54.
92. Khosravi R, Sodek KL, Faibish M, Trackman PC. Collagen advanced glycation inhibits its Discoidin Domain Receptor 2 (DDR2)-mediated induction of lysyl oxidase in osteoblasts. Bone. 2014;58:33–41.
93. Aoki C, Uto K, Honda K, Kato Y, Oda H. Advanced glycation end products suppress lysyl oxidase and induce bone collagen degradation in a rat model of renal osteodystrophy. Lab Invest. 2013;93:1170–83.
94. Saito M, Fujii K, Mori Y, Marumo K. Role of collagen enzymatic and glycation induced cross-links as a determinant of bone quality in spontaneously diabetic WBN/Kob rats. Osteoporos Int. 2006;17:1514–23.
95. Viguet-Carrin S, Roux JP, Arlot ME, Merabet Z, Leeming DJ, Byrjalsen I, Delmas PD, Bouxsein ML. Contribution of the advanced glycation end product pentosidine and of maturation of type I collagen to compressive biomechanical properties of human lumbar vertebrae. Bone. 2006;39:1073–9.
96. Saito M, Marumo K. Collagen cross-links as a determinant of bone quality: a possible explanation for bone fragility in aging, osteoporosis, and diabetes mellitus. Osteoporos Int. 2010;21:195–214.
97. Yamamoto M, Yamaguchi T, Yamauchi M, Yano S, Sugimoto T. Serum pentosidine levels are positively associated with the presence of vertebral fractures in postmenopausal women with type 2 diabetes. J Clin Endocrinol Metab. 2008;93:1013–9.
98. Schwartz AV, Garnero P, Hillier TA, Sellmeyer DE, Strotmeyer ES, Feingold KR, Resnick HE, Tylavsky FA, Black DM, Cummings SR, Harris TB, Bauer DC, Health, Aging, and Body Composition Study. Pentosidine and increased fracture risk in older adults with type 2 diabetes. J Clin Endocrinol Metab. 2009;94:2380–6.
99. Cai W, He JC, Zhu L, Chen X, Wallenstein S, Striker GE, Vlassara H. Reduced oxidant stress and extended lifespan in mice exposed to a low glycotoxin diet: association with increased AGER1 expression. Am J Pathol. 2007;170:1893–902.
100. Cai W, He JC, Zhu L, Chen X, Zheng F, Striker GE, Vlassara H. Oral glycotoxins determine the effects of calorie restriction on oxidant stress, age-related diseases, and lifespan. Am J Pathol. 2008;173:327–36.
101. Semba RD, Fink JC, Sun K, et al. Serum carboxymethyl-lysine, a dominant advanced glycation end product, is associated with chronic kidney disease: the Baltimore longitudinal study of aging. J Ren Nutr. 2010;20:74–81.
102. Semba RD, Ferrucci L, Sun K, et al. Advanced glycation end products and their circulating receptors predict cardiovascular disease mortality in older community-dwelling women. Aging Clin Exp Res. 2009;21:182–90.
103. Semba RD, Bandinelli S, Sun K, Guralnik JM, Ferrucci L. Plasma carboxymethyl-lysine, an advanced glycation end product, and all-cause and cardiovascular disease mortality in older community-dwelling adults. J Am Geriatr Soc. 2009;57:1874–80.

FSC
www.fsc.org
MIX
Papier | Fördert gute Waldnutzung
FSC® C083411

Kolibri 360 GmbH
Ferdinand-Jühlke-Straße 7
99095 Erfurt, Deutschland
produktsicherheit@kolibri360.de